THE QUEST FOR SEXUAL HEALTH

The Quest for Sexual Health

HOW AN ELUSIVE IDEAL HAS
TRANSFORMED SCIENCE,
POLITICS, AND EVERYDAY LIFE

+ + + + + + + + + + + + + + + + +

STEVEN EPSTEIN

THE UNIVERSITY OF CHICAGO PRESS
CHICAGO AND LONDON

The University of Chicago Press, Chicago 60637
The University of Chicago Press, Ltd., London
© 2022 by Steven Epstein
Published 2022
Printed in the United States of America

31 30 29 28 27 26 25 24 23 22   1 2 3 4 5

ISBN-13: 978-0-226-81814-6 (cloth)
ISBN-13: 978-0-226-81822-1 (paper)
ISBN-13: 978-0-226-81817-7 (e-book)
DOI: https://doi.org/10.7208/chicago/9780226818177.001.0001

Published with support of the Susan E. Abrams Fund.

Library of Congress Cataloging-in-Publication Data

Names: Epstein, Steven, author.
Title: The quest for sexual health : how an elusive ideal has
    transformed science, politics, and everyday life / Steven
    Epstein.
Description: Chicago : University of Chicago Press, 2022. |
    Includes bibliographical references and index.
Identifiers: LCCN 2021038755 | ISBN 9780226818146 (cloth) |
    ISBN 9780226818221 (paperback) | ISBN 9780226818177 (ebook)
Subjects: LCSH: Sexual health. | Sexual health—Social aspects.
Classification: LCC RA788 .E67 2022 | DDC 613.9/5—dc23
LC record available at https://lccn.loc.gov/2021038755

To Héctor, who makes so many things possible

Contents

Abbreviations

ASHA American Sexual Health Association

CDC Centers for Disease Control and Prevention

FDA Food and Drug Administration

HHS US Department of Health and Human Services

ICD International Classification of Diseases (in full, the International Statistical Classification of Diseases and Related Health Problems)

ICPD International Conference on Population and Development (held in Cairo in 1994)

LARC Long-acting reversible contraception

LGBT Lesbian, gay, bisexual, and transgender

LGBTQ Lesbian, gay, bisexual, transgender, and queer

NIH National Institutes of Health

PrEP Preexposure prophylaxis (to prevent HIV infection)

SDGs Sustainable Development Goals (of the United Nations)

SIECUS Sex(uality) Information and Education Council of the United States (since 2019 called SIECUS: Sex Ed for Social Change)

SRHR Sexual and reproductive health and rights

STD Sexually transmitted disease

STI Sexually transmitted infection

STS Science and technology studies

WAS World Association for Sexual Health (formerly, the World Association of Sexology)

WHO World Health Organization

Illustrations

Figures

Tables

Introduction: Catching Sexual Health

"Move Sexual Health Forward" is the slogan of the 2019 National Sexual Health Conference, which opens on a sweltering Chicago summer day, in the over-air-conditioned recesses of the Marriott Downtown Magnificent Mile. A volunteer hands me my registration materials, which include a name badge, a program, and a T-shirt in my preselected size, inside a bag displaying the conference logo on one side and the logo for the pharmaceutical company Gilead (the Diamond sponsor of the conference) on the other.[1] No relation to the sexually repressive "Republic of Gilead" (the brutal, theocratic police state depicted in Margaret Atwood's dystopian fantasy novel The Handmaid's Tale), Gilead Sciences Inc., is especially known in this setting for selling drugs that can prevent or treat HIV infection.[2]

I take advantage of the time left before the opening session to peruse the already-crowded exhibition hall, where the representatives of thirty-nine companies and groups—Modern Sex Therapy Institutes, Say It with a Condom, the Society for the Scientific Study of Sexuality, Walgreens—have their tables and booths. As I make my way around the room, I help myself to an array of printed materials and souvenirs: numerous branded condoms; the 2019 Pocket Edition Positively Aware HIV Drug Chart; and a cardboard coaster for the Wondrous Vulva Puppet®, which (as I learn later from the website) is "the #1 Anatomical model used for education, therapy, OB/GYN clinicians and schools worldwide" and is "taking the shame, mystery & porn out of the conversation of women's sexuality & sex education."[3] While many conference-goers chat with eager reps behind tables on the room's perimeter, others check out the poster presentations in the interior of the hall that summarize findings from a diverse assortment of academic studies: "She Speaks: Intersections of Intimate Partner Violence and HIV," "Overview of Sex Therapy and the Diagnosis of Sexual Functions and

Disorders," and "Research, Impact & Empowerment! Reaching Marginalized Youth through Evidence-Based Intervention to Reduce Teen Pregnancy."

As I traverse this space, surrounded by manifestations of the remarkably varied ideas and activities all somehow located at the meeting point of "sexuality" and "health," it strikes me that this is a domain of action, investment, and intervention: the commercial interests, the service providers, the consultants, the academics, and various others have all come to the Chicago Marriott to explain what they have been doing or figure out how to do things. They all, indeed, seek to "move sexual health forward."

The fourth such conference to be held biennially in the United States, this one has been planned by a consortium of nonprofit organizations and coalitions.⁴ In the large, crowded banquet hall where the conference officially opens, a representative of one of the local hosting organizations greets the crowd enthusiastically and announces that around nine hundred people have registered for the conference, of whom about seven hundred have traveled from outside the Chicago area. Those numbers constitute a 44 percent increase over the attendance at the previous conference in 2017.⁵ To my eyes, the crowd appears to skew female as well as young, with a median age perhaps in the low thirties and plenty of tattoos and piercings on display. It also seems relatively multiethnic. Data posted on the conference website, apparently obtained from preregistration forms, indicates that nearly a quarter of the attendees are affiliated with state and local health departments and just under a fifth work with community-based organizations; others are educators, researchers, activists, health providers, and service providers of various sorts.⁶

Over the course of three days, attendees take their pick of over one hundred sessions and roundtables. There is plenty to choose from: topics include clinical concerns ("Everything You Ever Wanted to Ask a Genital Reassignment Surgeon but Didn't Know How"), political debates ("Human Trafficking, the Truth about Modern Slavery in America"), and sexual exploration ("KamaSutra Café"). The session titles call out a diverse array of identities and constituencies: conservative Christians ("Jesus and Sexual Health"), Muslim Americans ("Allah Loves Consent"), and schoolchildren ("School Dress Codes: The Politics of Shame, Stereotypes, and Sexualization"), as well as elderly people, transgender people, and disabled people.

After immersing myself in the conference, I come away with a distinct impression of some especially salient themes. First, presenters regularly and routinely remind the audience that sexual health is something "more than" just the absence of disease. This formulation does not surprise me: as I will explain, it is a riff on the World Health Organization's (WHO) definition of health in general, and it also reflects the more specific "working definition" of sexual health that was developed under that organization's auspices. Yet precisely because a high proportion of those drawn to this particular conference (more so than at some of the others convened under the rubric of sexual health) are people who work in the area of prevention of sexually transmitted infections (STIs) and HIV,[7] it seems especially important for attendees to reject a narrowly disease-based approach. Sexual health is an imprecise "positive," imagined against the backdrop of the fight to wipe out various specific "negatives."

Second, speakers repeatedly invoke the importance of "telling one's story." This injunction sits, perhaps uneasily, alongside the assumption that claims should be "evidence based." That sexual health promotion should be an evidence-based activity is among the listed goals of the conference,[8] and conference speakers regularly reinforce the idea. For example, Dr. Debby Herbenick, in an engaging plenary on the changing sexual behaviors of Americans, makes clear that her facts are grounded in the methodology of the nationally representative probability sample. Yet this emphasis on evidence appears to coexist with exhortations about the "absolute importance of all of you raising your voices and telling your personal stories" (in the words of David Harvey, the executive director of the National Coalition of STD Directors, who adds, "We learned this from the HIV community"). Without questioning the importance of good science and hard evidence, the discourse of the conference seems also to insist on the power of truths that are deeply personal, authentic, and validated by the self. The motive behind this storytelling is presented as a practical one related to the dynamics of advocacy work: the personal is political. Yet I leave the conference with a sense of a vital, if underspecified, link between science and selfhood—and between facts and experiences—in the forging of sexual truths.

Third, the HIV/AIDS epidemic, with its vast toll of lives lost, stands out as a historical turning point in the evolution of activities centered on the promotion of sexual health. Again, this is partly because the threat of HIV is simply the concrete, workaday focus of many of the attendees of this particular conference. Yet there is much more to it than that, as speakers reference how the fierce political and biomedical crosswinds of the AIDS epidemic swept aside older approaches to issues of sexuality and health, ushered in new forms of health advocacy, and changed the conventional discourse. "We never used to talk about sexual health," comments conference cochair Dr. Kees Rietmeijer in his opening remarks; he goes on to attribute the destigmatization of the entire domain to the profound effect of the AIDS epidemic and the consequent increased attention to sexual rights and sexual justice. Yet while the epidemic transformed the landscape of sexual politics, the idea of sexual health has also broadened

the discussion of HIV and connected it to other concerns. At a lunchtime sym-
posium sponsored by Gilead, the presenter, Dr. Paul Benson, explains that he
"used to be an HIV doctor" but has come to consider himself a "sexual health
doctor."

Finally, the idea of "moving sexual health forward"—and the action orienta-
tion that motivates the proceedings—is tightly intertwined with contemporary
politics and topical debates. The Affordable Care Act and health insurance, the
#MeToo feminist movement, sexual consent on college campuses, the Black
Lives Matter movement, the opioid epidemic, restrictions on abortion—the dis-
course of the conference is inflected by the burning social issues of the day. As
speakers draw connections to these and other concerns and criticize dangerous
political trends, many conference participants snap fingers in audible displays
of solidarity. The point is not simply that conference-goers are reacting to all
the anxieties and uncertainties of a political moment characterized by the per-
sistent threats and incessant tweets of the Trump administration. More spe-
cifically, the claim is that sexual health is implicated, directly and indirectly,
in all these hot-button topics: anyone who cares about sexual health should
care about these issues, and anyone who thinks about these issues should be at-
tentive to sexual health. As I will describe, this treatment of sexual health as a
bridge to other concerns turns out to be not just the prerogative of those on the
political Left but also may characterize those on the Right.

The Ubiquity of Sexual Health

Two deceptively simple and ordinary words, spliced together in an unlikely pairing: the conjoining of "sexual" with "health" does an enormous amount of work, referencing a wide array of people and problems.
At least since the 1970s, health professionals, researchers, governments,
advocacy groups, foundations, and commercial interests increasingly
have embarked on the quest for something called sexual health. Programs have been launched, organizations founded, initiatives funded,
products sold—yet critical scrutiny has not kept pace with this flurry
of activity. How and when did people come to imagine that there might
be a form of health called sexual health? What might it mean to be sexually healthy or unhealthy? Which groups in society are deemed more
or less capable of achieving sexual health? Why has the achievement
and safeguarding of health become a relevant—and unavoidable—
consideration when evaluating one's sexual desires, capacities, and
behaviors? How did sexual health become the gateway to addressing a

host of social harms and reimagining both private desires and public dreams?

Sexual health, as I have already suggested, is a domain of action, investment, and intervention, undergirded by evidence as well as stories, shaped by contingent historical developments like the AIDS epidemic, yet serving as a pathway to an ever-widening range of contemporary concerns. At stake are the very real health needs and personal desires of individuals around the world, as well as the interests of many corporations and professional groups. The happenings at the National Sexual Health Conference reveal at least a portion of the sweep of activities, the diverse scientific agendas, and the broad political, economic, intellectual, and practical stakes—all premised ultimately on the idea that there is a form of health called sexual health.

That idea should not be taken for granted. While the precursors of what we now call sexual health can be traced back a ways (and I will do so in chapter 1), the contemporary understandings of sexual health date essentially to 1974, when the WHO convened a panel of experts who proposed the term and offered a definition. Refashioned over the years, the working definition, as it is called—never officially claimed by the WHO, yet posted on its website all the same—now stands as follows: "Sexual health is a state of physical, emotional, mental and social well-being in relation to sexuality; it is not merely the absence of disease, dysfunction or infirmity. Sexual health requires a positive and respectful approach to sexuality and sexual relationships, as well as the possibility of having pleasurable and safe sexual experiences, free of coercion, discrimination and violence. For sexual health to be attained and maintained, the sexual rights of all persons must be respected, protected and fulfilled."[9]

This, at least, is one definition of sexual health—an especially influential one, though not the only contender. Even on first glance, the definition seems all over the map—ranging, as noted, from the physical to the emotional to the mental to the social. It aligns with very contemporary emphases on promoting health and wellness (as expressed in regular exhortations from the human relations departments of today's corporations[10]), but it treads far beyond the usual connotations of "health," zooming off toward destinations that include pleasure, safety, freedom, and rights. Yet for all its apparent capaciousness, even vagueness, the "WHO definition" fails to capture the remarkably varied ways in which people, groups, organizations, and governments have taken up the term or thought about the concept. However authoritative, this definition has not come close to resolving the question of what sexual health might mean. As a sexual health consultant in a Department of Sexual Health at a UK hospital observed in the pages of a medical journal: "No seminar or conference on the subject of sexual health seems complete without a presentation or debate rhetorically titled 'What is sexual health?'"[11] It seems that a defining feature of the discourse on sexual health, then, is the recurrent question of how to define it.

Sexual health is the topic of thousands of scientific journal articles, and, according to Google, if one searches for the English-language term, "about 41,900,000" web pages.[12] The phrase appears in the names of professional associations, journals, research centers, treatment centers, conferences, protocols, and statistical surveys. The University of Michigan's School of Social Work offers a certificate program in sexual health.[13] The University of Minnesota has an endowed "Chair in Sexual Health," as well as the "Joycelyn Elders Chair in Sexual Health Education."[14] Sexual health is a marketing category for selling products like vibrators and lubricants; it describes the agendas of agencies and governments; it is something that, according to a promotional campaign by Gilead, one may be encouraged to "own" by knowing one's HIV status.[15] Sexual health also merits its own day on the calendar: September 4 is World Sexual Health Day, an event recognized by the WHO.[16]

Around the world, there are reports, agendas, agencies, and offices devoted explicitly to the promotion of sexual health, and the presence, absence, degree, or quality of sexual health is deemed a knowable characteristic of individuals, groups, and whole societies. A striking indication of the global salience of sexual health involves the new edition of the WHO's influential International Classification of Diseases, which goes into effect in 2022: the fifty-five thousand health conditions coded in the ICD—the full gamut of human suffering of body and mind—will be grouped into just twenty-six chapters, and, for the first time, one of those will be "Conditions Related to Sexual Health."[17] People seem increasingly to care about sexual health; people fight over sexual health—even the attempts to ban the term during the Trump administration testify to its significance. That is (as I discuss in chapter 9), the US State Department under Secretary of State Mike Pompeo fomented controversy by seeking to proscribe the very use of phrases like "sexual and reproductive health" in international health policy documents.[18] Reminiscent of how Victorian society, in the philosopher

Michel Foucault's well-known account, "[spoke] verbosely of its own silences" about sexual matters,[19] one of the things we now discuss about sexual health is whether we can discuss it.

Yet because sexual health is still so relatively new—but perhaps also because so much stigma continues to surround sexuality—the current hypervisibility of sexual health seems at times to coexist with its invisibility. I have learned through researching this book that many people have never heard the phrase and can only guess at its meaning. "Sexual health" lacks a Wikipedia page, and a search for the term on Wikipedia redirects automatically to "reproductive health." In 2010, when two physicians published a call in *JAMA* for a national strategy to improve sexual health, they complained that "'sexual health' does not appear once" in the more than one thousand pages of the Affordable Care Act.[20] The National Library of Medicine did not assign a Medical Subject Heading code to catalog sexual health until 2018.[21] How can sexual health be both everywhere and nowhere at the same time?[22] And how can we make sense of something that has those characteristics?

The Returns on an Investment

This book provides an entryway into the distinctive worlds of sexual health. The chapters to follow traverse the distance between many venues: the research and treatment domains where sexual health is assessed, measured, and improved; the "sex expos" that invite attendees to "leave their inhibitions at the door and explore today's top intimacy products"; the headquarters of Focus on the Family, where the group's "sexual health analyst" explains what a healthy sexuality entails from a conservative Christian standpoint. The quest for sexual health turns out to encompass wildly disparate agendas, and it comes to ground in relation to innumerable concerns—from sexual dysfunction to sexual violence, from HIV prevention to reproductive freedom to the practicalities of sexual contact in the COVID-19 pandemic. Rather than a thing apart, sexual health is intertwined with nearly every conceivable topical debate—more of them every day, which explains why sexual health has become ever more salient.

For that reason, my point in writing this book is not just to survey these various worlds, as fascinating as they might be. Rather, I set out to show that the growing attention to something called sexual health *matters*, and that the generative idea of sexual health has carved out new and important routes by which people make sense of their lives and along which societies seek to organize themselves.

The term "sexual health" signals a wide range of investments: financial, intellectual, practical, moral, and—of course—libidinal. It is also a concern of some urgency. When over one million cases of sexually transmitted infections such as chlamydia, gonorrhea, and syphilis are reported each day around the world, with the greatest burden of disease in those countries with the fewest resources to confront it (and when cases in the United States reached a record high in 2019); when nearly two million people become newly infected with HIV across the globe each year; when the rise of the #MeToo movement has ruptured the long silence surrounding sexual harassment and assault in the United States; when the debate over access to abortion and birth control casts a shadow across the terrain of domestic politics in the United States as well as its foreign policy; and when the global market in "sexual wellness" products was estimated at nearly $75 billion in 2019, there can be little doubt that the question of what it might mean for sexuality to be "healthy" is increasingly unavoidable.[23]

Yet the consequences of these various investments in something called sexual health spill out beyond the domains of immediate topical concern. I argue that "sexual health" has been *put to use* in ways that help give form to how we imagine what it means to be a citizen, achieve happiness or well-being, secure social order, or work collectively toward a better future for the society. What is at stake here exceeds the domains of both sexuality and health: promoting sexual health, I suggest, proves surprisingly valuable on the way to other goals.

Following the assertion that the burgeoning attention to sexual health is more consequential than generally recognized, it might be expected that I would immediately pronounce on whether the undertaking of activities under the banner of sexual health is therefore to be judged as being either "good" or "bad." Yet I maintain that we cannot and should not make such broad declarations. Indeed, sexual health has come to mean so many different things that blanket assessments are unhelpful and misleading. We need, instead, to consider the many alternative possibilities, as well as the tensions, that lie embedded within the idea of sexual health.

As will become clear, the proponents of sexual health have directed attention, marshaled resources, and propelled action in ways that are easy to applaud. Most immediately, they have championed sexuality as something important and valued—conferring legitimacy on a core dimension of experience that too often remains stigmatized and feared—and they have promoted better cures and techniques of prevention for a host of unwanted outcomes. In the face of devastating diseases such as HIV/AIDS, sexual health initiatives are life affirming and essential. These efforts have also helped to install a new vision of doctoring (however imperfectly realized to date) that includes attention to sexual matters. And they have given license to new voices, expanding our conception of who might constitute a credible expert about matters relating to sexual desires and health needs. At a broader level, sexual health projects have expanded popular understandings of what may be encompassed under notions of human rights and social justice. Such efforts do more than cure disease, as important as that may be: they expand the scope of freedom and capacity for fulfillment available to many individuals.

Yet sexual health initiatives also confront us with intractable dilemmas and pointed questions:

- Do these initiatives take normative judgments about what sex should be like and dress them up in the (perhaps less easily contested) language of scientific truth? Do they translate moral convention into scientific visions of "normality"? Alternatively, might they provide more differentiated understandings of what "the normal" can entail, and offer new pathways to challenge and redefine moral codes and cultural practices?
- Similarly, by reframing sexual matters in the language of health, do sexual health projects "leave it up to the experts" to draw conclusions about how our lives should be lived? Or, perhaps, does the unbounded nature of sexual health discussions effectively grant a license to a far more diverse set of authorities, many of them with less conventional claims to expertise?
- Do visions of sexual health impose purportedly universal and global solutions that fail to acknowledge the remarkable diversity in how sexuality, health, and other key dimensions of everyday life are construed and pursued around the world? Or, does the flexibility in meanings attributed to sexual health facilitate adaptation and innovation of agendas within diverse locales, settings, and populations?
- Do sexual health projects conceive of the management and exploration of sexuality and the quest to be healthy as purely individual

concerns? Or, do such projects support the rise of new communities and promote collective action to pursue political goals?

- Finally, is sexual health ultimately a "sex-negative" pursuit that construes sexuality as infused with risks and dangers that must be properly managed or averted? Or, is sexual health compatible with a "sex-positive" valorization of sexuality as a domain of freedom, self-expression, the actualization of rights, and the pursuit of bodily pleasures, social connections, and possibilities for cultural development?

Although it might be satisfying to provide a simple answer to such questions, my claim is that my analysis is improved by taking a step back from them. First, this book will help the reader understand why "sexual health" has come to serve as the ground on which these kinds of debates play out—a place where we skirmish around matters of morality, normality, expertise, universalism, globalization, collective action, risk, responsibility, rights, passion, and pleasure. Second, the book will show how sexual health has proved capacious enough, and contradictory enough, to allow for many possibilities—and how it therefore presents choices about which potential internal tendencies to endorse and which to resist. Third, the book will consistently remind us that the stakes of sexual health are positioned differently for different groups, who may not run the same risks or reap the same benefits—and that the possibilities to navigate among the various tendencies afforded by sexual health projects may depend on where one sits within hierarchies of many kinds, such as the racial, gender, and class order, or one's position within global power relations. Needless to say, the stakes of sexual health also cut differently for those whose sexualities differ from the mainstream, not excluding those who define themselves as asexual.

Given this complex and double-edged character of sexual health, how should we survey its varied topography and make our way across this landscape?

Catching Sexual Health?

It is painfully easy to catch a disease, yet it is harder to "catch health." Sexual health, in particular, is hard to catch hold of. We struggle to *apprehend* it—that is, to understand it, but also to capture it and take it into custody, so to speak. Yet discourses and practices of sexual health "catch" us in various ways: they compel us to take action and to consider our bodies and selves from new and different angles. Investigating how sexual health gets "caught" means studying all the ways that sexual health, as a way of thinking about and acting on people, bodies, and societies, is brought into being and enacted, and all the ways that people have been trying to latch onto it—discursively, materially, practically, and politically.[24]

Stitching sexuality to health does powerful work—for both terms.[25] Yet a fundamental starting point in understanding that work is to recognize the very different moral valences of the two words in the compound phrase. On the one hand, health is a virtue, an obligation, an aspiration. On the other hand, sexuality suffers from a legitimacy deficit. It is hard to think of any social practice as widespread and as generally popular as sexuality would seem to be that is, at the same time, so routinely stigmatized, burdened by moral controversy, freighted with metaphorical baggage, and perceived as a threat to the foundations of the moral and social order.[26] Thus sexuality (and especially certain kinds of sexuality seen as problematic, irresponsible, or taboo[27]) stands in special need of legitimation—and this is what the concatenation with health provides in abundance. Against the backdrop of this preoccupation with legitimacy, sexual health has emerged as a distinctive, evocative, and especially resonant way of visioning what it means to be a healthy citizen of the modern world. It offers people a screen onto which they can project their aspirations and imaginings, their anxieties and their envy—that is, people are interested in knowing not just whether they are sexually healthy but also how their sexuality "measures up," and how what they experience may compare to what they expect others may be doing and feeling.

This book explains how and why sexual health has become entwined with complicated histories of understanding and directing human desires; how and why it has become a buzzword fueling diverse attempts at problem solving; how and why it has provided a basis for new scientific projects of classification, measurement, and evaluation; how and why it has denoted the targets and goals of individual efforts at self-optimization as well as government projects of social improvement; and how and why it has become a political battleground where the stakes are competing visions of the future. Along the way, I consider how sex has become a growing topic of health advice; how norms about "healthy sex" emerge and change; how sexual health has become intertwined with ideas about human rights; how a consumer market for health-promoting sexual commodities has expanded; how the prospect of achieving pleasure either has or has not become incorporated into sexual health projects; and how the sexual threats imagined to be posed by various marginalized groups affect health promotion agendas. In traversing this complex terrain, the book provides critical tools to bring into focus the different faces of sexual health and to assess the range of potential consequences described earlier—to parse the debates about the defining of normality, the role of experts, the universality of claims, the individualizing and collectivizing tendencies, and the "positive" and "negative" ways of addressing sexuality and health.

MEDICALIZING SEXUALITY?

This is a big agenda, and an important implication is that the developments I track in the chapters that follow are too varied to be shoehorned into any single theoretical framework. For instance, much ink has been spilled about the phenomenon of "medicalization"—and it might seem natural to suppose that the rise of sexual health is a story of how sexuality has become medicalized—yet this book is only very partially about that.

Certainly, a defining feature of modernity is a tendency for societies to characterize social problems as medical concerns, or invite medical professionals to exercise jurisdiction over them, or endorse medical treatments as solutions.[28] Scholars have had much to say about new drivers of medicalization in recent years, such as direct-to-consumer pharmaceutical advertising;[29] about the impact of biomedical research developments in transforming medical authority and the illness experience in a new era of "biomedicalization";[30] and about the countervailing tendency for some conditions to be demedicalized.[31] More specifically, scholars have usefully traced how diverse aspects of modern sexuality have been brought under the sway of the medical, including sexual performance (as yesterday's "impotence" has become today's "erectile dysfunction"), sexual predilections (deemed normal or abnormal), and the very look and shape of genitals.[32] From a critical perspective, scholars have rightly worried about the implications of the very long tradition, in the West and elsewhere, of viewing sexuality as fundamentally connected to disease (though also to sin).[33]

This is undeniably part of the story of sexual health. Yet as the sociologist Nikolas Rose has argued more generally, reliance on medicalization as an explanatory concept may lead too quickly to generalizations across time, place, and context, in ways that are insensitive to the heterogeneity of modern medicine. There are many kinds and degrees of medicalization (and demedicalization), and the term may simply bring together too many diverse kinds of relationships to health and medicine under a single banner. Therefore the idea of medicalization is best seen as "the starting point of an analysis [or] a sign of the need for an analysis, but . . . not . . . the conclusion of an analysis."[34]

More specifically, with regard to the view of sexual health as a case of medicalization, three points of qualification are worth making. First, if sexual health, in the words of the WHO's working definition, "is not merely the absence of disease, dysfunction or infirmity," then the concept seems to escape the confines of the narrowly biomedical. To be sure, one important subset of sexual health is a field called *sexual medicine* that focuses quite specifically on the diagnosis and treatment of disease, dysfunction, and infirmity. Yet sexual health involves so much more, and those who speak authoritatively about it come from many different fields, professions, and walks of life. Put a bit grandly, sexual health has taken on characteristics of a full-fledged "regime of living," to borrow a term developed by the anthropologists Stephen Collier and Andrew Lakoff. According to these scholars, a regime of living is "a tentative and situated configuration of normative, technical, and political elements that are brought into alignment in situations that present ethical problems—that is, situations in which the question of how to live is at stake."[35] Sexual health fits the mold: it raises vital questions about what it means to live as a good and proper subject of a modern world.[36]

If sexual health exceeds the biomedical, then perhaps the story is less one of medicalization than of the process sometimes (inelegantly) called "healthicization," or of the corresponding ideology called "healthism." These terms describe the transformation of health into a moral imperative, indeed a key injunction in contemporary societies—a fundamental obligation of modern citizens to live up to standards of what constitutes good health.[37] As Jonathan Metzl and Anna Kirkland nicely illustrated through the title they gave to a volume dedicated to this theme, it seems almost unthinkable nowadays to stand "against health."[38] Yet the boundaries of health continue to expand, to encompass not just the prevention of disease and the reduction of risk but also the embracing of specific ways of behaving—which foods to consume when, how often to drink alcohol, how best to exercise, and so on. Indeed, the very concept of health has increasingly functioned to demarcate not only the bounds of "normality" but also that which is considered good, proper, and moral.[39] Nowadays, "health" functions much like "freedom" in the sociologist Orlando Patterson's history of that concept: "People may sin against freedom, but no one dares deny its virtue."[40]

The prospect of healthism does raise important questions about attitudes and practices relating to sexual matters in particular. I share with many scholars what Theo Sandfort and Anke Ehrhardt, in an article on the concept of sexual health, term a "'healthy' suspicion against promoting the use of a health perspective in relation to sexuality," given how often "'health' has been the pretext for suppressing or regulating sexual practices in the past."[41] Therefore, an analysis and critique of healthicization seems essential for any careful consideration of the worlds of sexual health.

Yet (and this is the second qualification), even the more expansive idea of healthicization may not be either broad or flexible enough to "capture" sexual health. As I describe, the notion of sexual health provides a vehicle for (and sometimes a cloak of legitimacy to) the pursuit of a very wide range of goals: pleasure, rights, responsibility, autonomy, freedom, desire, integrity, religiosity. To view the attainment of such ends solely through the prism of healthism is to risk a reductive account that begins with the presupposition that all other values are necessarily, in the end, subordinated to that of health. Moreover, many sexual health activities are put forward in contexts relatively far from the direct control (either administrative or definitional) of either health professionals or researchers of any sort. I argue that as sexual health expertise has become omnipresent, it has become increasingly hard to say what sort of person gets to be called a sexual health expert.[42] Thus, to analyze sexual health from the standpoint of medicalization and healthicization alone is also to risk restricting our attention to a circumscribed set of actors. Finally, to propose that the healthicizing of sexuality has reinforced normative conceptions of sexuality—while certainly correct in particular instances—runs the risk of granting a solidity, coherence, and enduring uniformity to "the normal" that it may never actually possess. As Peter Cryle and Elizabeth Stephens have observed in their "critical genealogy" of normality: "The normal is not monolithic. It is not an inexpugnable edifice towering over the intellectual landscape of our modernity. Its power derives from the very looseness that allows it to be everywhere available even as it continues to be questioned."[43]

The third limitation inherent in reading sexual health as a matter of either medicalization or healthicization is that doing so assumes the causal arrow runs in a single direction, from health to sexuality. The implication is that what requires assessment is the effect that the former has on the latter.[44] Yet I argue that the conjoining of "sexual" with "health" changes the meanings of both terms.[45] To treat sexuality as a key dimension of what we mean by health is to change what health *means*—potentially to expand the very idea of health to encompass new conceptions of rights and pleasures. To mandate that health professionals concern themselves with the domain of the sexual is to call for a redefinition of professional identity, with implications for how such professionals are trained and how they go about their daily work. Of course, such aspirations may prompt significant pushback. But the point is that an overemphasis on the healthicization of sexuality can preclude sufficient attention to the "sexualization of health."[46]

These various initial reflections about the limits of the medicalization framework for understanding how health and sexuality have become connected are also meant to signal my own distance from a certain kind of moral critique. To be sure, scholars of medicalization rightly observe that extending the domain of the medical to cover new arenas or problems is neither inherently good nor inherently bad: it all depends on the case, as well as on the values of those doing the judging. Yet it is not uncommon for scholars to position themselves as exposing the insidious creep of medical authority, health institutions, or pharmaceutical marketing into new domains where it may not belong. This critique makes sense in many suspect cases where ordinary ways of being different (say, children who are shorter than others their age) are converted into diseases ("idiopathic short stature"), with medications prescribed to correct the "problem."[47] Yet sexual health is a much more complicated and much more interesting case, precisely because it has come to mean so many things and promote so many different goals. This book describes the significant benefits that accrue from the concatenation of "sexual" with "health," and it also points to the risks. There may certainly be more helpful and less helpful ways of conceiving of, and pursuing, sexual health. But as I have already observed, it makes little sense to ask whether linking sexuality with health is, in itself, "good" or "bad."

THE PLAN

This book shows, first, how the invention of a new historical object called sexual health has reverberating effects on contemporary understandings of both sexuality and health—effects that remain significantly up for grabs. Indeed, the rise of sexual health has refracted and multiplied the meanings of both "sexuality" and "health," furthering the confusion over both terms. Second, despite—or because of—this indeterminacy, "sexual health" has proved useful in all sorts of ways: performing medical diagnosis, quantifying social trends, selling commodities, and promoting political agendas, among others. But here again, the visions are multiple: "the question of how to life," referenced by Collier and Lakoff, is answered in diverse and starkly competing ways. "Sexual health" in fact comes to signify, and propel, some of the most intractable ideological divides of the current moment. Thus, to ask whether the project of sexual health is radical or conservative—or whether it disrupts or reinforces "normality"—is to miss the point that "the project" is not singular and has been made to serve many political ends, and is also to beg the question of how "the normal" continues to evolve.

Indeed, nothing about this story is fixed, as "sexual health" remains an object in formation. We do not yet know how the very meaning of what it means to be healthy may change via the rise of a new kind of health called sexual health, and we do not yet know how the very meaning of sexuality may change with the spread of sexual health activities. The future of sexual health remains to be written. But we can begin to understand the interactions of sexuality and health—and the broad effects of this conjunction—by examining how the discourses and practices of sexual health are transforming how and what we know, how societies are governed, how people imagine their potentialities, and how political struggles are joined. By undertaking that analysis, we also acquire a better handle on the competing tendencies at play within sexual health projects: between leaving judgments about health and sex up to the experts and expanding the range of voices that can weigh in on them; between imagining paths to sexual health that are universally applicable and recognizing a diversity of goals and values; and between treating sex and health as domains of freedom, pleasure, and self-realization or as landscapes of risks to be skirted or negotiated.

Part 1, "Making Sexual Health: Invention, Dispersion, and Reassembly," analyzes how "sexuality" and "health" have been brought together in new ways that end up affecting the meanings of both. It leads off with the story of the relatively recent invention of what we now call sexual health (chapter 1); traces the growth, diversification, and splintering of sexual health (chapter 2); and then examines how key actors have tried to reassemble the different "pieces" of sexual health into new combinations (chapter 3). I argue that both dispersion and recombination create new possibilities for projects and initiatives under the banner of sexual health.

Chapter 1 takes a genealogical approach. I sketch the conditions of possibility for the rise of sexual health in the 1970s, and I identify relevant precursors over the past few centuries, such as medical advice about sexuality, the rise of the field of sexology, and the reform efforts of the social hygiene movement. I then pay close attention to the first promulgation of a definition of sexual health at the meeting organized by the WHO in 1974. I examine, in particular, how proponents sought a "positive" conception of sexual health while skirting troublesome issues relating to the normative status of the definition—should we judge people as being sexually "healthy" or "unhealthy"? and its presumed universal applicability.

As the term subsequently began to travel, it also experienced a remarkable diversification in meaning. Chapter 2 (based on scholarship I undertook with Laura Mamo and drawing on our coauthored work) tells this story of mutability and ambiguity, focused on the period from the 1990s forward. In the context of a specific historical conjuncture in the 1990s that gave the term prominence, the semantic flexibility of "sexual health" permitted it to make its way across a wide range of domains. As the phrase "sexual health" has taken on the qualities of a buzzword, its vagueness and flexibility have permitted the term and concept to spread across domains, as well as to mobilize attention and resources. Along the way, the capacity of "health" to sanitize and legitimize "sexuality" has granted sexual health a wide-ranging appeal, yet the different organizations and institutions that have taken up the concept have found it useful in quite different ways.

Chapter 3 concludes the historical analysis of part 1 by tracking the attempts by various organizations, particularly including the WHO and the World Association for Sexual Health but also various advocacy groups, to reassemble the components of sexual health into new combinations and thereby connect the worlds of medicine, science, and advocacy. This effort has included repeated attempts to revisit and refine the working definition of sexual health—and thereby bring together many of the various disparate meanings and projects under what I call a "sexual health umbrella." In addition, various actors have sought to create new constructs and projects—such as "sexual and reproductive health and rights"—that unite what might otherwise be distinct concerns. Along the way, advocates of sexual health have continued to grapple with vexing issues: the normative stakes of their definitions and the role of scientific expertise (Should we specify what constitutes "healthy sex"? And if so, who gets to say?), the problem of universalism (Is there just one way to be sexually healthy?), and the relative emphases placed on the pleasures and dangers of sexuality.

If the focus, in part 1, is largely on how sexuality and health have become conjoined and what effect this has on each, then the remainder of the book asks, What *else* does this conjoining facilitate? Part 2, "Operationalizing Sexual Health: Enabling Science, Medicine, and Health Care," considers what work sexual health authorizes for health care providers and their patients, researchers and their publics, and experts and their clients. It examines both "subjects" and "objects"—that is, both the people who intervene (or are intervened on) and the efforts to create stable objects of scientific investigation and medical treatment. How is sexual health made knowable and manageable? The four chapters in part 2 examine, in turn, projects that adopt four different means of operationalizing: standardizing, classifying, enumerating, and evaluating. Here, bonding sexuality and health functions not just to sanitize sexual issues but also to "scientize" them by converting them into questions that ostensibly are answerable by experts. Normative concerns are never too far from the surface, as operationalizing often leads to evaluating and judging sexualities, and defining and redefining what is normal—though not without resistance.

Chapter 4 begins this story by considering how medical practice is being reimagined via the engagement with sexual health but also how sexual health, in the process, is transformed into a manageable object of medical scrutiny. I focus on two examples: the standardizing of the sexual health history and its incorporation into medical care, and the development and use of standardized scales and inventories to assess sexual health function and dysfunction.

Next, in chapter 5, I analyze the recent process of revising the WHO's International Classification of Diseases to incorporate sexual health concerns. More than simply a major advance in formal recognition of sexual health concerns at the transnational level, this effort reflects a concerted project of progressive reform. In the context of close scrutiny and critique by advocacy groups and heightened attention to human rights considerations, diagnostic reform has brought about the depathologization, destigmatization, or "de-psychiatrization" of various behaviors and identities related to gender and sexuality. But it has also raised questions about the ability of a putatively universal tool to transcend local particularities and about the rights of the "diagnosed" to weigh in on global systems of diagnosis.

Chapter 6 turns our attention from the biomedical to the social sciences, and from the level of the individual to that of the population, as I examine the dynamics of survey research. I show how efforts to survey the sexual health of the population result in the dissemination of ideas about the sexual characteristics of subgroups of the population while also promoting, and challenging, ideas about what it means to be sexually "normal" or "average."

Part 2 concludes with chapter 7, which focuses broadly on the transformations in the kinds of professions involved in giving voice to claims about sexual health. I examine the remarkable diversification of sexual health expertise: just as the worlds of health nowadays extend far beyond the purview of the medical profession, so the kinds of people who make claims about how we should be sexually healthy range very far afield, from nutritionists to massage therapists to practitioners of kink to porn stars. Of course, some voices speak more authoritatively than do others. Yet this blossoming of expertise constitutes a kind of democratization of knowledge and advice giving, while also raising perplexing questions about who should be trusted and why.

Part 3, "Under the Sign of Sexual Health: Beyond the Worlds of Science and Medicine," pushes the question of consequences in new directions that transcend health and biomedical domains. Here, the focus is on the ripple effects that spread outward, altering the broader culture, economy, and polity.

I begin, in chapter 8, by examining projects of self-improvement and self-optimization. Here, the "will to sexual health" is expressed through various efforts, often linked to consumption, that encourage individuals to maximize their sexual health (or "sexual wellness") and lead more sexually healthy lives. While much previous analytical attention has focused on the specific case of men's use of Viagra and its pharmaceutical cousins, I turn to a broader range of examples, spotlighting women's sexual health consumerism and gay men's use of preexposure prophylaxis against HIV. I call attention to the contradictory tugs in these projects of self-betterment, examining the complex and open-ended relations between the commodification of sexuality and the construction of new political projects around sexual freedom.

Chapter 9 also considers exhortations to be sexually healthy, but it turns to the question of how this motivation has become a feature of modern governance. I examine some of the concrete projects by which state agencies have made sexual health an object and tool of governance over the past two decades—how notions of responsibility have become linked to rights and how conceptions of sexual health have become tied to ideas about who properly "belongs" as a member of the political community. In tracing the trajectory of sexual health governance from the Clinton administration to the eve of the Biden administration, I also consider how governmental plans, actions, and imaginaries have varied depending on changes in historical and political circumstances.

Then, chapter 10 expands the conception of politics to consider how programs for sexual health are mobilized to imagine and install competing political visions of the future. I examine specific, illustrative efforts on both the political Right and the Left in the United States to use sexual health as a bridge—a way of drawing connections in order to frame a political agenda for education and social change. For Christian conservatives, for example, the concept of sexual health holds strategic utility in developing a moral critique of modernity and defending traditional family forms, even while valorizing certain forms of sexual expression. Meanwhile, for those on the left in the era of #MeToo feminism, sexual health provides a language to intervene in debates about sexual assault and consent while elaborating a progressive vision of gender relations. This juxtaposition of examples demonstrates why societal consensus on sexual health topics will likely continue to be elusive—yet also how sexual health figures centrally in the reproduction of key political divides.

Finally, in the conclusion, I connect the threads of this analysis. I consider the possible futures of sexual health, and I examine the central tendencies and countertendencies that seem to run alongside one another within it. The diverse projects to advance sexual health have materialized multiple, competing visions of both health and sexuality, as well as competing projects of asserting and establishing conceptions of what it means to be normal. Moreover, these visions implicate different groups in society differently—according to gender identity, race, nationality, and so on—and therefore shape both the contours of social belonging and the character of social hierarchies. The effect is to raise questions of "how to live" (in Collier and Lakoff's terms) that "sexual health" cannot readily answer. However, the point, I suggest, is not to reject or repudiate sexual health but to find strategies to work both "with" it and "beyond" it.

A THING OF THIS KIND

In some respects, all of my previous empirical studies over more than three decades—of the politics of the HIV/AIDS epidemic, of lesbian, gay, bisexual, and transgender (LGBT) health advocacy, of struggles to make medical research more inclusive, of the debates surrounding vaccines to prevent HPV infection[40]—have prepared me to take up the broad topic of the rise of sexual health. Yet I have confronted unique challenges in "catching" it and pinning it down. From an analytical standpoint, the problem is not merely that sexual health is hard to define. More profoundly, it is difficult to say what sort of thing sexual health *is*, such that we can place it with like things within the right categorical bin.

Sexual health has characteristics of a medical specialty area—think "women's health," "occupational health," or "veterans' health"[49]—but it is claimed by many professions both medical and nonmedical. It has features of a social movement, marked by mobilization and advocacy,[50] although I have also called it a regime of living in light of the ethical injunctions that it seems to entail. In the chapters of this book, I label it a "genealogical outcome," a "buzzword," an "unruly object," a "mode of governance," a "constituent of citizenship," an "aspect of self-formation," and a "bridge to political futures." Across the chapters, I invoke a range of theoretical constructs with the goal of refracting light on the different dimensions of sexual health.

As a professor who regularly mentors doctoral students, I have learned to push them to generalize—to think beyond the confines of the particular issue or episode that fascinates them. "Yes, but what is this a *case* of?" is the challenging and often acutely frustrating question that people like me routinely put to those seeking to join the academic tribe.[51] So, what is *this* a case of? Perhaps it is a case of those things whose very "caseness" is at stake. If so, I hope my approach proves helpful as a guide to others studying objects and concepts of social import whose qualities and connections cause them to spill across the boundaries of the categories that might seek to contain them—or whose very emergence and diffusion is tied to the generation of new categories and new boundaries.[52]

Lines of Approach

FOUCAULT AND BEYOND

A necessary starting point for this analysis is the philosopher Michel Foucault's account of the transformation of sexual cultures in Europe in the eighteenth and nineteenth centuries. Foucault described how emergent scientific and medical conceptions of sexuality, which defined putatively normal and abnormal ways of being sexual, provided ordinary people with a new vocabulary to understand their sexuality. At the same time, as governments became concerned with "the population" as a vital resource to be administered, the control of sexuality and fertility emerged as a critical gateway to the political management of the citizenry. In these respects, Foucault's work prefigures central themes of this book. It therefore seems reasonable to ask, Can the story he told be brought forward into the recent era of sexual health?

In taking discourses about sexuality as his chief example of the productive character of the operation of power in modern Western societies, Foucault made two related arguments that challenged conventional wisdom. First, rather than viewing power as primarily constricting, confining, and negating—as that which "says 'no' to sex"— Foucault emphasized how the modern exercise of power could cultivate and shape sexual desires, meanings, and identities in profound and impressive ways, particularly through the propagation of discourses about sexuality, both among experts and in everyday life. In relation to sexuality, modern Western societies had witnessed a "discursive explosion": "Rather than a massive censorship, what was involved was a regulated and polymorphous incitement to discourse."[53] Second, rather than imagining that the power relations surrounding sexuality take a singular aim—for instance, as is so often bemoaned by critics of social convention, the goal of restricting sex to the sacred purpose of reproduction within monogamous heterosexual marriages—Foucault insisted on the diversity of agendas that sexuality has been called on to serve. In the social relations of modernity, sexuality has proved "useful for the greatest number of maneuvers and capable of serving as a point of support, as a linchpin, for the most varied strategies."[54]

Both of these observations retain a clear relevance. First, the recent proliferation of sexual health recalls the explosion of discourses surrounding sexuality in the eighteenth and nineteenth centuries— particularly those of a medical and scientific nature. Second, Foucault's observation about the range of political aims connected to the deployment of sexuality likewise remains helpful in thinking about the implications of the rise of a commitment to sexual health. As will become clearer as the book proceeds, the discourses and practices of sexual health are adaptable to a host of political goals, from protecting the population from harm, to governing and sanctioning irresponsible conduct, to promoting the betterment of the individual, to pursuing pleasure as a human right. There no single biopolitical "strategy" to which sexual health corresponds.

At the same time, recent developments suggest important differences from Foucault's account of an earlier era and underscore those considerations that Foucault may have failed to appreciate. As a preview of what will follow, I offer several caveats to signal the importance of qualifying and supplementing a Foucauldian account.

First, it will become clear that what especially distinguishes sexual health is not what, following Foucault, we might call its "discursive explosion," but rather the combination of that impressive spread with the mutability of its meanings. The spread of sexual health has depended on the productive ambiguity of the term itself, which seems to permit almost anything remotely connected to sexuality to be deemed a matter of sexual health. Moreover, the international reach of the concept of sexual health, both in English and in translation, suggests the more thoroughgoing impact of globalization on both sexual and health matters in recent decades, as compared to the time period that Foucault mostly considered.[55]

Second, in considering sexual health, it should be emphasized that neither sexuality nor health stand apart, as isolatable features of modern societies. On the contrary, the varied entanglements of sexuality and health are themselves profoundly shaped by other defining aspects of contemporary societies—and in particular, by the interweaving of sexuality with differences of race, social class, gender, and gender expression.[56] While this point is one that Foucault also recognized, he has been justly criticized for not having considered such issues in much detail.[57]

Third, Foucault's overall "take" on the modern deployment of sexuality was one of suspicion, and he was especially attuned to the policing of bodies and curtailment of pleasures that he associated with the rise of new forms of knowledge and power in relation to sexuality. When considering the more recent rise of sexual health, by contrast, I argue for a more open-ended appraisal of the consequences of its pursuit—one that recognizes trends that move in opposing directions and that is cautious about drawing sweeping conclusions or generalizations.[58]

STUDIES OF SEXUALITY, SCIENCE, AND HEALTH

Yet perhaps the most important caveat is the simple point that Foucault is not enough: we need to insert his insights into a broader theoretical framework shaped by studies of sexuality, health, and science. In the first place, then, this book fits in the tradition of "critical sexuality studies."[59] As the sociologist Ken Plummer framed it in 2012, that project assumes not only that "sexuality is a profoundly social matter" but also that "human sexualities are multiple, varied, and contradictory," and the range of "practices, meanings, identities, and worlds" is "mind-boggling." The analytical work needed to comprehend this "seething matrix of desires and practices"[60]—an effort that is, or ought to be, resolutely interdisciplinary[61]—resists taking constructs such as attraction, desire, the body, and identity for granted. Instead, it explores the cultural and historical processes that give them specific meanings in different places and times.[62] Drawing on feminist theory, queer theory, and critical studies of race, critical sexuality studies also takes a perspective from the margins; it seeks to reveal various forms of power and privilege that have structured the experience of sexuality and have obscured some forms of experience or rendered them socially invisible.[63]

At least in my version of it, critical sexuality studies treats sexuality (and therefore sexual health) as being, simultaneously, materially embedded in organizations and infrastructures, culturally expressed in symbols, artifacts, and practices, and physically enacted and experienced in bodies—and this book moves across these levels of analysis. As the sociologist Héctor Carrillo has observed, to study sexuality in this fashion "is simultaneously to shed light on culture, power, social interaction, social inequality, globalization, social movements, science, health, morality, and public policy"—all of which, in turn, also affect "the varied meanings, embodied experiences, power relationships, and personal and collective identities that take shape in relation to sexuality."[64]

Over time, critical sexuality studies has also become more attentive to the significance of sexual matters in the formation and operation of modern nation-states and the constitution of citizenship.[65] And it has likewise become more attuned to the transnational flow of bodies, meanings, categories, and practices across the borders of those states, and the place of sexuality within complex global histories of colonialism and postcolonialism.[66] Finally, a growing number of scholars in sexuality studies have emphasized the study of passion, desire, pleasure, and the "carnal" aspects of embodied experiences.[67] These various directions in sexuality studies provide important context for studying how sexual health becomes important to debates about who counts fully as a citizen, how sexual health is mobilized by transnational agencies such as the WHO, and whether sexual health promotion makes sufficient room for such matters as pleasure.

At the same time, an important premise of this book is that the various entanglements of sexuality and health are shaped by the interweaving of sexuality with differences of gender and gender expression, race and ethnicity, social class, religion, and (dis)ability. Sexual health, in short, is a fully intersectional construct whose meanings emerge in the fields of power within which various social identities, differences, and inequalities are organized and expressed.[68] Gender relations are a perfect example: perhaps most obviously, sexual health may have different stakes for people of different genders.[69] More subtly, but just as important, many ideas about sexual health have been powerfully shaped by the presumption that there are exactly two genders and that everyone identities with one or the other, as well as by assumptions about the naturalness of cisgender and heterosexual experiences.[70] The academic literature on these topics helps us analyze how, from the standpoint of sexual health discourses and practices, sexuality and gender may come to be construed either in appropriately broad or in problematically narrow ways.

The racial dynamics of sexual health bear out Ghassan Moussawi and Salvador Vidal-Ortiz's recent contention that an adequate sociological theorization of sexuality (or queer theory) is impossible without centering race and processes of racialization.[71] One theme that recurs over the course of this book is the racialization of sexual health— expressed sometimes in the implicit whiteness of ostensibly race-neutral discourse, and at other times by the ways in which nonwhite racial and ethnic groups become explicit targets of concern, intervention, and (sometimes) stigmatization and coercion. Race and racism affect who is considered capable of achieving sexual health (and of what sort), which kind of body is deemed healthy, and who is seen as possessing agency in pursuing sexually healthy outcomes.[72] My thinking here is informed by much scholarship on the mutual constitution of race and sexuality, including studies of how definitions of proper sexuality have been invoked to consolidate understandings of whiteness.[73]

These considerations suggest the richness and usefulness of critical sexuality studies as applied to the topic of sexual health. Yet no matter how comprehensive critical sexuality studies may become, that field alone cannot do justice to the terrain of sexual health. As an analysis of medical knowledge and health practice, this book is also deeply rooted in a second interdisciplinary field: social, cultural, and historical studies of science, technology, and medicine. Science studies (for short) has focused attention on how scientific practitioners organize their work activities; make claims about knowledge and strive to endow those claims with credibility; and defend, or extend, the boundaries of their practice.[74] However, over time such work has progressively broadened the scope of analysis and cast of characters to consider much more expansive arenas. These include the political, organizational, and infrastructural dimensions of knowledge production; the cultural meanings and effects of tools, objects, standards, and categories; the manufacture and deployment of expertise; and the dynamics of citizen engagement and social movement activism in debates surrounding knowledge, risk, and innovation.[75]

Increasingly, scholars working from a science studies tradition have turned their attention to understanding the diverse worlds of health and medicine, as well as the ways in which human bodies, in all their organic, cellular, and genetic distinctiveness, appear to take on an ever more central role in defining our selves, our identities, and our places within the society and the polity.[76] Such work has both borrowed from, and invigorated, long traditions of discipline-based scholarship in fields such as the sociology of health and illness, medical anthropology, and the history of medicine. I take from this broad literature a number of emphases that are especially salient when thinking about sexual health. First, in the words of Annemarie Mol and Marc Berg, "medicine is not a coherent whole [but], rather, an amalgam of thoughts, a mixture of habits, an assemblage of techniques."[77] Studying this multiplicity and diversity is challenging but crucial. Second, the worlds of research and the worlds of health care have become interconnected in ever more substantial ways—as suggested by the compound word "biomedicine," a twentieth-century invention that signals the necessarily joint study of the "normal" and the "pathological."[78] Finally, biomedical and health practices and processes increasingly have shaped how people make sense of who they are in the world and have also contributed to new understandings of "biocitizenship"—the varied ways in which one's relationship to one's own body, particularly including issues of health and disease, becomes a basis for political claims or for the assertion of rights or assumption of responsibilities.[79]

In its formative years, science studies was slow to take up the topic of sexuality. However, that such work can be made broadly compatible with what I have called critical sexuality studies is suggested by recent moves to "queer" science and technology studies.[80] More specifically, a review essay by Jennifer Fishman, Laura Mamo, and Patrick Grzanka on "sex, gender, and sexuality in biomedicine" goes a long way toward articulating a synthetic theoretical backdrop for studies such as this one.[81] These authors emphasize how sex, gender, and sexuality function as key categories of difference in biomedicine: they serve as objects of biomedical analysis, but such analysis also helps to generate, or transform, the very meanings of those categories.[82] To be sure, the persistent emphasis (at least nominally) on "biomedicine" in their essay is somewhat at odds with my goal here of connecting the study of biomedicine with that of the broader terrain of health. However, the approach is important for its insistence on the embodied and material aspects of both sexuality and health and its rejection of a dualistic opposition between "biological facts" and "social constructions."[83] In this book, I seek not to sever nature from culture or biology from society, or reduce one side of the pair to the other, but to examine their complex intertwining.

Tracing the Worlds of Sexual Health

Of course, I am not the first to wonder about the rise of the term "sexual health" and the ways of organizing social, political, and biomedical activities that the term has engendered. While most literature on sexual health simply takes the term for granted (or, perhaps, ponders the definitional complexities), some scholars have taken a more historicist approach. I build on four perceptive, article-length analyses of sexual health that all appeared in the early 2000s—by Alain Giami, Theo Sandfort and Anke Ehrhardt, Weston Edwards and Eli Coleman, and Richard Parker and coauthors—as well as an encyclopedia article on the topic by Laura Carpenter published in 2007.[84] By sharing the presumption that there is nothing obvious about the fact that a form of health called sexual health has come into being, these scholars prompted me to undertake a more broad-ranging analysis of the rise, proliferation, and effects of sexual health discourses and practices.[85]

Even with the benefit of exemplars, it is challenging to systematically research an object or concept when, as I have noted, part of what needs to be investigated is what the thing *is*—how it is defined, how it is bounded, and how it has come into being. I have had to sample widely in order to capture different conceptions and instantiations of sexual health. In this regard, my approach bears similarities to Elizabeth Bernstein's "ethnography of a discourse," which she describes as being "deliberately mobile and multisited, traveling with its empirical object across varied political and cultural domains."[86] My thinking about the study of discourse is influenced by what Reiner Keller calls "the sociology of knowledge approach to discourse," a research program that examines "the discursive construction of symbolic orders which occurs in the form of conflicting social knowledge relationships and competing politics of knowledge." This approach, according to Keller, treats discourses as "performative statement practices which constitute reality orders and also produce power effects in a conflict-ridden network of social actors, institutional dispositifs, and knowledge systems." By this reading, as Keller emphasizes, "discourse is concrete and material, it is not an abstract idea or free floating line of arguments."[87]

Concretely, conducting the research for this book has meant reconstructing histories of sexual health activities and tracing those activities across a wide range of institutions and locations. I collected and analyzed a very substantial body of diverse sources, both print and electronic, in which sexual health was a topic of discussion, including medical and public health journal articles, reports and documents from local and federal governments, reports and documents from transnational agencies such as the WHO and the United Nations, news media articles and editorials, and documents obtained from websites of organizations including advocacy groups, nongovernmental organizations, professional associations, and foundations. My analysis emphasized not only tracing developments over time but also juxtaposing and comparing the portrayals of the same issues found in different social worlds, organizational spaces, informational platforms, or communities of practice.

For the conclusions presented in chapter 2 about the proliferation of the discourses and practices of sexual health, I draw on an earlier article coauthored with Laura Mamo. With the assistance of our research assistants, Mamo and I adopted a more systematic mode of analysis: we subjected specific bodies of data, including more than one thousand journal article abstracts and nearly five hundred newspaper articles, to formal content analysis.[88]

In addition, to research sexual health, I conducted interviews with selected leaders in the field, and I undertook ethnographic work at conferences, such as the National Sexual Health Conference and an annual meeting of the World Association for Sexual Health. Qualitative research of these kinds helped me to observe interactions in real time among key participants in the worlds of sexual health, and helped me to confirm or disconfirm the understandings I reached from reviewing literature.

Both to generate hypotheses and to illustrate trends, I made use of "Google Ngrams," which I created using the Google Ngram Viewer,[89] and a number of these appear in the book. Ngrams are produced through an algorithm that searches the Google Books database, an extensive collection of digitized books (through the publication year 2019, as of the time of this book's completion). Each Ngram takes the form of a graph over time of all occurrences of specified phrases, expressed as a percentage of all phrases of the same word length cataloged in the Google Books database, with results normalized by the total number of such books published each year.[90] The utility of these graphs in demonstrating trends and suggesting angles of investigation outweighs, in my view, the potential pitfalls of the tool.[91]

My Path Forward

This book tells many of the key stories of sexual health, but it cannot be comprehensive. In some respects, the book is "kaleidoscopic," to borrow the science studies scholar Karin Knorr Cetina's characterization of her book *Epistemic Cultures*. Like Knorr Cetina, I examine "conjunctions of activities by means of a succession of shifts in focus, as someone might turn a kaleidoscope." Although this book charts historical processes of development, and while each chapter builds on preceding ones with key themes recurring across them, I share with Knorr Cetina the disavowal of any pretense "that the combination of patterns I discuss somehow adds up to all that could be said" about the topic.[92]

To write a book on sexual health, I have had to make strategic choices. My focus is on the conjoining of sexuality with health—what happens at their intersection. Therefore, readers seeking a more general treatment of the current landscape of sexuality politics, or health politics, will need to consult additional sources. A research dilemma along the way has concerned whether to trace "sexual health" (the term) or the various ideas and practices encapsulated by the concept, whatever those might end up being called. I have done some tacking back and forth between term and concept, although mostly I have "followed the term,"[93] and in fact, some of my research strategies (such as the content analysis of all medical journal articles containing the phrase "sexual health" in the title) have necessarily required me to do just that. In following the term, I was influenced by Stefan Helmreich and Sophia Roosth, who, in their keyword analysis of the term "life form," emphasized the constitutive effects of language as "a crucible in which ideas take shape." They noted: "Our aim is to use *life form*, the term, as an index through which to gauge what 'life,' the concept, has meant at different moments."[94]

Another set of strategic and practical choices concerns the geographic range of my data collection and analysis. Sexual health traverses various global fields of action, raising important methodological and theoretical questions about how to trace activity that is distinctively transnational or global.[95] At the same time, this characteristic of sexual health generates practical dilemmas for any researcher not prepared to devote multiple lifetimes to a study of the topic. Moreover, my own focus on the term itself prompts thorny issues of language translation. I reflect on the global spread of concern with sexual health in several chapters, but suffice it to say for now that there are many stories to be told about *salud sexual* (in Spanish), *santé sexuelle* (in French), *sexuelle gesundheit* (in German), and *seksuelle gesondheid* (in Dutch). Undoubtedly, "sexual health" has also been translated into many other languages besides these, though in addition the English-language term crops up regularly in many non-Anglophone settings.

I have not tried to tell all those stories in this book. Nor have I tried to determine whether the translated terms connote "the same" or "different" constructs, or to trace what might be "lost in translation." While I bring in examples from various parts of the world along the way, my focus is mostly on the United States (about which I possess relevant scholarly expertise),[96] as well as on the important transnational actors that have helped the concept to circulate globally both in English and in translation—especially the WHO, a key player in many of the chapters in this book.[97] My hope is that the investigation presented in these pages opens up space for others to conduct finer-grained explorations of sexual health in many different places and at different geographic scales. Such scholarship, in turn, would shed needed light on the broader concept as well as on developments in the United States.

I now turn to the story of how this multifaceted thing called sexual health came into being as a widespread object of concern. What is its provenance? What circumstances gave it birth?

Part 1: Making Sexual Health

INVENTION, DISPERSION, AND REASSEMBLY

Nowadays, "sexual health" is everywhere. It is a term that heads government websites; a marketing category for selling condoms and sex toys; a topic of scientific investigation and survey research; a set of medical diagnoses; and the name given to journals, conferences, organizations, and popular magazines. Why is this, and how did it come to be? Through what processes did sexuality and health come to be joined? What *is* sexual health—and who gets to define it? How does the rise of sexual health affect our visions of sexuality and our images of health?

Chapters 1 through 3 reconstruct the history while exploring the paradox of dispersion and reassembly. Sexual health first built on pre-existing ways of thinking about bodies and desires, but then it took on a life of its own. As sexual health evolved into a way of addressing a range of social problems, it seemed to become a buzzword, capable of application in the most diverse circumstances, at the risk of losing any specific meaning. Yet the very diversity of sexual health projects has created new possibilities to stitch together the meanings to form a comprehensive sexual health umbrella.

These developments all hinged on the ability of the definers and promoters of sexual health to wrestle successfully with several conundrums: Is sexual health a scientific concept or a moral judgment? Is sexual health the same everywhere, or is a universal approach the wrong way to think about it? Can concepts of sexual health be invoked without privileging the experiences of some groups in society and devaluing others? The intractability of these questions has framed debates over the definition, purposes, and utility of sexual health.

1 A New Definition and the Backstory

INVENTING SEXUAL HEALTH

"Happy Birthday, Sexual Health," proclaimed the headline of a magazine article, published in 2016, that marked the passage of "100 years since the first Planned Parenthood clinic was opened by women's health advocate Margaret Sanger in Brooklyn."[1] The idea of marking birthdays is appealing, but can we really speak of "sexual health" as having such a well-defined origin point in the course of history? It can be a tricky enough matter even to locate an organization's birth: in fact, what Sanger (not alone, but working with others) founded in 1916 was a clinic that, in 1921, became part of the American Birth Control League, which changed its name to Planned Parenthood in 1942.[2]

Even more problematic is the suggestion that a concept like sexual health might have a specifiable birthdate (let alone one that coincides neatly with the history, or prehistory, of Planned Parenthood). The point is not merely that neither Sanger nor any of her collaborators in 1916 would have been likely to call what they were doing the pursuit of "sexual health." More profoundly, "sexual health" is, at one and the same time, the conceptual progeny of diverse ways of imagining the intersection of sexuality and health that went under various names, and a specifically recent way of thinking about this intersection that was first codified in the form of a definition hammered out in Geneva, Switzerland, at a meeting convened by the WHO in 1974. In other words, sexual health is, simultaneously, older than one hundred years and a fair bit younger as well.

This chapter examines the defining of sexual health in 1974, but it first provides a summary genealogy of sexual health. Doing so takes me into a brief review of nineteenth- and twentieth-century manuals of marital and sex advice; the rise of a modern global science of sexology; and the influential late nineteenth- and early twentieth-century public health initiatives and activism undertaken under the rubric of "social hygiene."

This prehistory of sexual health matters. The ideas and motivations that fueled the invention of what we now know as sexual health did not appear suddenly, out of nowhere, in the 1970s. Nowadays, as I have already indicated, "sexual health" is an omnipresent concern. But to make sense of the invention of sexual health and the explosion of interest in it, we need to examine the immediate precursors—medical and cultural projects that bequeathed to the modern definers of sexual health, and their successors, particular ways of thinking. These include not just the general belief that the proper management of sex is central to healthy living, although that is certainly important. In addition, our contemporary perspectives appropriate and rework a number of more specific assumptions that circulated in the nineteenth and twentieth centuries—for example, that we should turn to experts to tell us about our sexual natures as well as for advice about how to manage sexual risk and experience a more healthy and fulfilling sexuality; that individuals may possess rights in relation to their sexualities; that healthy sexuality is something that governments might seek to promote; and that the sexuality of some groups in society might be deemed "problematic" and in need of social management. In these respects, the genealogical precursors of sexual health set the stage for the discussion that follows in the rest of this book.

The topics of medical sex advice, sexology, and social hygiene have been considered carefully by historians and other scholars. My goal is more specific: I extract particular ways of thinking and acting that set the stage for recent-day approaches to sexuality and health—indeed, ways of thinking and acting that helped to solidify the very understanding that sexuality and health are to be seen as indissociable concerns. Of course, I could go back further: there is a longer history—in Western societies and elsewhere—of associating sex with disease and, often simultaneously, with sin.[3] But the developments I trace here share the specific presumption that the proper management of sexuality is crucial for health, broadly construed—and not only for individual health but also for marital and relationship health, as well as for the health and functioning of the society as a whole. While these projects demonstrate the influence of medical expertise in speaking credibly about sexual matters, some of them also place a spotlight on nonmedical experts as well as other sorts of advocates and activists.

I therefore begin by describing the forging of consequential links between the domains of health and sexuality in the century and a half preceding the WHO-sponsored meeting. I focus on the United States, but I also consider developments elsewhere that directly prefigured that definitional process. Then, I turn to the events and social transformations of the 1960s and 1970s that led up to and surrounded the defining of sexual health in 1974 at a WHO-sponsored meeting. This is followed by a close reading of portions of the report from that meeting that was published the following year.[4] I consider why the act of defining something called sexual health came to make sense at this historical moment, but also how it built on and brought together aspects of earlier ways of connecting sexuality and health. Finally, I explore some of the specifics, and peculiarities, of the definition and examine how it presaged and prepared the way for future developments and debates.

Studying the "Coming into Being"

How do we best study and describe how something like sexual health has made its way into the world? To be clear, in describing the "inventing" of sexual health, my goal is by no means to suggest that sexual health is somehow "not real"—that it is, perhaps, a fanciful concoction whose very legitimacy as a thing in the world we might call into question or debunk. Rather, the point is to trace the set of meanings that have come to adhere to the term and the concept as they have come into being.[5] The profound effects of the discourses and activities connected to sexual health are sufficient in themselves to establish sexual health as something real but also as an entity with a discernable history that warrants investigation.

My exploration in this chapter of the historical emergence of sexual health is guided by the theories and examples of scholars, studying other topics, who have taken broadly "genealogical" approaches to trace the origins and trajectories of various terms, concepts, or objects.[6] Often influenced by the work of Michel Foucault, such genealogies are concerned with the simultaneous constitution of new entities and new historical actors; they examine conditions of possibility for emergence and link those conditions to power relations of diverse sorts.[7]

A useful offshoot of the genealogical approach that specifically considers the emergence of new entities is called "historical ontology"—a
term borrowed from Foucault by the philosopher Ian Hacking to refer to the methodological tracing of the "space of possibilities" of a
concept in formation.[8] While this method often focuses attention on
processes of emergence, it is equally useful, as David Ribes and Jessica
Polk have described, in examining how objects change over time, even
as they appear to remain "the same thing."[9]

Tracing the trajectories of new entities is especially challenging,
however, when they evolve through interactions across multiple social
worlds, both expert and lay, and when the terminology used to describe
them appears to consist of everyday words—like "sexual" and "health"—
that may take on specialized meanings within distinct communities
of practice. As the analysts of science Evelyn Fox Keller and Elisabeth
Lloyd noted in their dissection of familiar terms in evolutionary biology, such as "competition," "adaptation," and "fitness," these ostensibly
scientific terms cast long "semantic shadows." They observed: "Words,
even technical terms, have insidious ways of traversing the boundaries
of particular theories, of historical periods, and of disciplines—in the
process contaminating the very notion of a pure culture."[10]

Sexuality, Medical Authority, and Sex Advice

In the nineteenth century, a significant precursor of what we now know
as the promotion of sexual health was the provision of advice about
sexual matters in book form, typically, though not always, by medical
doctors, to ordinary people eager for a clearer understanding of human
sexuality and reproduction.[11] On rare occasions, advice books of this
sort even identified themselves using the very term "sexual health"—as
in the title of New York physician Henry G. Hanchett's volume, *Sexual
Health: A Plain and Practical Guide for the People in All Matters Concerning
the Organs of Reproduction in Both Sexes and All Ages*, published in New
York City in 1887.[12] More often, however, those proffering advice used
other labels to characterize their concerns, though many shared with
Hanchett a certain sensibility reflected in the latter's assertion that
"the author has no apology to make for the plain and outspoken manner in which he has treated the delicate subjects considered."[13]

As the historian Helen Horowitz has emphasized, nineteenth-
century Americans engaged in a "complex conversation about sex" that

reflected multiple and competing understandings of sexual topics—indeed, sexuality was "among the matters about which Americans disagreed most sharply."[14] One important flavor emerging from within the stew of "sexual cultures" that Horowitz has described was an understanding of sexuality rooted in "new notions of the body, nerves, and the relation of mind and body." Lecturers and writers concerned with health and disease promoted a vision of sexuality that united a focus on the nervous system with "new notions of romantic love that put feeling and its expression at the center."[15] The authors presenting this "new science of the body" to an expanding middle-class audience were invested in offering "prescriptions for living": in some cases, they "[insisted] on the naturalness of the body's sexual appetites and desires," but in others—exemplified by the aggressive campaign against masturbation—they "counseled sobriety and habits of order."[16]

The historian Charles Rosenberg has examined the prolific work of one widely read US writer and lecturer of this sort: Frederick C. Hollick, whose mid-nineteenth-century books and pamphlets offered advice on sexual behavior interspersed with advertised opportunities to obtain, via mail order, such products as condoms, aphrodisiacs, and a device intended to increase penis size.[17] Hollick (who may have lacked formal medical training) ranged widely, addressing methods of birth control, the ills caused by masturbation, and the secrets of marital bliss. His approach was one that sought, on the one hand, to treat sexual desire as normal and legitimate, and, on the other hand, to help individuals learn how best to manage and structure that desire in socially appropriate ways. Perhaps what is most intriguing, Rosenberg suggests, is that Hollick's work prefigured a future-directed orientation to risk management and a desire to "optimize" one's sexuality that many would associate more closely with the present day: "Hollick was particularly attuned to the needs and perceptions of a rapidly urbanizing, economically labile, society anxious to predict its future in a challenging world. How to think about oneself? How to think about the number and prospects of one's children? . . . Managing sex was managing future social risk—for oneself as well as one's family."[18]

In the decades that followed, and indeed into the early to mid-twentieth century, "marriage manuals" continued what the historian Jessamyn Neuhaus has described as enunciating a "sexual ideal," stamped with the imprimatur of the expert.[19] With the ostensible goal of improving marital harmony, these prescriptive guides sometimes set forth "very detailed instructions for sexual activity"—like the assertion by one author that, during coitus, the penis should be inserted at "a forty-five degree angle downward."[20] Matters of timing were also addressed in the pages of these manuals, as Annamarie Jagose has described in her analysis of the promotion of the virtues of the simultaneous orgasm.[21] In some cases, as Jane Ward has observed, the authors sought to recuperate heterosexual marriage by teaching women and men how they might accomplish the goal of physical attraction, which was presumed not to arise naturally. These experts "made explicit that heterosexual marriage was no longer a labor contract in which both parties showed up 'as is' but an ongoing affective project requiring access to precise tools and information that would build mutual affection."[22]

The authors of these guides were prophets of normality—indeed, in their "critical genealogy" of the concept of normality, Peter Cryle and Elizabeth Stephens have suggested that it was particularly in sex advice books of this time "that the word 'normal' gradually came into more regular use in professional discourses and then moved into the public sphere."[23] But the idea of the normal was noteworthy both for what it endorsed and for what it left unsaid. In the latter category, as Julian Carter has argued, was the implicit whiteness, as well as heterosexuality, of the normality placed on offer in these books. Absorbing earlier ideas of "civilization" and "evolution," the new discourses of normality "made it possible to talk about whiteness indirectly, in terms of the affectionate, reproductive heterosexuality of 'normal' married couples."[24]

Such volumes also proved to be remarkably popular with consumers. In the United Kingdom, by far the most important marriage manual was *Married Love: A New Contribution to the Solution of Sex Difficulties.* Published by Marie Stopes in 1918, the book had sold more than half a million copies by 1925, offering these readers a vision of a healthy and satisfying erotic life.[25] In the United States, the gynecologist Theodoor van de Velde's *Ideal Marriage: Its Philosophy and Techniques* (translated into English from the Dutch original) first appeared in 1930 but remained in print until the mid-1960s; one edition alone sold more than half a million copies.[26] Van de Velde's title-page epigraph from Balzac—"Marriage is a science"—captured the philosophy of a volume that sought to bring contemporary knowledge to bear on intimate matters.[27]

We know little about how readers made sense of what they encountered in the pages of nineteenth- and twentieth-century sex advice books or whether or how the prescriptions they found there made their way into their everyday sexual practices or social relationships. But we can glean from their popularity that these books served as important touchstones. In their manifest concern not only with the well-being of individuals but also with the proper functioning of societies, these guides both reflected and furthered changing social norms about sexuality, gender, race, reproduction, and the body. Most important for my purposes, the market for these publications demonstrates the emergent solidity of two relationships: first, that between sexuality and health, now perceived as linked, in part by a preoccupation with "normality"; and second, that between the self-proclaimed experts speaking of this unified domain of inquiry and the eager consumers of their knowledge and commodities.

The Advent of Sexology

While sexual matters have long been considered to fall under the purview of medicine, the late nineteenth century saw the rise of broader-ranging attempts to develop a scientific study of sexuality.[28] Reflecting a shift in interest, as the historian Chris Waters has described, from "the classification of the vices" to "the psychology of the perversions,"[29] this emergent science went on to adopt broader goals· beyond the understanding and treatment of sexual "pathologies" to the identification of the very "laws of Nature." But the effects were imagined to be even more profound. In the words of the historian Jeffrey Weeks: "The early sexologists perceived themselves as engaged in a symbolic struggle between darkness and light, ignorance and enlightenment, and in this 'science' was their surest weapon."[30]

Once scholars such as Richard von Krafft-Ebing had proposed increasingly elaborate taxonomies of sexual "perversions," physicians, scientists, and other scholars began to address the question of how to understand "normal" sexuality.[31] In 1906, the Berlin scientist Iwan Bloch coined the term *Sexualwissenschaft*—"sexual science," or sexology—to characterize this new field of inquiry.[32] In 1908, together with German physician and scholar Magnus Hirschfeld, Bloch established the new field's first journal, the *Zeitschrift für Sexualwissenschaft*.[33] While most histories of sexology have emphasized male scholarly figures, the

historian Kirsten Leng's recent account traces the surprisingly extensive links between sexological research and the feminist movement
in Germany in the prewar and interwar periods, and she examines in
detail how a group of women drew on diverse scientific writings of
the time period to establish their credibility within, and reshape the
nature of, a distinctive field of knowledge production.[34]

But in fact, the knowledge base of sexology was hybrid from the
start—"interdisciplinary avant la lettre," as Leng puts it—encompassing
findings from natural science fields such as endocrinology alongside
more humanistic investigations into broadly psychological, sociological, and ethnographic concerns.[35] This variety was also reflected in sexology's global spread, which, according to Waters, was already evident
by 1914.[36] While sexological developments most typically have been
associated with scholars and physicians in Germany and England,
Veronika Fuechtner, Douglas Haynes, and Ryan Jones have argued
that "sexual science . . . was a global formation that simultaneously
emerged in multiple sites and that took multiple shapes."[37] Although
sexology took root "in places like Shanghai, Mexico City, Tokyo, Bom-
bay, Windhoek, Santiago, Casablanca, Tel Aviv, and Buenos Aires,"
there was "no tendency toward intellectual homogenization in the
views put forward."[38] Rather, not only did local sexologies reflect local
preoccupations but also the ideas that bounced around from place to
place traveled by diverse pathways, in ways that belie any simple notion of transmission from "core" to "periphery."[39]

The golden age of sexology corresponded roughly to the interval
between 1919, when Hirschfeld founded the world's first Institute for
Sexology in Berlin, and 1933, when a Nazi mob ransacked the institute
(deemed degenerate) and its papers were burned.[40] Hirschfeld and others worked to convene a series of world congresses on sexology, beginning in 1921 with the first such congress held in Berlin. In 1928,
Hirschfeld also launched an advocacy organization, the World League
for Sexual Reform.[41] As the sociologist Gert Hekma has described,
the league's practical goals encompassed a wide range of themes that
would be recognized as "progressive" today, including the equality of
women and men, access to birth control, and systematic sex education, but also others that "would be out of place in a contemporary progressive organisation" such as "racial betterment through eugenics."[42]

Over the course of the first three-quarters of the twentieth century
(that is, in the period preceding the defining of sexual health), sexology

also became intertwined with other influential approaches to the study of sexuality and treatment of sexual problems. While Sigmund Freud at times collaborated with sexologists and engaged with their work, psychoanalysis took the study of sexuality in different directions. Freud presumed a biological basis to the sexual drive, but in practice he rooted his developmental theory of human sexual maturation in an analysis of the vicissitudes of interpersonal relationships and intrapsychic processes.[43] After the Second World War, the United States became a center of sex research, but Alfred Kinsey's survey research moved that field in a more empirical and sociological direction.[44] Subsequently, as sexual science in the United States veered toward applied sex therapy—epitomized by the work of William Masters and Virginia Johnson—the focus turned to the physiology of the sexual response and the possibilities of using behavioral interventions to treat sexual dysfunctions.[45]

By the second half of the twentieth century, in Europe and the United States, sexual science had lost any claim to status as a well-defined field.[46] Moreover, in the 1960s, the status of sexology in the United States was eroded by various challenges to psychiatric authority, certainly including the vigorous protests by gay liberationists of the classification of homosexuality as a mental disorder.[47] Elsewhere, sexology developed in other directions—for example, as Fuechtner, Hayes, and Jones have noted, "in Mexico and Argentina, sexology remains a prominent discipline tied to human rights initiatives, as well as to fields like anthropology and psychoanalysis."[48]

Like the sexological projects promoted by pioneers earlier in the century, these various forms of twentieth-century sexual science have lent themselves to a wide variety of political, social, and moral stances, ranging from the advocacy of sexual freedom to the preaching of sexual restraint. Each of them has inspired new techniques of diagnosis and classification and new understandings of what it might mean to be normal. And each of them, in different ways, has also continued the practice of offering advice to laypeople—the curious and the worried alike—about how to solve sexual problems and live a healthier sexual life.[49] These various attributes and inclinations would carry forward into the worlds of sexual health. Indeed, as will become clear in subsequent chapters, the rise of the idea of sexual health in the 1970s and its spread in subsequent decades has been propelled in part by sexologists even while providing them with a crucial opportunity to repackage and relabel their concerns.

But in addition, as the historian Dagmar Herzog has described, the increasing professionalization of sex research has proceeded "in dialectical interaction with the self-representations of sexual minorities."[50] As the groups that were named and classified by sexologists came to assert, and insist on, the authority to speak for themselves—what Foucault had called a "reverse discourse"[51]—the political consequences were, at least potentially, profound: "Ordinary people increasingly understood and represented themselves not only as beings with sexual identities, but also as beings with sexual rights—whether to privacy or to public attention, to 'normal' functioning or to the transgression of norms perceived as illegitimate, to intensity of experience or to safety from sexual harm."[52] Thus, as Weeks has also emphasized, the experts who divided the sexual world into the "normal" and the "deviant" and named new identities encouraged social and political changes that increasingly called into question the very idea of the normal.[53] This view perhaps risks overstating the real-world impact of sexological thinking or understating the extent to which sexology itself incorporated, and emerged in response to, ordinary people's self-understandings.[54] Yet it offers an important suggestion: in considering more recent developments billed as connected to sexual health, we should examine how categories and norms emerge out of the space of interactions between credentialed experts and laypeople of various sorts.

The Era of Social Hygiene

A particularly relevant historical predecessor to the present-day conception of sexual health, as Theo Sandfort and Anke Ehrhardt have also observed, was the social hygiene movement, visible in the United States especially from the latter years of the nineteenth century through the First World War.[55] Social hygiene united the efforts and interests of physicians, social workers, public health officials, military leaders, and other government bureaucrats with those of "predominantly female moral reformers, heirs to the tradition of the 'purity crusade.'"[56] As the sociologist Kristin Luker has noted, "Together, the two traditions created the quintessentially Progressive blend of moral zeal and technical expertise."[57] The name of this movement is revealing: while "social" functioned as much as a euphemism for "sexual" as a reference to social issues, "hygiene," according to Luker, "was a magical word": it "encompassed health in all its dimensions: social, mental, spiritual, and physical."[58]

As the historian of medicine Allan Brandt has emphasized, social hygiene was the imagined solution both to the moral contamination of modern urban society and to the "venereal diseases" that seemed to be the physical embodiment of a fraying moral fabric.[59] In line with the eugenic discourses that were ubiquitous at the time, reformers associated this moral decay with the infusion of immigrants to US urban centers at the same time as those people of Anglo-Saxon descent were committing "race suicide" through their failure to reproduce at the same rates as newcomers.[60] In addition to race and nationality, hygienists also focused on the category of age. The body of the child—the target of sex instruction—"functioned as a metaphor for larger social concerns," according to R. Danielle Egan and Gail Hawkes: "childhood sexuality within the social hygiene movement was constructed as a site in need of precautionary interference and as a justification for wider social intervention."[61]

Social hygienists focused on diverse strategies of sex education, disease prevention, and legal regulation to carry out their moral campaigns, assert a normative vision of social order, and draw boundaries around social belonging.[62] In public lectures about venereal disease, "social hygienists stressed the physical horrors of syphilis with such vigor that it was common for listeners to faint where they sat."[63] But the point was not simply to warn of consequences but also to emphasize the moral imperatives of healthy behavior. According to Dr. Prince Morrow, the founder in 1905 of the American Society for Sanitary and Moral Prophylaxis (a group that consisted mostly of physicians), "venereal disease seeks no man . . . ; it must be sought in order to be acquired."[64] US Surgeon General W. C. Gorgas, like the movement generally, placed the blame for venereal disease on the looser morals of men and argued against the sexual double standard, yet in practice it was female sex workers who bore the brunt of reformers' energies.[65]

Legislation promoted by reformers created a new category of laws against "morality crimes" that focused particularly on penalizing commercial sex workers, including, in some jurisdictions, the detention of prostitutes found to be infected with a venereal disease.[66] In addition, a concern with "male perversion" prompted new scrutiny of male same-sex activity in urban areas.[67] Laws promoted by social hygiene advocates combined in their effects with earlier laws on the books, such as the 1873 federal Comstock Act, ostensibly an anti-obscenity bill that also outlawed the dissemination of birth control, or information about it, across state lines.[68] Thus, legal social controls extended well beyond the domains of sex work and sexually transmitted diseases to envelop a wide range of sexual and reproductive concerns.

The campaign against venereal disease took on new urgency with the entry of the United States into the First World War, for, as Secretary of the Navy Josephus Daniels observed, "men must live straight if they would shoot straight."[69] Or as one reformer claimed, "It is generally recognized that a bad and diseased woman can do more harm than any German fleet of airplanes that has yet passed over London."[70] Of course, anxieties about the moral fiber of soldiers coincided with more prosaic concerns about manpower: government officials characterized syphilis as the primary cause of lost workdays within the US military during the war.[71]

The twin impetuses of moralism and science existed in some state of tension within the social hygiene movement; and especially with the advent, by midcentury, of antibiotic treatment for sexually transmitted infections, moral campaigners and health professionals pushed toward different practical solutions.[72] While some of the discourse of social hygiene continued to find expression through the Second World War and beyond, the energy of the reform wave subsided. However, the social hygiene era anticipated that of sexual health in several important respects: it brought together, under one platform, new forms of activism, social regulation, and normative judgment with regard to sexuality and health, and it combined state governance of sexuality with exhortations for the governance of the self. I will return to these ideas particularly in chapter 9, where I will point to continuities but also important differences between social hygiene and what I will there call "sexual health governance."

Setting the Stage for the Defining of Sexual Health

The historical developments in the nineteenth and first half of the twentieth centuries that I have summarized in the preceding pages did not lead in any direct or inexorable way to the present-day pursuit of sexual health. But, together, these episodes suggest the accretion of a series of connections between sexuality and health—connections that were not altogether new in themselves but were new in their intensity and their historical simultaneity. Sex as a flourishing topic of health advice; the rise of a consumer market around sexual knowledge and commodities seen as health promoting; the impetus to manage sexual risks and optimize one's sexuality in a healthy or scientific direction; the emergence of ideas about sexual rights as an intrinsic human possession; the growing power of science to define the nature of sexuality (and the growth of resistance to that power); the shaping of sexual norms out of interactions between expert and lay actors; the increasing differentiation of expertise about sexual topics; social attention to the imagined sexual threats posed by various marginalized groups, including people of color; the link between political governance in relation to sexual threats and the governance of the sexual self: these became the building blocks for recent conceptions of sexual health, and these are themes that recur over the course of this book.

In the decades following the decline of the social hygiene movement, these trends continued to develop, with some of them, such as the provision of sex advice, becoming increasingly widespread.[73] But if such ideas had been percolating for some time, the promulgation of a definition of sexual health in 1974 also responded to more specific developments—social, cultural, political, and health related—in the second half of the twentieth century. These conditions of possibility for the emergence of a new object included, first, important changes in the social organization of sexuality over the course of the twentieth century and, most immediately, in the 1960s and 1970s.[74] The sexual revolution, fueled by political, cultural, and technological developments—including the invention and mass marketing of new modes of contraception such as the pill[75]—had put sex on the agenda as an important and prized dimension of human experience, which experts, professionals, and governments were expected to take into account.[76] Moreover, new social movements, including second-wave feminism and the emergent gay rights movement, were, by the 1970s, foregrounding questions of sexuality and sexual freedom in new and profound ways around the globe.[77] As Janice Irvine has described, these movements, together with other organizational byproducts of the sexual revolution, have helped to transform the emotional culture of Western societies in favor of new forms of expressiveness.[78] At the same time, along with the rise in attention to "reproductive health" (itself an invention of the time period[79]) also came "First World" concern with the economic consequences of "Third World" population growth.[80]

On the one hand, these various social changes marked an important moment in the historical disembedding of sexuality from the domain of procreation and the emergence of the sexual as a domain with its own scientific questions and practical concerns, including assertions of women's as well as men's bodily autonomy. On the other hand, these changes reflected the continued intertwining of sexual and procreative issues in practice (particularly including a focus on the risks that those in "developed" countries imagined to be stemming from uncontrolled sexuality, and hence rapid population growth, in the "developing world"[81]). Increasingly, as reformers and advocates took stock of these varied social changes that, importantly, now seemed to take on a global character, "sexual health" seemed like an appropriate thread to stitch together many of these concerns.

A good example of this new packaging of an overlapping set of salient issues is the lecture on "sexual health and family planning" delivered in 1967 at the annual meeting of the American Public Health Association by the physician, sex educator, and activist Dr. Mary Calderone, president of the Sexuality Information and Education Council of the United States (SIECUS) and former president of Planned Parenthood.[82] Calderone's talk began with a discussion of family planning, the pill, the intrauterine device (or the IUD), and the growing awareness of population growth as a concern, but then segued to the process by which a child builds a sexual identity, and from there to the theme of sex education. Advocating "sex education as preventive medicine" that encompassed the total sexual development of the individual, Calderone united the goals of what she called sexual fulfillment, sexual responsibility, and sexual health.[83] Thus Calderone, in 1967, was already well on the way to promoting the kind of expansive definition of sexual health that would be put forward a few years later—at the WHO-sponsored meeting in which she, in fact, participated.

To be sure, when speakers in this period, such as Calderone, referred to something they called sexual health, they were gesturing at an entity that lacked formal institutionalization. The term could not be found in medical dictionaries, for example, nor was it an indexing term used by the Library of Congress.[84] Yet the phrase seemed evocative, and its apparent simplicity made it appealing in diverse quarters.

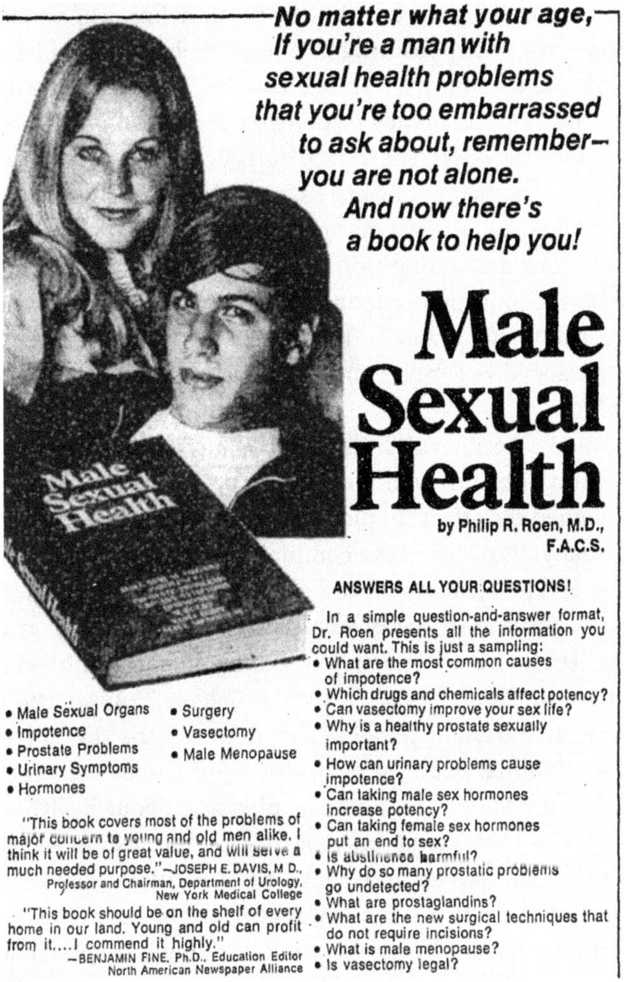

Figure 1: "Male Sexual Health" in the *New York Times*, 1974

Display ad in the *New York Times*, October 12, 1974, for *Male Sexual Health*, by Philip R. Roen. Copyright 1974 by Philip R. Roen. Used by permission of HarperCollins Publishers.

For example, a display advertisement in the *New York Times* in 1974 promoted, for "only $6.95," a book "that could protect your happiness and perhaps save your life," and that, "with illustrations and an easy-to-understand style, . . . gives the facts about the internal structures that control a man's sexual life and health" (fig. 1). Perhaps predictably, the title of the book, by Philip R. Roen, MD, FACS, was *Male Sexual Health*.

A second crucial factor contributing to the defining of sexual health was the presence of a sponsoring body with global reach and an investment in big ideas about what it means to be healthy. Founded in 1948 as the United Nations agency responsible for health policies and programs around the world, the WHO, in its constitution, expressed the commitment to a vision of health as "one of the fundamental rights of every human being without distinction of race, religion, political belief, economic or social condition."[85] But what, exactly, was "health"? In its influential definition propounded at the time of the organization's founding, the WHO declared: "Health is a state of complete physical, mental, and social well-being and not merely the absence of disease or infirmity."[86]

As the medical ethicist Daniel Callahan has observed, such a sweeping definition of health could not fail to be controversial. Supporters have applauded the effort "to place health in the broadest human context." Its many detractors have complained that the definition's "very generality, and particularly its association of health and general well-being as a positive ideal, has given rise to a variety of evils," principally including "the cultural tendency to define all social problems, from war to crime in the streets, as 'health' problems."[87] As we will see, the subsequent definition of *sexual* health followed the tracks laid down by the foundational defining of health itself three decades earlier—not only via the adoption of similar phrasing about health as being something *more than* the absence of disease, but also in its considerable ambition and sweep. Indeed, by the late 1960s, key figures had already begun to think about the implications of the WHO definition of health for understanding sexuality. Calderone, in a speech delivered at the Seventeenth Annual World Health Forum of the American Association for World Health and US Committee for WHO, in Philadelphia in 1969, described the very goal of her organization, SIECUS, as being "to establish man's *sexuality* as a health entity, always remembering the W.H.O. definition of health and thinking of sexuality as a part of man's total well-being."[88]

Meanwhile, for many reasons, and certainly not just because of the influence of the WHO, "health" had become a master term in contemporary discourse. Figure 2 shows a Google "Ngram"—a graph of word usage in books in English—for the word "health" over the course of the twentieth century. The graph reveals an impressive upward growth beginning in the late 1960s and continuing to the mid-1990s. But cer-

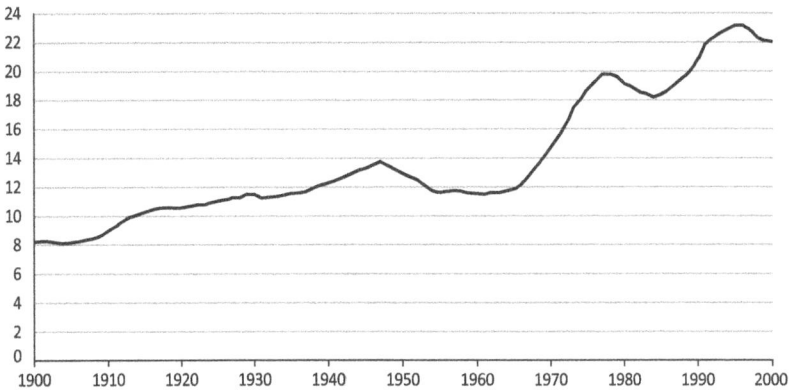

Figure 2: "Health" in Google Books, 1900–2000

The y-axis describes occurrences of the word "health" as a percentage of all single words cataloged in Google Books (normalized by the number of books published per year), multiplied by 1,000. Generated January 2021 at https://books.google.com/ngrams and reconstructed by Exactus Servicios.

tainly one aspect of this increase in "health speak" has been the emergence and institutionalization of various new "subspecies" of health in the final decades of the twentieth century. The National Library of Medicine created a Medical Subject Heading for "world health" (later "global health") in 1977; for both "family health" and "urban health" in 1978; for "holistic health" in 1979; and for both "occupational health" (which, since 1966 had been "occupational medicine") and "women's health" in 1990. The more work the idea of health seemed to perform, the more it became possible to imagine distinctive subtypes.[89]

The expansion of "health" discourses also reflects, or benefits from, the corresponding decline in the once-popular language of "hygiene." As the latter term fell out of favor—coming to sound both quaint and unduly moralistic, and too closely associated with ideas of purity and cleanliness—"health" became available as a more all-encompassing substitute. (Figure 3, which tracks usage in books of the phrases "social hygiene," "sexual hygiene," and "sexual health" since 1900, suggests this shift.) In some cases, "health" absorbed meanings directly connoted previously by "hygiene"—for example, the US Library of Congress subject heading for sexual health, which dates to 1985–86, replaced the earlier "Hygiene, Sexual."[90] Interestingly, the most important organization to be formed during the social hygiene era, the American Social Hygiene Association (founded in 1914), changed its name to the

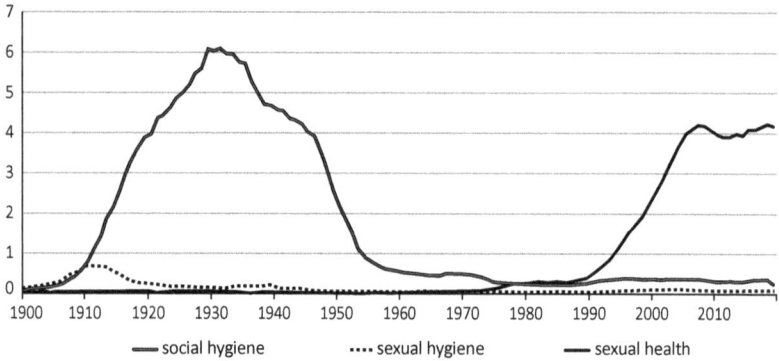

Figure 3: "Social hygiene," "sexual hygiene," and "sexual health" in Google Books, 1900–2019

The y-axis describes occurrences of each phrase as a percentage of all two-word phrases cataloged in Google Books (normalized by the number of books published per year), multiplied by 100,000. Generated January 2021 at https://books.google.com/ngrams and reconstructed by Exactus Servicios.

American Social Health association in 1959 and then to the American Sexual Health Association in 2012.[91]

This shift in nomenclature is not altogether surprising: Just as "hygiene," during the social hygiene era, was (as noted earlier) a capacious and "magical word" that could fuse medical and moral concerns, so "health" nowadays is the likely term of choice when one seeks to describe how bodies, selves, and societies are best meant to be. It is not surprising that various concerns once described as matters of "hygiene" are now referenced by "health"—for example, "mental health" has almost completely displaced "mental hygiene," and the National Library of Medicine recataloged the latter as the former in 1966.[92]

In addition to the factors discussed so far—broad social changes, the presence of the WHO, and the rise of both "health speak" and health "subtypes"—the modern "invention" of sexual health also reflected the work of motivated actors. Specifically, academic sexologists, who sought to revitalize and professionalize the field, restore its diminished prestige in the wake of challenges, and set it on a firmer scientific footing on an international basis, played an important role, particularly in the actual crafting of the definition of sexual health.[93] As Alain Giami has noted, this new wave of sexology was marked by a renewed emphasis on scholarly research, exemplified by the founding of key journals, such as the *Archives of Sexual Behavior* in 1971.[94] The first World Congress of Sexology, held in Paris in 1974, reflected an explicit attempt to revive the sexological congresses of the early twentieth century.[95] The sexological profession received a further boost in 1978 with the founding, at a meeting held in Rome, of what would prove to be the leading international organization of sexologists: the World Association of Sexology (WAS). Yet, eventually, the discourse of sexual health would provide a strategy for rebranding, as the profession sought to assert its continued relevance, insist on the legitimacy of studying sex, and align itself with broader social and public health concerns:[96] As I describe in chapter 3, in 2005 the WAS, while retaining its acronym, changed its name to the World Association for Sexual Health.

Promulgating a "Working Definition"

On February 6–12, 1974, the WHO convened a meeting in Geneva, Switzerland, on the topic "Education and Treatment in Human Sexuality," and they invited a group of medically oriented sexologists and other experts on sexuality to discuss the training of health professionals about sexual matters.[97] The widespread perception was that most health professionals were woefully unprepared to address sexual matters that arose in their clinical practice. (A WHO consultation held two years earlier "had called attention to the lack of opportunity for health practitioners to study human sexuality" and had recommended further attention to this issue.[98]) The goals of the meeting, therefore, were to develop recommendations on the role of sexology in health programs, the "content and methodology" for teaching health professionals about human sexuality, and improved international coordination within the field of sexology, among other topics.[99] A technical report, issued by the WHO the following year, summarized the discussion and listed the conclusions.

In other words—and this point bears notice—the WHO did not convene the meeting for the purpose of defining sexual health. Although commentators on the history of sexual health have rightly treated the meeting as a formative moment, as we will see, participants did not arrive at a definition because they were tasked to do so, but rather because the meeting provided them with an opportunity, and because doing so seemed to them a necessary precondition for advancing the stated agenda of the meeting: training health professionals about human sexuality. Thus, in the pages of the technical report, the first mention of something called sexual health (aside from in the table of contents) is, in fact, the definition of it, on page 6. In the remainder of the thirty-three-page report, the term is then invoked repeatedly— for example, in reference to identifying sexual health needs, providing sexual health care services, and providing sexual health education.[100]

Another clarification: What emerged from the meeting was not, technically, a "WHO definition." Although it has become common to refer to the published report as providing "the 1975 WHO definition of sexual health,"[101] the WHO did not officially claim it at the time, nor has it done so since. Indeed, the title page of the report displays a careful, if legalistic, disclaimer: "This report contains the collective views of an international group of experts and does not necessarily represent the decisions or the stated policy of the World Health Organization."[102] To this day, because the WHO has never seen fit to seek (or has shied away from seeking) approval of the definition by vote of the 194 member countries that comprise the World Health Assembly, the official categorization of the language on sexual health is that it is a "working definition": it "does not represent an official WHO position and should not be used or quoted as such."[103]

The participants at the 1974 meeting constituted a "Who's Who in sexology," in the evaluation of Eli Coleman, a sexologist who later emerged as a leading figure in the development of sexual health.[104] They included twenty-one sexologists and other experts on sexuality from Belgium, Colombia, Czechoslovakia, Denmark, England, France, India, Italy, the Netherlands, Switzerland, the United States, and Yugoslavia. Nearly all were medical doctors, specializing in areas ranging from psychiatry to gynecology to pediatrics, and only one—identified as Mrs. Lorna J. Sarrel, the codirector of the Human Sexuality Program at Yale University Health Services—was neither a doctor nor a professor. Most of the participants were affiliated with universities, either in conventional departments such as Medicine or, in some cases, in specialized research institutes devoted to human sexuality or related fields, such as the Institute for Sex Research (the Kinsey Institute) at Indiana University. Aside from those named as participants, the meeting also included representatives from two other organizations: the International Planned Parenthood Foundation and the International Task Force on World Health Manpower. Finally, there were five attendees from the WHO Secretariat, including the chief medical officer in the area of family health and the senior medical officer for mental health.[105]

Participants presented and considered background papers on topics ranging from the programmatic ("Developmental prospects for sexological teaching in Italy") to the highly technical ("Phyletic and idiosyncratic determinants of gender identity").[106] By the end of the meeting, the participants had reached consensus on many issues relating to research, education, and policy. Yet in retrospect, what made the meeting memorable and gave it historical significance was not any of the above but, rather, the definition of something called sexual health.

DEFINITIONAL LOGICS

As the subsequent report made clear, defining sexual health was deemed a satisfactory first approximation of what would be a far more difficult task to accomplish: arriving at "a universally acceptable definition of the totality of human sexuality." Given the meeting's specific concern with the training of health professionals and its sponsorship by the WHO, it seemed reasonable to focus the definitional task not on sexuality writ large but rather—"as a step in this direction"—on the intersection of sexuality with the domain of health.[107] The participants thus declared, in a separate, indented sentence meant to attract attention: *"Sexual health is the integration of the somatic, emotional, intellectual, and social aspects of sexual being, in ways that are positively enriching and that enhance personality, communication, and love."*[108]

To this short but capacious definition the report added several elaborations. First, in an abrupt one-sentence paragraph, the report tied the definition of sexual health to the idea of rights in relation to sexuality: "Fundamental to this concept are the right to sexual information and the right to pleasure."[109] How those rights were themselves to be defined—or secured—and what made them "fundamental" to an understanding of sexual health was not explained. (The word "right" does not recur in the report, except in the conclusion where the definition is recapped.) As I have noted, the notion of a basic right to health was affirmed by the WHO, while the social movements of the 1960s and 1970s had extended the idea of rights to ever more aspects of human life and kinds of social groups (including, for example, people with nonnormative sexual identities).[110] Still, the reference to a "right to pleasure" is striking. Elsewhere in the document, the term "pleasure" appears occasionally, but in a more clinical or physiological sense, essentially as a synonym for orgasm or its precursor states—as in a reference to the use of hypnosis "to induce positive sensations such as a feeling of heat at the base of the abdomen to induce easier achievement of sexual pleasure."[111] Here, though, "pleasure" (unmodified by "sexual") is treated as a more basic and more general concern, and as an individual's presumed inalienable "right."

Second, the authors maintained that their definition of sexual health "implies a positive approach to human sexuality." Consistent with the WHO's long-standing emphasis on characterizing health as more than simply the absence of disease, they proposed that "the purpose of sexual health care should be the enhancement of life and personal relationships and not merely counselling and care related to procreation or sexually transmitted diseases."[112] In this regard, the document aligned itself not only with the WHO definition of health from a quarter century earlier but also with a growing cultural investment in health and wellness, increasingly understood to be the province and concern of many professions beyond physicians.[113]

THE IDEAL OF "POSITIVITY"

Several dimensions of these passages are worth drawing out. To begin with, given the predominance of medical doctors at the meeting, it is striking how little the definition has to do with a biologically based conception of disease processes. The core, one-sentence definition does not even refer to disease, illness, or pathology (and the closest it gets to biology is the term "somatic"). The additional text that follows does refer to "organic disorders, diseases, and deficiencies," but this is quickly followed by a reminder that sexual health is not "merely" a matter of "counselling and care related to procreation or sexually transmitted diseases." While, as I have noted, these emphases bear the imprint of the WHO's definition of health in general, the simultaneous introduction of vocabulary in quite a different register—"personality," "communication," "love"—suggests just how far the meeting participants had traveled from the terminology and ontology normally found even in the more expansive embrace of the WHO, let alone in ordinary medical practice. (As a test, I searched the more than two hundred thousand items in the WHO's online database to see how many used the word "love" in their titles; I retrieved only three publications.[114])

One implication is that the proposed goal of educating health professionals about sexuality—the ostensible purpose of the meeting—was potentially an uphill battle, if the discussion of even those aspects of sexuality most relevant to health was being undertaken in a language somewhat foreign to modern medicine. A second implication is one to which I have already alluded to in the introduction: however we want to read the effects on modern sexuality of its present-day alliance with health, a simple story of the "medicalization" of sexuality will not suffice. As the psychologist Leonore Tiefer has observed, the WHO-sponsored definition "represent[ed] a nonmedicalized approach" and an "alternative rooted in political rights, rather than evolutionary biology."[115]

What was an international group of experts convened by the World Health Organization doing grappling with intangibles like "love"?[116] To be sure, several of the participants were psychiatrists, a group whose discourse is sometimes markedly different from that of most other medical specialty areas. More generally, many of the participants, whatever their formal training, moved in sexological circles that, from the origins of that field into the present, had embraced a broadly interdisciplinary approach to their subject matter. The idea that sexual health had fundamentally psychological, social, and ethical dimensions, in addition to biological— that "the purpose of sexual health care should be the enhancement of life and personal relationships"—made sense to the attendees.

These inclinations led the participants to put forward a vision of sexual health that was "positive" in a triple sense. When they proposed that "the notion of sexual health implies a positive approach to sexuality," this meant that, as something more than the absence of disease, sexual health could not just be defined negatively, by what it *was not*; that the moral and political valences of the definition were "sex positive," to use a term that subsequently became more popular[117]—sex was something beneficial and worth defending, not dangerous or harmful in the first instance; and that, as something "positively enriching," sexuality had a purpose, or purposes—a presumed utility and function beyond reproduction, especially in solidifying intimate relationships and serving as the natural accompaniment of love.

In short, a "positive" conception of sexual health brought into alignment a medically progressive embrace of health and wellness, a political agenda of treating sex as a social and personal good, and a psychological model of the productive and appropriate employment of sexual desires. Yet part of the semiotic complexity of "positivity" involves the fact that these various expressions of it were, at least potentially and to some degree, in tension with one another. After all, a conception of sexuality that is invested in how sexual expression can be "positively enriching" is likely to label as "unhealthy" those varieties of expression deemed frivolous, irresponsible, or dangerous. Yet a radically sex-positive politics of sexuality would be suspicious of just such attempts to draw symbolic boundaries between "good" and "bad" sex and would question the authority of those seeking to do so.[118] On the one hand, the definition presupposed the conceptual vocabulary of the sexual revolution, such as the invocation of a right to pleasure. But on the other hand, by tying sexual health to love and relationships, it also stood in conflict with the basic premise, derived from that revolution, that sex should be defended as a form of pleasure, pure and simple.

In different combinations and to different degrees, this triadic conception of "positivity"—along with its internal tensions and instabilities—would inform many subsequent endeavors authorized by the idea of sexual health. Moreover, these conceptions of sexuality are broadly consistent with assumptions that my genealogy has identified as having underlain other projects tying sexuality to health over the preceding hundred years—namely, that the proper management of sexuality is crucial not only the health of individuals, but also for that of marriages and relationships and, indeed, the larger society.

IMPLICATIONS OF A DEFINITION

Three additional features of the working definition deserve mention. First, a noteworthy aspect is that the report took for granted that the construct being defined should be called "sexual health" and not something else entirely. Scholars' subsequent references to the meeting and the report have not problematized the nomenclature, perhaps precisely because the term has become so commonplace. Why "sexual health"? To be sure, the term seems like a pithy way of referring to those aspects of sexuality that are relevant to health, and therefore appropriate for a WHO-sponsored meeting discussing the training of health professionals about sexual matters. Moreover, the term had been introduced in passing at the WHO meeting two years earlier, although, there too, without an explanation of why *that* name, as opposed to any other, was best suited to the purpose.[119] But these contingent factors do not fully explain why a term without a clear medical provenance or institutionalized presence within public health was adopted at this moment.

While the question may be difficult to answer in any definitive way, the genealogical approach of this chapter offers a series of clues. By the 1970s, the phrase "sexual health" was beginning to circulate as a way of pointing to the historical descendants of various nineteenth- and twentieth-century projects that yoked health to sexuality, from sex advice, to social hygiene, to sexology. And at a time when health, in general, was increasingly being treated as a predominant social value; when compound terms denoting health "subtypes" were on the rise; when alternative terms, such as "hygiene," were falling out of fashion; and when the WHO's definition of health suggested the breadth of concerns that potentially might fall under that rubric, the designation "sexual health" does seem, if not inevitable, then perhaps overdetermined as the linguistic choice in this case.

A second point concerning the text of the report has to do with the universal and the particular, or more specifically, the tension between an implicitly universalistic framing of the concept of sexual health and an occasional recognition of the significance of social identities and differences. For the most part, in the eyes of the attendees, sexual health was sexual health, and it presumably took the same form for everybody, regardless of their gender, sexual identity, nationality, race, ethnicity, religion, or age. As Calderone had expressed it a few years earlier: "The functioning of a human being as a sexual individual is as universal and continuous as the functioning of his heart."[120] And the rather obvious concern that a definition emphasizing such things as the enhancement of "personality, communication, and love" might privilege culturally specific (read: modern Western) ways of envisioning both sexuality and health appeared not to register, at least at this moment.[121] Yet in contrast, scattered through the report were occasional mentions of social differences that were deemed relevant to the practical goal of securing sexual health. For example, the report maintained that "although sexual health is of concern to both sexes, in most of the existing health and family planning programmes the approach is directed mainly to women."[122] Moreover, sex education efforts may be hampered by "negative attitudes" about the sexual desires expressed by "older people, the mentally retarded, the physically handicapped, prison inmates, and certain racial groups."[123] Finally, the report observed that there are distinctive sexual health problems corresponding to different age groups across the life cycle.[124] While by no means an emphasis of the report, these considerations presaged a much more fine-grained focus on the sexual health "risks" of specific social groups—especially racial, ethnic, and sexual minorities—that would emerge in subsequent decades.

A third and final point that also merits attention concerns the open-ended and inclusive character of the definition and the accompanying text: this prose from the 1970s already suggested, or presaged, the polyvalent discourses and multiform practices that sexual health has since come to represent.[125] Disorders and deficiencies; well-being; enrichment and enhancement; sexual as well as reproductive functions; love and relationships; rights and pleasures: on the one hand, the definition seemed to lay claim, in an almost totalizing fashion, to all aspects of the person and, indeed, set as its goal "the integration of the somatic, emotional, intellectual, and social." But on the other hand, by revealing the range of concerns that must have been voiced around the table, the definition seemed to invite future appropriators to pick and choose, from among the diverse components, those specific aspects that spoke to them. For example, the terse and awkwardly inserted single-sentence paragraph about "rights"—one senses a bureaucratic compromise designed to placate a vocal minority—served, in retrospect, as a promissory note for elaborations that would follow. Indeed, we might call it a beachhead for the future establishment of a crucial hub of sexual health activity.[126]

The door had thus been opened to many different callers, both expert and lay. A narrower definition of sexual health might have been more precise, and hence more cleanly translatable into specific scientific, medical, or public health initiatives. By contrast, the expansive definition paved the way for a surfeit of possibilities in a way that threatened, by the 1990s, to strip the term of any clear meaning even while guaranteeing its overall success. That proliferation of activities and understandings is the topic of the next chapter.

2 *Proliferation and Ambiguity*

THE BUZZWORDING OF SEXUAL HEALTH

From understanding the parts, to making sex hotter: Here's what you need to know for using a penis pump. #sexualhealth

Safe sex is great sex! If you are over 16, live in Ohio, and need condoms, the Free Condom Project has got your back. #OHIO #safesex #FreeCondom-Project #sexualhealth

Sex and intimacy can be a struggle for folks with embodied trauma, join us for this workshop on creating space for pleasure #traumainformed #sexualhealth

What makes a car? An outfit? A man cave? The answer is ACCESSORIES! See how they can make everything better, including sex! #sexualhealth[1]

In 1975, when the WHO published the report from the conference at which a definition of sexual health was first promulgated, two subsequent developments would have been nearly impossible to predict. First, even the most eager advocates of promoting sexual health would have been unlikely to imagine just how successful the term would become, simply as measured by its use. Second, no one would have anticipated how many different things sexual health might come to mean

This chapter developed out of, and expands on, arguments and text found in Steven Epstein and Laura Mamo, "The Proliferation of Sexual Health: Diverse Social Problems and the Legitimation of Sexuality," *Social Science & Medicine* 188 (2017): 176–90. It reflects the collaborative work between Mamo and myself that was crucial to my early formulation of this book project.

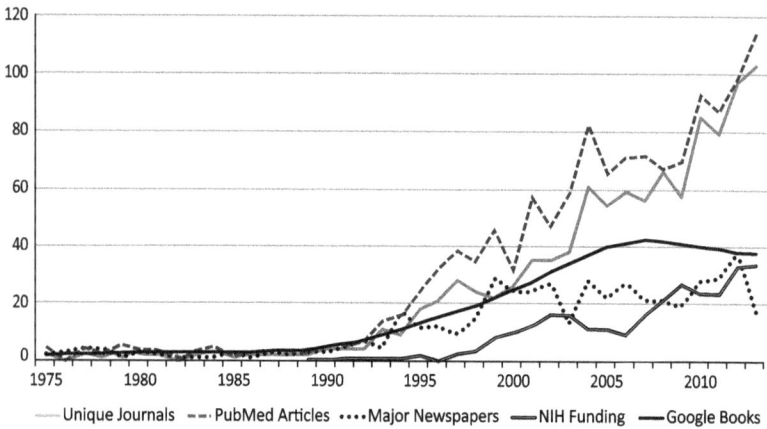

Figure 4: Expansion of "sexual health": Various indicators, 1975–2013

The y-axis describes the following: (a) PubMed articles: the number of PubMed articles with "sexual health" in the title, per every 500,000 articles published in PubMed that year; (b) unique journals: the number of unique journals in PubMed publishing articles with "sexual health" in the title; (c) NIH funding: funding by the US National Institutes of Health to projects with "sexual health" in the title or abstract, in increments of US $500,000; (d) Google Books: occurrences of the phrase "sexual health" as a percentage of all two-word phrases cataloged in Google Books (normalized by the number of books published per year), multiplied by 1 million; and (e) major newspapers: occurrences of "sexual health" in the body of articles published in the *New York Times*, *Washington Post*, and *Los Angeles Times*. Adapted by Exactus Servicios from Steven Epstein and Laura Mamo, "The Proliferation of Sexual Health: Diverse Social Problems and the Legitimation of Sexuality," *Social Science & Medicine* 188 (2017): 181.

and therefore how many kinds of activities it would productively enable. This chapter delves into—but also provides a rough classification of—the manifold ways in which sexual health has become ubiquitous, and it seeks to understand why and how it did.

We can start with some indicators of success. Research that I conducted together with Laura Mamo and our research assistants reveals an impressive trajectory, measured in multiple venues (fig. 4). The markers include the increase over time in medical journal articles that have used the phrase "sexual health" in their titles, the growth in the numbers of unique journals publishing those articles, the increase in funding by the National Institutes of Health to projects with "sexual health" in the title or abstract, the increase in occurrences of the phrase "sexual health" in the books cataloged in Google Books, and the increase in uses of the phrase in the body of articles published in the *New York Times*, the *Washington Post*, and the *Los Angeles Times*.[2]

Across these various indicators of the growing use of the term, the trend is substantially similar, and two points stand out. First, uptake was gradual and fairly slow for the first decade and a half after the 1975 definition, as the term "sexual health" began to take root. Second—and quite striking—the early to mid-1990s marks the turning point between the phase of gradual emergence and that of rapid expansion: it was in that period that sexual health began to "go viral."[3]

But the story I want to develop goes well beyond the simple idea of growth. In fact, attending to the *quantitative* explosion of sexual health projects risks missing what proved to be the most consequential development: the *qualitative* expansion of meanings as the term became dispersed across social space. When Mamo and I, together with our research assistants, analyzed a wide range of materials—particularly, journal articles, newspaper articles, and websites—we found a remarkably diverse set of speakers giving voice to sexual health matters, including scientists, doctors, public health officials, pharmaceutical companies, foundations, religious organizations, sex-toy manufacturers, activists, and advocacy groups across the political spectrum. Just as significantly, our analysis revealed a divergent, if sometimes overlapping, set of practical concerns: sexually transmissible infections, sexual dysfunction, sexual compulsivity, reproductive health and rights, rights to sexual expression and self-definition, sexual violence, sex aids and toys, sex education, sexual responsibility, and sexual morality, among others.

Sexual health, it seems, is not a unitary construct.[4] As the flexible term has traveled through social and professional networks that only partially overlap, a range of quite different sorts of activities, unfolding in different social worlds, have been labeled sexual health "concerns," with varied and complicated results. Unlike the kinds of diffusion often described by sociologists that result in isomorphism or the spread of similar forms,[5] discourses and practices of sexual health have come to be widely available yet in a range of distinct flavors.

The point is that tying sexuality to health has proved a generative process that has opened the door to a host of new biomedical, social, and cultural possibilities. Sexual health now seems to show up nearly everywhere, at least as suggested by dissemination of the specific phrase (both in English and in translation). But its meanings seem remarkably plastic across diverse contexts of use. Rather than a convergence on a homogeneous understanding of sexual health, we find a dispersion of possibilities for pursuing and enacting it.

The differentiation of sexual health projects and programs is what prevents me from providing a kind of account that might have been expected in this case: the story of the formation of a new medical specialty area, with its own recognized concerns and organizational structures. Such histories have proved useful in describing the trajectory of many other health-related topics, and they point to the indisputable significance of specialization as a hallmark of modern medicine.[6] This case certainly has some of the defining features: it's not hard to find examples of professional associations, journals, research centers, treatment centers, conferences, protocols, courses, and training programs, all with the words "sexual health" in the title. But the point is that, even within the worlds of biomedicine and public health, sexual health is not a single, unified, common project. Indeed, as we will see, sexual health contains within it at least one, relatively well-bounded, new biomedical specialty area—"sexual medicine," involving the treatment of sexual dysfunction—while also cutting across multiple others. Moreover, the worlds of sexual health extend well beyond the specialized arenas of modern medicine and public health, spilling out into many other domains of contemporary social existence.

This chapter develops that story of the appeal of the idea of sexual health as the scaffolding for diverse scientific, political, and lifestyle projects. It examines the fate of a semantically flexible term as it has journeyed through various social and professional networks within which various distinct interests can be served.[7] To make sense of proliferation and diversification, I proceed in three steps. First, I decompose sexual health into specific kinds of activity associated with particular social problems to which "sexual health" has been presented as the solution. Then, I step back to ask why sexual health has emerged as an all-purpose solution to social problems, and why, in particular, it seemed to "go viral" in the 1990s. Finally, I examine the productive character of the polysemy of sexual health—how it can mean so many different things. I argue that imprecision and ambiguity have facilitated the "buzzwording" of sexual health, giving it a distinctive capacity to travel and take root.

By suggesting the generativity of sexual health, this chapter begins the work taken up systematically in the rest of the book: indicating the consequences of the rise of sexual health for medical and scientific practice, social management, individual development, and collective existence. The chapter also introduces a paradox that surrounds the growth of sexual health. On the one hand, sexual health activities have diversified and splintered, even as the term has become more popular. On the other hand, as shown in the chapter that follows this one, the ambiguous character of sexual health also permits the stitching together of new hybrid objects that may connect the different worlds of sexual health. Therefore, this chapter and the next focus our attention on the powerful tension between dispersion and recombination that characterizes sexual health.

Social Problems, Action Plans, and Six Ways of Framing Sexual Health

To better understand the profusion of activities undertaken under the banner of sexual health, Mamo and I, aided by research assistants, performed a content analysis of various materials: biomedical journal articles (in the PubMed database), three major newspapers (the *New York Times*, *Los Angeles Times*, and *Washington Post*), and websites.[8] We found that people were taking up numerous important goals in the name of sexual health, and moreover that these activities, though varied, clustered in noticeable ways.[9] We grouped the projects into six clusters—six ways of characterizing sexual issues such that "sexual health" is the proposed solution to a problem. Each of these groupings demonstrates a particular way of framing sexuality as being a matter of health.[10] Yet in each of these cases, both "sexuality" and "health" effectively mean different things, and therefore "sexual health" fuels different kinds of projects, programs, and initiatives.

What follows is a schematic summary of these six "solutions" to social problems.[11] I emphasize how they matter but also how they differ. To get a handle on their distinctiveness, I consider how each such of these solutions implies a specific conception of both "sexuality" and "health." To further characterize each approach, I also answer a question that offers insight: From this standpoint, what would be the *opposite* or negation of sexual health? (That is, what counts as being "sexually unhealthy"?)

Although these six social problems may intersect in practice, the point is that each frame corresponds to an "ideal type" of sexual health.[12] We can distinguish among a meaningful set of sexual health subtypes, even if they sometimes overlap or appear in combination.

First is containing the spread of sexually transmissible infections. According to the logic associated with this social problem, sexual health is construed as the solution or resolution brought about by programs of surveillance, prevention, or treatment of STIs. This is a dominant understanding of sexual health that is well represented in the disciplines of infectious disease and epidemiology, as well as at public and private clinics and at US federal health agencies such as the Centers for Disease Control and Prevention (CDC). The salience of STIs as a global health problem—and especially the continued devastating global impact of the HIV/AIDS epidemic—ensures the prominence of this way of thinking about sexual health. New understandings of how STIs may cause cancer have furthered the commitment to work in this area—as reflected, for example, in efforts to vaccinate young people against human papillomavirus (HPV) to prevent the development of cervical and other cancers.[13]

In this sexual health frame, sexuality is understood essentially as a risky behavior, health is construed as risk reduction, and the opposite of sexual health is the spread of disease. Sexual health is promoted by interrupting transmission networks and developing the proper messaging to reach and motivate at-risk individuals to seek treatment or restructure their sexual practice. Yet while this conception of sexuality largely emphasizes the negatives that are to be avoided or treated, a sexual health approach may indicate the adoption of a positive spin. As a report issued in 2021 by the National Academy of Sciences noted, after quoting the WHO's working definition of sexual health, "STI control that is viewed within a healthy sexual life is likely to be more successful than the traditional medical and public health model that is steeped in blame, stigma, marginalization, and discrimination."[14]

Second is addressing failures of sexual functioning. Here sexual health is understood to be the reparative solution to biomechanical and/or neurological failure—a solution engineered by "sexual medicine," a field that dates to the 1970s in Germany, the United Kingdom, the United States, and Japan and that has its own journals, professional societies, and academic conferences.[15] This expression of sexual health cuts across several biomedical specialties, particularly including urology, gynecology, neurology, and endocrinology, as well as sex therapy.

As described in the aims of the *Journal of Sexual Medicine*, the field seeks to develop the "multidisciplinary basic science and clinical research to define and understand the scientific basis of male, female, and couples sexual function and dysfunction."[16] Yet the activities in this sexual health frame are most clearly reflected in the development and marketing of pharmaceutical and biotechnological products for male sexual performance and female sexual function—products that, especially since the 1998 introduction of Pfizer's blockbuster drug Viagra and the simultaneous redefinition of impotence as erectile dysfunction, have traveled seamlessly from medical specialty areas into everyday life.[17]

While the WHO working definition of sexual health is at pains to insist that health is more than just the absence of disease or dysfunction, from the standpoint of this social problem frame, a "negative" definition of sexual health (as essentially just the absence of disease or dysfunction, or the overcoming of deficits) is fairly typical. "Remember, sexual medicine is the field that helps people regain their sexual health," explained Sue Goldstein, clinical research manager and program coordinator for San Diego Sexual Medicine, in response to my research assistant's query about the relation between the two terms.[18] However (as I discuss in chapter 8), efforts in this field invoke a broader vision of fulfillment and the extension of potency, reflected most notably in the marketing of Viagra and related drugs and the associated quest to reverse the effects of aging.

In this domain, sexuality is understood largely in mechanical or neurological terms as a matter of physiology, whereas health is viewed as a matter of potency and performance. The opposite of sexual health, therefore, is the inability to perform (or the presence of pain or discomfort during sexual activity). The injunction here is to strive for presumed normal (or perhaps better than normal) sexual performance, defined typically by the model of heterosexual penetrative sex, often through the use of pharmaceuticals and devices designed to attain these lifestyle goals.

Third is controlling population growth and promoting procreative autonomy. The paradoxical nature of what has become known as "sexual and reproductive health" lies in the way the two terms—"sexual" and "reproductive"—stand in a complex relation of simultaneous merging and differentiation. On the one hand, the contemporary discourse of sexual health presumes the historical disentangling of the procreative (or reproductive) and the erotic aspects of people's lives: only when sexuality is permitted to escape subordination to the goal of reproduction does the sexual fully emerge as a domain of concern in its own right, central to self-definition, social interaction, and human enjoyment. On the other hand, since the time of the initial WHO working definition, sexual and reproductive concerns have in fact often been tightly entwined in projects of sexual health promotion.[19] Even today, some sources completely subsume sexual health under reproductive health: as I have noted, a Wikipedia search for "sexual health" automatically redirects to "reproductive health."[20] However, many other sources use the compound phrase "sexual and reproductive health" or "reproductive and sexual health" without distinguishing further.

This conception of sexual health as the solution to problems of population, procreative autonomy, and fertility nowadays characterizes activities within a wide variety of settings, including clinics for teen health, family planning services, and fertility biomedicine. In an era when non-procreative sexual activities are no longer defined presumptively as perversions, dysfunctions, or disorders, heteronormative reproduction nonetheless remains a widespread assumption in this understanding of sexual health.[21]

In general, from the vantage point of "sexual and reproductive health," sexuality is understood as a pathway to reproduction, whereas health is defined as the capacity to control, direct, and enhance reproductive functions. Therefore, depending on circumstances, the opposite of sexual health might be excess population growth, unwanted childbearing, failure to achieve one's reproductive potential, or lack of empowerment or autonomy with regard to procreation.

Fourth is solving injustices linked to the absence of sexual rights. In this rendering, sexual health is both the solution to the denial of sexual rights and an idealized state that cannot be achieved unless rights are valorized and recognized. Like sexual health itself, "sexual rights" is a term whose meanings are both contested and under development— what Rosalind Petchesky described in 2000 as "the newest kid on the block in international debates about the meanings and practices of human rights, especially women's human rights."[22] I shall defer until chapter 3 a proper genealogy of the concept of sexual rights and a discussion of some of the debates surrounding its employment. However, from the beginning, sexual rights have been closely tied to sexual health, in part because organizations such as the World Association for Sexual Health, Planned Parenthood, and SIECUS have avidly promoted both terms.[23]

Here, the goal is to address threats such as social restriction of the freedom to express a sexual or gender identity or choose a sexual partner, and the denial of health care related to sexual matters. However, as Richard Parker and colleagues have noted, activists around the world representing the feminist, LGBT, and HIV/AIDS movements have sought "to extend the definition of sexual rights to the enablement and even the celebration of sexual diversity and sexual pleasure."[24] Meanwhile, the linkage of sexual health and sexual rights has also encapsulated a growing concern with protection from sexual violence.[25] This development is consistent with a broader recent trend in which matters of violence and injustice have been recoded as matters of health, often through the conceptualizing of violence as physical or mental trauma that leaves its mark on the body.[26]

Frequently advanced by foundations, nonprofits, and civil society organizations, projects that conceive of sexual health as a matter of rights also emphasize goals such as social equality and justice and valorize ideals such as agency, autonomy, bodily integrity, self-actualization, and pleasure. The point, though, is that the more scientific and neutral-sounding language of "sexual health" has often been invoked precisely as a disguised way of talking about rights (including human rights in general or sexual rights in particular), as the latter are presumed to be more controversial in certain circles or to raise "red flags."[27]

In short, "sexual health" became either the adjunct or replacement term of choice adopted by a range of social movements that sought to promote sexual rights in the 1990s and beyond, including international women's health activists, reproductive rights and reproductive justice activists, and the global LGBT movement. Overall, in this social problem frame, sexuality is understood as an integral component of personal identity, and a state of health involves freedom from unwarranted external constraint or coercion. Therefore, the opposite of sexual health is a state of subjugation and inequality.

Fifth is containing threats of irresponsible sexual behavior. The idea here is that promoting sexual health solves the problem of sexual irresponsibility or immorality. Of course, the concern with responsibility overlaps some of the other social problems already discussed, such as the spread of STIs. However, in particular institutional contexts, responsibility or morality are the dominant considerations. A key example is sex education—particularly for adolescents but also for college students—now often labeled "sexual health education." This rebranding, in turn, reflects a longer history in which, since the 1960s, "sexual education activists [have] sought to redefine sexuality as a 'health entity.'"[28]

In addition, much discourse related to sexual health and responsibility addresses the sexuality-related concerns of social conservatives, around issues such as abortion, sexualized material in popular culture, young people's use of the internet, and many others. Online, conservative commentators have applied the term sexual health to a range of topics, from the appropriate level and type of sexual outlet within marriages or romantic relationships to the development of a sexual identity over the course of childhood and adolescence.[29] In their practical work, conservatives sometimes adopt the terminology strategically—such as when a Christian ministry opposed to abortion opened the "Mosaic Sexual Health Clinic" across the street from Planned Parenthood in Tallahassee, Florida, in 2021.[30]

Certain professional projects also find a home under the broad rubric of sexual responsibility, coded as sexual health. The treatment of "sex addiction" or "sexual compulsivity" is one example: while many mental health groups are skeptical of the diagnosis,[31] some organizations treat it as a paramount sexual health concern. According to a "conservative estimate" put forward by the Society for the Advancement of Sexual Health, between 3 percent and 5 percent of the US population may meet the criteria for sexual addiction and compulsivity and may merit treatment for the condition.[32] While the professional discourse around sex addiction dates back to the late 1970s,[33] the explicit billing of such concerns as a sexual health matter is more recent.[34]

Generally speaking, from the standpoint of this social problem, sexuality is conceived as a morally charged social practice that demands regulation, whereas health is seen as intrinsically connected to social betterment. The opposite of sexual health is sexual and social anarchy or anomie.

Sixth is promoting sexual self-expression. This is an approach found largely outside the domains of government, public health, and biomedicine. The emphasis here is on self-fulfillment and (as I describe in much more detail in chapter 8) the pursuit of "wellness," largely through the purchase and employment of various toys, devices, drugs, and other products that enable sexual pleasure and diversion. Such technologies nowadays are promoted endlessly, particularly on the internet but in brick-and-mortar stores as well, often under the banner of sexual health. For example, CVS Pharmacy's website uses the marketing category of sexual health to sell condoms, "sexual enhancers," vibrators, and "adult toys," and eVitamins' list of "Best Sexual Health Products" includes items for sale such as "M.D. Science Lab Max Hard," "Irwin Naturals Steel Libido for Women," and "Now Foods Horny Goat Weed Extract."[35]

From this general standpoint, sexuality is understood as a self-actualizing practice, and health is defined largely from the standpoint of wellness and lifestyle. The opposite of sexual health, in this sense, is a lack of enjoyment. These sexual health discourses interpellate individuals as self-enterprising consumers. They preach the virtues of bodily pleasures, yet the realization of that potential may require not just an openness to experimentation but also access to the requisite funds.

DISCURSIVE TRAJECTORIES

From the 1970s onward, and especially since the 1990s, "sexual health" has served as a kind of discursive engine furiously propelling diverse and multivalent initiatives. As a result, sexual health is not unitary—and the analysis of the different social problem frames brings this point into relief. Whether advocates characterize the problem as the spread of sexually transmissible infections, the difficulties caused by sexual dysfunction, inadequate control over population growth or insufficient reproductive autonomy, the injustices linked to the absence of sexual rights, the threat of sexual irresponsibility, or the lack of sexual self-expression, key actors invested in these declared problems are all promoting solutions under the banner of something they call sexual health. Moreover, all these actors might point plausibly to aspects of the WHO's working definition to justify their approach. The overall increase in sexual health discourse documented in figure 4 in fact reflects the combined effect of attention to these individual social problems.

Of course, the point is not that those invested in any one of the six social problems are necessarily blind to the existence of the others. There are clear and obvious examples of people and organizations who simultaneously invoke more than one social problem and may even see them as connected—for example, those who insist on the linkage between HIV prevention and LGBT rights. As scholars such as Dennis Altman and Richard Parker and colleagues have argued, the globally

Table 1: Social Problem Frames for Sexual Health

Social problem frame	Meaning of sexuality	Meaning of health	Opposite
Containing the spread of STIs	Risky practice	Risk reduction	Spread of disease
Addressing failures of sexual functioning	Set of mechanical and neurological mechanisms	Potency; performance	Inability to perform; pain or discomfort
Controlling population growth and promoting procreative autonomy	Pathway to reproduction	Capacity to control, direct, and enhance reproductive functions	Excess population growth; unwanted childbearing or failure to achieve reproductive potential
Solving injustices linked to the absence of sexual rights	Integral component of identity	Freedom from unwarranted external constraint or coercion	Subjugation and inequality
Containing threats of irresponsible sexual behavior	Morally charged social practice	Social betterment	Sexual and social anarchy or anomie
Promoting sexual self-expression	Self-actualizing practice	Wellness	Lack of enjoyment

palpable impact of the HIV/AIDS epidemic has made demonstrably clear the important connections between the spread of STIs and the development of sexual rights.[36] The relations between those two social problem frames are therefore not surprising—and the virtues of making connections are clear. In chapter 3, I provide additional examples of intentional linkage work in my discussions of the WHO and the World Association for Sexual Health.

Yet to address each of these various social problems, professionals and other moral and commercial entrepreneurs are, for the most part, busily engaged in doing relatively specific things: disseminating STI prevention messages, prescribing drugs to treat erectile dysfunction, advocating for the rights of the sexually disenfranchised, selling commodities. Each of these framings comes with its own set of behavioral injunctions and materializes distinct bodies and action plans—and as a result each framing travels with values, assumptions, and prescriptions about what it means to live a sexually healthy life. Therefore, from the vantage point of each social problem, whether explicitly or implicitly, both "sexuality" and "health" take on distinctive meanings (table 1). As we have seen, sexuality may come to mean a risky practice, a set of physiological mechanisms, a pathway to reproductivity, an integral component of identity, a morally charged social practice, or a self-actualizing practice. And health may be understood as risk reduction, potency, control over reproductive functions, freedom from unwarranted constraint, social betterment, or wellness. That is, each social problem frame not only propels work but also construes the world in a different way.[37]

Some additional indication of how the overall discourse around sexual health comprises meanings developed within multiple social problem frames can be gleaned from searches of Google Books. Figure 5 traces the trajectories of various terms related to sexuality from 1975 (the publication year of the initial WHO working definition of sexual health) through 2019. For the most part, sexual health is "greater than" its various component parts, although several of these component terms, such as "sexual and reproductive" and "sexual rights," have also been rising over time in frequency of use. Certain terms, such as "sexual dysfunction" and "sexual pleasure," initially were more prevalent than "sexual health" in Google Books but now have converged with it.

While this analysis based on Google Books is certainly not conclusive, it provides further suggestive evidence that the proliferation of

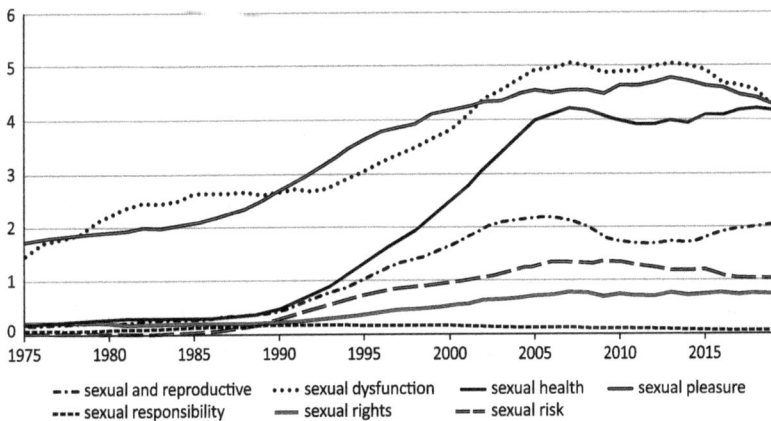

Figure 5: Terms related to sexual health in Google Books, 1975–2019

The y-axis indicates occurrences of each phrase as a percentage of all phrases of the same word length cataloged in Google Books (normalized by the number of books published per year), multiplied by 100,000. Generated January 2021 at https://books.google.com/ngrams and reconstructed by Exactus Servicios.

sexual health reflects not just a quantitative increase but also a diversification of usage. On the one hand, sexual health appears to have drawn on the increasing currency of terms, such as sexual rights, that are on the rise for their own reasons. On the other hand, sexual health appears to have gained visibility as a respectable substitute or replacement term. Indeed, there are plenty of examples of how sexual issues are being formally "rebranded" as matters of sexual health, especially since the year 2000. For example, in 2001 the Female Sexual Function Forum became the International Society for the Study of Women's Sexual Health, in 2003 the National Council on Sexual Addiction and Compulsivity became the Society for the Advancement of Sexual Health, in 2005 the World Association of Sexology became the World Association for Sexual Health, and in 2007 the *Journal of Psychology and Human Sexuality* became the *International Journal of Sexual Health*.[38]

Thus, with the rise of sexual health, older terminology has been absorbed and often replaced. In 2017, when New York City Health Commissioner Mary T. Bassett announced that the city's eight "STD clinics" would be renamed as "sexual health clinics," she effectively acknowledged the more general tendency to understand the prevention of sexually transmissible infections as a defining characteristic of sexual health. At the same time, the nomenclature of sexual health offered strategic advantages: Guillermo Chacón, the president of the Latino Commission on AIDS and founder of the Hispanic Health Network, applauded the renaming of the clinics for "reducing the stigma in our diverse communities."[39]

To be sure, the term "sexual health" has not imperialistically laid claim to *all* discussions of sexual matters. A "wildcard" search in Google Books for two-word phrases beginning with "sexual" revealed a number of common terms—"sexual abuse," "sexual orientation," "sexual assault," "sexual harassment," "sexual intercourse," and others—that significantly outpace "sexual health," at least in Google Books.[40] Thus, while "health" is offering legitimacy, respectability, and "cover" to many discussions of particular social problems related to sexuality, it is by no means the only possible language for characterizing sexual matters.

IDENTITIES, DIFFERENCES, AND INEQUALITIES OF ACCESS AND SCRUTINY

Several additional dimensions of the proliferation of sexual health merit attention. First, discourses of sexual health target or describe an ever more diverse set of specific social identities. In the previous chapter, I described how early discussions of sexual health in the 1970s occasionally made reference to social differences and how they might affect outcomes. Nowadays, one can find scholarly publications addressing the sexual health concerns of military veterans, tenth graders, stem-cell transplant recipients, women with schizophrenia, Latino migrant day laborers, Chinese sex workers, Polish elderly men with coronary artery disease, Deaf American Sign Language users, and students at historically Black colleges and universities, among many, many others.[41] On the one hand, sexual health increasingly is seen as being at stake for people of many different sorts. On the other hand, their distinctive group identities are perceived as relevant for understanding and addressing their sexual health concerns.

At a time when biomedicine is increasingly attuned to the specific needs of categorical identities—when doctors are trained in "culturally competent care," and when researchers are enjoined to consider diversity goals when enrolling subjects in clinical trials[42]—sexual health often becomes a targeted enterprise. There may be no general recipe for the achievement of sexual health: one size does not fit all. Practitioners may also organize themselves in ways that reflect the concern with group-specific needs. For example, the Association of Black Sexologists and Clinicians, "an interdisciplinary professional organization dedicated to improving the sexual expression and lives of persons of African descent," not only seeks to "build and sustain Black professional community involvement" but also seeks "to formally address the intersection of race and sexuality through research, clinical practice, and social discourse."[43]

The implication is not just that diversity in society changes the nature of sexual health practice. At the same time, conceiving of specific groups as having distinctive sexual health profiles, risks, and requirements potentially changes the social understanding of what such groups are fundamentally like. Certainly this happened with gay men in the wake of the HIV/AIDS epidemic, as the group was depicted in various ways, both pejorative (as victims of an "unhealthy" lifestyle) and affirmative (as dedicated caretakers and courageous resisters of social injustice).[44]

That attention to social differences and inequalities can have either beneficial or pernicious effects is evident within the social problem frame that addresses risks of STIs. In response to epidemiological

patterns, researchers, public health officials, grant agencies, and community activists often focus on specific groups deemed to be at higher
risk of infection, but the valences of attention vary considerably. In
some cases, sexual health prevention activities (often undertaken
from within the communities positioned at risk) have been tied to
projects of empowerment and challenge to structural inequalities.[45] In
other cases, specific groups—such as Black and Latino men who have
sex with both men and women and who have been the objects of moral
panic concerning "down low" sexual practices—are deemed threats to
the social body that necessitate strategies of containment.[46]

Other social problem frames likewise demonstrate sharp distinctions with regard to who benefits and who is subjected to scrutiny.
The sexual dysfunction frame may often presume a White,[47] middle-
class, heterosexual subject—particularly a male subject who has access
to the funds or health insurance to afford medications such as Viagra.
In the case of sexual and reproductive health, the target population is
often limited to women's bodies, as men continue to lie largely outside
of reproductive health care, politics, and responsibility.[48] With regard
to women, however, the effects of sexual and reproductive health attention are highly uneven, sometimes manifested as hypervigilance
and sustained intervention and at other times leaving many women
without access to needed services such as contraception, abortion, or
maternal health care.

Moreover, the promotion and provisioning of sexual and reproductive health often reflects entrenched biases about the dangers of
"excessive" reproductivity. At a global level, such concerns may invoke
long-standing tropes, in countries of the global North, about the threat
posed by the fertility of the world's nonwhite poor.[49] In countries like
the United States, family planning campaigns sometimes presume
that higher rates of pregnancy among young, unmarried women of
color is a consequence not of structural inequalities and lack of access
to abortion and contraception, but rather of supposed lifestyle choices
shaped by deficient cultural values and an underdeveloped ethic of responsibility—or, as in the racist and sexist myth of the Black "welfare
queen," a desire to "game the system" and reap reward for excess procreation.[50] Such biases may shape the particular kinds of sexual and
reproductive health services offered to specific social groups. As Jenny
Brian and coauthors have described in an analysis of the promotion

of long-acting reversible contraception: "The implicit focus on low-income young women of colour . . . forecloses a consideration of how such [targeting] invokes a long history of population control and the denial of agency for those with the fewest resources."[51]

Similarly, the social problem frame that associates sexual health with sexual responsibility is also very often freighted with assumptions about the social meanings of racial and class (and other forms of) difference. Projects of sexual health education may tend to pathologize racial and ethnic minority youth and poor youth by associating them with a sexuality that is imagined as out of control (or as shaped by cultural deficits) and that can be managed only through tight regulation.[52] Somewhat similarly, proponents of sexual health for people with intellectual and developmental disabilities complain that far too many approaches to the sexual education of such individuals begin with the implicit assumption: "You shouldn't be doing this anyway, so therefore we're not going to teach you about it."[53]

In short, studying the diversification of sexual health activities also calls attention to the differentiated ways in which specific groups are positioned or position themselves. Ideas about identities and differences of all kinds affect sexual health projects, making those projects more or less available to, and more or less judgmental of, distinct population groups. Those efforts, in turn, can have ramifying effects on the social identities of people in those groups, as well as on capacities to achieve social equality and justice.

THE GEOGRAPHY OF PROLIFERATION

Another characteristic of the spread of sexual health discourses and projects from the 1990s forward is the international uptake of the term, both in English and in translated forms. To be sure, the bulk of published sexual health scholarship comes from Europe, North America, and Oceania, which, in the content analysis sample that Mamo and I assembled, jointly account for 80 percent of the authors (with an additional 14 percent of unknown location, and thus only 6 percent from Asia, Africa, Central and South America, and the Middle East).[54] Yet our survey of sexual health activities on the internet revealed a very wide range of organizations and events: the Africa Conference on Sexual Health and Rights, the Australasian Sexual Health Conference, the Asia Pacific Coalition on Male Sexual Health, the Asia Pacific Con-ference on Reproductive and Sexual Health and Rights, the Estonian Sexual Health Association.

Of course, the use of English-language titles marks these events and organizations as operating in a transnational space, sometimes involv-ing the collaboration, backing, or funding of organizations such as the WHO or major foundations from beyond the borders of the country or region in question. Yet the currency on the internet of translated terms—*salud sexual* in Spanish, *sexuelle gesundheit* in German, *santé sexuelle* in French, and so on—suggests deeper engagements with the concept in ways that may resonate with local experiences in distinc-tive cultural settings. The point here is not to suggest that the con-cept stays the same as the term undergoes translation. Rather, it seems likely that the term (in whatever language) takes on distinctive shad-ings of meanings in different places—and that this, too, is evidence of the proliferative differentiation of sexual health.[55]

Data on web searches obtained from Google Trends provide further insight into the degree of popular interest in sexual health around the globe.[56] For the period 2004–19, the "density" of Google searches for "sexual health" (that is, the number of searches for the term in a given country relative to the total number of searches conducted in that country) was greatest for the United Kingdom,[57] followed by New Zea-land, Zimbabwe, Uganda, Australia, Ethiopia, and Canada. The United States ranked seventeenth in the list of countries. Although it is not surprising that countries with high English-language use would pre-dominate, it is interesting to find the United States so far down on the list, behind a number of countries with far less scientific and public health infrastructure.

A similar mapping of the density of Google searches for *salud sexual* shows the term to be fairly well disseminated through the Spanish-speaking world, particularly in Cuba, Nicaragua, Bolivia, Mexico, and El Salvador, in that order. In Mexico, *salud sexual* functions not just as an official term, used by government agencies and nongovernmen-tal organizations,[58] but also as a marketing category for condoms (as my photo taken in a supermarket confirms) (fig. 6). In short, while it would take considerable sustained research to examine the breadth and depth of uptake of sexual health projects and concerns in differ-ent places around the globe—and the subtle or not-so-subtle ways in which definitions and meanings likely shift even as the term itself

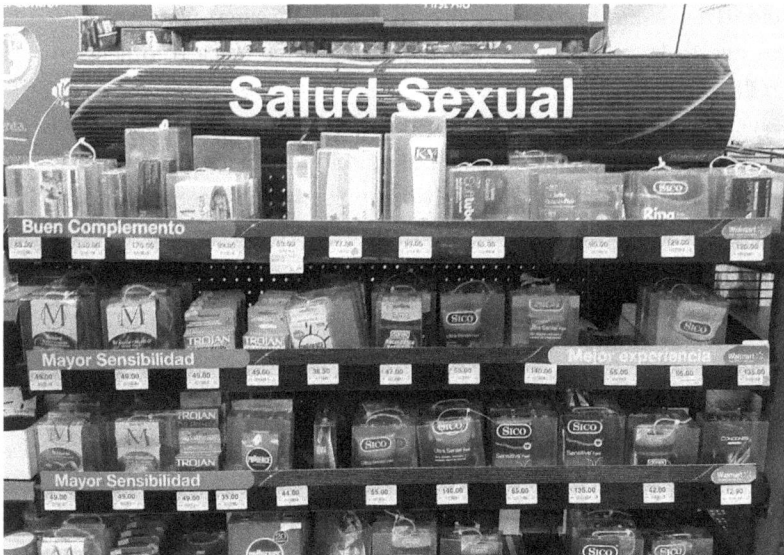

Figure 6: *Salud sexual* in a Mexican supermarket

Photo credit: Steven Epstein

travels, whether in English or in translation—it seems fair to point to the international reach of the term and concept as an important indicator of its success.

Accounting for Proliferation: Historical Causes and Correlates

During the period of explosive growth that began in the 1990s, sexual health has blossomed as a capacious grab bag of ideas, practices, and initiatives, and its meanings have extended across problem domains and geographic space to encompass the concerns of more and more social identities. Why has this happened? And why has sexual health become polysemous, or imbued with multiple meanings?

In part, the expansive character of the original WHO working definition set the stage—and, as I describe in Chapter 3, subsequent redefinitions have brought even more concerns under the sexual health umbrella. But fundamentally, as I suggested in the introduction, the answer turns on the precarious status of sexuality in so many societies around the world. In the compound term "sexual health," "health" sanitizes "sexuality," containing stigma, cleansing supposed dirtiness and messiness, and papering over moral panic.[59] In addition, "health" scientizes "sexuality": to suggest that sexual issues are matters of sexual health is to propose that experts may give voice to objective and credible truths about them.

Often, sanitizing and scientizing sexuality can then be a strategy for depoliticization and conflict avoidance. Individuals and organizations may assert that their positions on sexual matters should not be questioned because they are "evidence based" and required for healthy outcomes—not the product simply of values or ideology—and they may thereby hope to extinguish the flames of political and moral controversy that so frequently threaten to engulf sexuality.[60] For example, the sociologist Laura Carpenter has observed that "the increasing popularity of the term 'sexual health' may reflect an attempt by researchers worldwide to circumvent conservative opposition, under the assumption that research on sexuality is more likely to be deemed justifiable if it concerns health."[61]

Finally, "health" endows sexuality with seriousness of purpose as a legitimate concern of public discourse. In a recent example, an online post about the "sexual health and well-being of astronauts" insisted that the satisfaction of their sexual needs while isolated in space (perhaps by means of sex robots) was a "far from trivial" consideration.[62] Sexual health, in these various ways, overcomes the perceived illegitimacy of sexuality—which is what begins to explain why so many kinds of endeavors related to sexuality have come to be characterized as matters of sexual health.

This more or less functionalist explanation serves reasonably well in accounting for the broad appeal of sexual health as a "solution" to diverse social problems. But it does little to clarify why, specifically, sexual health entered a phase of rapid growth and proliferation in the 1990s. Locating the moment of proliferation necessarily directs attention to the kinds of questions I first raised in chapter 1, under the rubric of genealogy (or historical ontology). There, I considered the conditions of possibility for the initial emergence of sexual health and the definitional process that ensued in the 1970s. Now it is time to ask, What particular conjuncture of events and sensibilities facilitated the "virality" of sexual health in the 1990s? What were the conditions of possibility for the ramping up of attention to sexual health at that time? While the analysis builds on that presented in chapter 1, I argue that the factors that propelled the proliferation of sexual health activities differ somewhat from those that led to its initial rise.

It is impossible to prove precisely what caused a flourishing of "things called sexual health" in the 1990s. Yet the descriptions I have provided of the six social problems provide some important clues about a set of important developments.

AIDS CHANGED EVERYTHING

First, it seems especially plausible that the global HIV/AIDS epidemic functioned as a powerful relay to move the concept and term sexual health into broader circulation—just as the epidemic, more generally, has helped to usher in a new era of global health.[63] Perhaps more than any other single development in recent decades, the spread of AIDS— but also the political activism that emerged to confront it—has forced biomedicine and public health to grapple with sexuality as something that fundamentally matters.[64] Moreover, the language of sexual health offered crucial legitimacy to the necessity of zeroing in on sexual topics in order to address the epidemic. It is certainly true, as Petchesky, Corrêa, and Parker have argued, that "one of the strange ironies of the HIV pandemic [is] that it has created a space for more open talk about sexuality, sexual behaviour and erotic pleasure."[65] Yet at least in official venues, much more often than not, such discourse has been under threat except when it can be justified as a crucial ingredient of a public health approach made necessary by a deadly global pandemic. Similarly, AIDS has brought about the "sexual healthicization" of the condom, as the historian Dagmar Herzog has noted: "A major effect of the public awareness efforts was to transform the condom from a reluctantly used object with a still slightly tawdry aura into something commonly accepted and no longer controversial."[66]

In the United States, in the context of a stigmatizing illness that affected stigmatized populations, "sexual health" served critical functions. In response to claims from the radical right that the advent of AIDS proved the essential unhealthiness of gay sex,[67] "sexual health" affirmatively conveyed the idea that sex and health could properly be aligned. More specifically, "sexual health" could be mobilized as a respectable, if euphemistic, way of discussing gay sexuality, thereby offering the possibility of an end run around obstacles imposed by the homophobic and sex-phobic legal and political environment of the time. A legislative amendment put forward in 1987 by the virulently anti-gay Senator Jesse Helms of North Carolina, and supported by a large majority of the US Congress, prevented the expenditure of federal funds on AIDS prevention or education materials that would "promote or encourage, directly or indirectly, homosexual sexual activities."[68] While the wording was later modified, the CDC created strict guidelines for any activities it funded and tasked its program-review panels with ensuring that educational materials were not "offensive" or "indecent."[69] The policy was overturned by judicial order in 1992,[70] but the perception remained that AIDS educators working in gay communities had best fly under the radar if they wanted to avoid problems in getting access to federal funds. In this context, rebranding AIDS work as "sexual health promotion" helped to "de-gay" the discourse and escape unwanted scrutiny. Somewhat similar pressures confronted academic researchers studying sexuality in the context of the AIDS epidemic, and in 2003 the US House of Representatives came within two votes of revoking grants made by the National Institutes of Health (NIH) to four research projects on topics related to sexuality and health. For nervous NIH officials who sought to defend their funding decisions (and their institutional autonomy), the solution was precisely to rely on the sanitizing functions of "health" in relation to the putatively stigmatizing character of sexual matters; and program officers contacted dozens of researchers to ask them to explain the contributions of their work to the promotion of public health.[71]

Elsewhere around the world, especially where LGBT organizing has arisen during the AIDS epidemic rather than before it emerged, "sexual health" has provided a safe vehicle for promoting LGBT rights. In the context of Malawi, for example, Ashley Currier and Tara McKay have described the complex dynamics of "pursuing social justice through public health." As the authors noted, "using HIV/AIDS advocacy as a cover for reaching gender and sexual dissidents cloaks LGBTIQ activism in the safety of a pressing public-health concern"—yet in Malawi, it also created possibilities for activist groups to pursue creative fusions of public health and social justice.[72]

OTHER FACTORS IN THE 1990S

As transformative as the HIV/AIDS epidemic has been, other aspects of the time period also seem important to understand the spread and diversification of sexual health discourses and practices. As Sandfort and Ehrhardt noted in an earlier analysis, an additional impetus for the investment in sexual health was the discovery of Viagra and its marketing in 1998.[73] This development was crucial for sexual medicine in particular, but it brought attention to the whole domain of sexual health and the very idea of linking the two terms.

In addition, the 1990s was a time for consolidation of the links between sexual health and reproductive health at the global level, and this, too, helps us understand the timing of the proliferation of sexual health. Scholars have pointed in particular to the International Conference on Population and Development (ICPD) held in Cairo in 1994. The ICPD was a watershed event sponsored by the United Nations that involved twenty thousand delegates from around the world who discussed the agenda for family planning and reproductive health. Along with government representatives, it brought together a wide array of women's health and development nongovernmental organizations committed to feminism, human rights, and women's empowerment.[74] Jane Cottingham has helpfully recapped how "sexual health" entered the conversation in Cairo: "At one point during government negotiations on the Programme of Action of the [ICPD], someone suggested that the term 'sexual health' should be included in the definition of reproductive health. There was a flurry of activity. Representatives of the [WHO] were asked whether an official definition of sexual health existed and urgent messages were sent back to Geneva for people to comb the archives."[75] Thus, not only did the very existence of a WHO working definition of sexual health prove strategically useful, but, via its uptake in this context, the definition proceeded to circulate through a new set of global networks.

Despite opposition to discussion of sexual matters from a number of countries with religious fundamentalist representatives,[76] the official report from the ICPD declared that reproductive health "implies that people are able to have a satisfying and safe sex life and that they have the capability to reproduce and the freedom to decide if, when and how often to do so." A few sentences later, the paragraph closed with the explicit statement that reproductive health "also includes sexual health, the purpose of which is the enhancement of life and personal relations, and not merely counselling and care related to reproduction and sexually transmitted diseases." While this definition appeared to locate sexual health as a subset of reproductive health, the very next paragraph referred to "sexual and reproductive health," introducing the phrasing that places the two concerns on a par while establishing their intimate relation.[77] Subsequent transnational activity further solidified the juncture of sexual and reproductive health, including the 2004 adoption by the World Health Assembly of the WHO Global Reproductive Health Strategy. As Cottingham has noted, "Despite its title, which was deliberately created to be aligned with the ICPD Programme of Action, the Strategy uses the term '*sexual and* reproductive health' throughout the main text."[78]

In considering the conjuncture of developments in the 1990s that facilitated the proliferation of sexual health, it is worth observing that this period also witnessed the early blossoming of the internet and the World Wide Web—which may have provided the communication infrastructure that allowed many terms and concepts, including sexual health, to "go viral" at just this time. (Indeed, the very idea of the "computer virus" and the metaphor of viral spread in relation to new media of communication also date from this period and, of course, reflect the anxieties prompted by the global transmission of HIV/AIDS;[79] the "virality" of sexual health is overdetermined.) Technological developments in subsequent years, such as the rise of new forms of social media, have also transformed sexual expression while furthering an interest in sexual health.[80]

Taking place in the background, and intertwining with several of the specific concerns of the sexual health frames, are broader changes unfolding in the domains of biomedicine and health. For example, scholars such as Peter Conrad have emphasized the new "drivers" of medicalization that have emerged in recent decades, including the heightened role of the pharmaceutical industry in creating new conditions that it is positioned to treat, as well as the growing salience of medical consumers in demanding medical labels, explanations, and treatments for their conditions.[81] These phenomena have been well documented in relation to sexual issues and problems, particularly including the production and treatment of sexual dysfunction.[82] In addition, Adele Clarke and her coauthors, analyzing the technological and scientific reorganization of medicine since the 1980s, have described how the increasing sophistication of biomedicine has given rise to new regimes of risk, risk assessment, and risk management in biomedicine.[83] Again, sexual matters provide excellent examples of these trends, particularly including strategies for reducing risks of STIs.[84]

Finally, the period during which sexual health has proliferated has also witnessed what I and Stefan Timmermans have termed a consequential shift "from medicine to health."[85] That is, the overall landscape of healing has been reshaped by the influx of a diverse array of influential actors who nowadays make credible claims about the nature of disease, disability, and impairment and the pursuit of health and well-being. A varied assortment of authorities, invoking New Age ideas, pop psychology, nutritional and dietary strategies, self-help philosophies, and fitness regimens, now comment on fundamental aspects of existence: What substances should people consume, and what practices should they engage in, to stay well? What makes life meaningful, and when is it not worth living?[86] While some of these new actors advance biomedical perspectives, many others come from outside of biomedical worlds: rival and adjunct semiprofessional groups, new experts who speak about how to pursue health and wellness, and nonexperts and social movements that advance their own arguments and frames of reference about health and medical topics. Collectively, but often in competition, these diverse and proliferating manifestations of cultural authority speak in the name of health.[87] They seek to shape the understandings about bodies, illnesses, and health that inform decisions about how to go about the business of living—not just what treatment to pursue for illness but also how to eat healthily, how to sleep well, and (of course) how to have healthy sex. In short, while the cultural authority of biomedicine in the US remains impressive, a growing portion of the cultural authority of health now lies outside the purview of the medical profession.[88] Developments in sexual health have tracked a broader transformation in which more and more actors and institutions have involved themselves in offering advice, diagnoses, and cures that promote the goal of healthy living.

Thus, a series of large-scale social, cultural, biomedical, epistemic, and technological developments created possibilities for the expansion of concern with sexual health, especially beginning in the 1990s. We can now deepen our analysis of how this process has unfolded by considering the productive character of the ambiguity and polysemy that has come to characterize sexual health.

The Productivity of Ambiguity and the Power of Buzz

In some respects, the proliferation of sexual health recalls the "discursive explosion" around sexuality that Michel Foucault described for an earlier historical moment.[89] However, other aspects of the advent of sexual health call out for different explanatory tools. Specifically, the combination of proliferation and polysemy—and the resulting fact that such a diverse array of activities can be undertaken under the ambiguous banner of sexual health—suggests that sexual health has moved into the ranks of contemporary buzzwords (or buzz phrases, in this case). The phenomenon of the buzzword, that is, calls attention to aspects of sexual health discourses and practices that the Foucauldian story does not fully capture. And it points us to the surprising ways in which conceptual fuzziness can be the key to success.[90]

The term "buzzword," along with the broader idea of "buzz," is well entrenched in popular culture. In addition, scholars have taken up the "buzzy" characteristics of many individual terms: "development," "diaspora," "diversity," "empowerment," "globalization," "identity," "interdisciplinarity," "intersectionality," "NGO," "resilience," "social capital," "sustainability," and "wellness," to name a few.[91] The idea of buzz draws on a sonorous mix of metaphorical associations taken from both nature and technology, including the fierce sound of bees swarming in a hive,[92] the hiss of electrical current, the imagined hum of brain activity, and the jarring noise generated by devices like alarm clocks.[93] Of course, some sexual devices also buzz, as suggested by advertising for the San Francisco–based feminist sex shop Good Vibrations; in 2014, in addition to selling vibrators, the company also produced an online magazine called "The Buzz" and offered coffee mugs that read: "Creating a BUZZ since 1977."[94]

Buzzwords no doubt have a longer history than the term itself, and they bear a family resemblance to other long-standing cultural phenomena—catchphrases, keywords, slogans, brands, memes, "ideas that stick," things that "go viral," and so forth.[95] Yet the common perception that contemporary life is flooded with buzzwords may reflect actual characteristics of changes in global communications and the consequent compression of time and space. Especially with the rise of new communication technologies such as the internet, it may be that people increasingly speak in shortcuts to give their ideas a certain robustness that makes them well packaged to travel, and that they seek new modes of discourse that will stand out in an ever-crowded "attention space."[96] Buzzwords also seem connected to present-day emphases on hype and the generation of expectations about technological and other forms of progress. They are often used to promote what Adam

Hedgecoe has called "promissory sciences," and they function to generate imaginable futures.[97]

In marking sexual health as a buzzword, I invoke these sonic and temporal associations, but I suspend the typical judgment that buzzwords are necessarily "bad." Certainly the term "buzzword" tends to have pejorative connotations: it often suggest a transient importance if not utter triviality—the sense that the term in question is, after all, "*just* a buzzword."[98] According to Merriam-Webster, for example, a buzzword is "an important-sounding usually technical word or phrase often of little meaning used chiefly to impress laymen."[99] The suspicion of buzzwords also reflects their association with the manipulative promotion of "buzz" in marketing and advertising, where buzz, understood as "explosive self-generating demand," is something one invents and cultivates in a deliberate fashion for profit.[100] In the face of this hostility and dismissiveness toward buzzwords, it is worth emphasizing the meaningful and consequential character of sexual health discourses and activities—a practical efficacy that has persisted even as the term "sexual health" has become more elastic and slippery. We might therefore view the "buzz" around sexual health in a different light, and even adopt a less uniformly negative assessment of the buzzword phenomenon itself.

Part of what often prompts suspicion about buzzwords is just how vague they can be. According to science and technology studies (STS) scholar Bernadette Bensaude Vincent, "fuzz and buzz work together." Rather than conveying clear meaning or a precise agenda, buzzwords function "more like signposts, pointing to a direction and inviting us to move."[101] And many analysts of specific buzzwords see fuzziness as precisely the problem. For example, Lars Grönvik, writing of "disability" as a "fuzzy buzz word," has portrayed the field of disability studies as stymied by a lack of definition clarity.[102] But such laments of the ill effects of ambiguity contrast sharply with Kathy Davis's analysis of "intersectionality"—its "spectacular success as well as the uncertainties which it generates." According to Davis: "I shall not be providing suggestions about how to clarify the ambiguities surrounding the concept, nor how to alleviate uncertainties about how it should be used. Quite the contrary, I shall be arguing that, paradoxically, precisely the vagueness and open-endedness of 'intersectionality' may be the very secret to its success."[103] Rather than policing usage of the term,

Davis argued that "intersectionality," for all its messiness, merits praise because it "encourages complexity, stimulates creativity, and avoids premature closure."[104]

Ambiguity, in short, is culturally productive, and the exploitation of ambiguity is a pathway to social change.[105] Several other scholars have likewise pointed to ambiguity as the key to a buzzword's success. Tarleton Gillespie has located the resonance of "platform" in the term's capacity to seem "specific enough to mean something, and vague enough to work across multiple venues for multiple audiences."[106] Jeremy Greene, writing of "essential medicines," has described "the flexibility of the essential medicines concept within increasingly plastic conceptualizations of global health." For Greene, "the essential medicines concept, like global health itself, has taken on somewhat of a moral universality, as a thing that has acquired enough stakeholders and commonsensical status that it is increasingly difficult to argue against and even more difficult to define."[107]

To the extent that buzzwords like sexual health can profit from ambiguity and mean different things in different contexts, they resemble other kinds of objects that STS scholars have described. The historian of science Ilana Löwy, adapting a phrase from the sociologist Mark Granovetter, has written of the "strength of loose concepts" in facilitating collaboration and inter-group alliances within large scientific fields.[108] Given that buzzwords have a greater reach—extending beyond the professional domains of science into everyday worlds of varied sorts—they may therefore more closely resemble what Susan Leigh Star and James Griesemer called "boundary objects," which possess a flexibility of definition that allows them to traverse social worlds, both expert and lay. Boundary objects, according to Star and Griesemer, "are objects which are both plastic enough to adapt to local needs and the constraints of the several parties employing them, yet robust enough to maintain a common identity across sites."[109]

Yet as apt as the connection to boundary objects might seem,[110] it is important to observe that Star and Griesemer (like Löwy) are fundamentally concerned with the possibilities for communication and coordination of work across disciplinary and social boundaries. While some buzzwords certainly do seem to function this way, the analysis of the distinctive social problems associated with sexual health suggests, alternatively, that the same buzzword can sometimes be used simultaneously by different groups in distinct social worlds, without much meaningful communication or coordination taking place across those worlds. As a prelude to the next chapter, which considers attempts to forge connections across the problem domains of sexual health, I would propose that adopters and spreaders of buzzwords sometimes aim to coordinate activity and other times seek to let the proverbial hundred flowers bloom—and that over the course of its usable life, a buzzword might first take one of those two paths and then the other.

Of course, there is also a third, important possibility: rather than cooperative consensus or peaceful, noncommunicative coexistence, buzzwords may be stakes and weapons in overt ideological warfare. In such cases, the animating question is who succeeds in monopolizing the symbolic power needed to say what the buzzword "actually means."[111] To the extent that individuals and groups fight over the meanings of buzzwords, then those terms may more closely resemble what W. B. Gallie called "essentially contested concepts"—concepts whose use "inevitably involves endless disputes about their proper uses on the part of their users."[112] This is also part of the story of sexual health, at least some of the time. In chapter 10, I return to the topic of conflict and consider competing attempts to specify meanings of sexual health across the political spectrum.

The tensions and paradoxes inherent in buzzwords like sexual health are now apparent. On the one hand, buzzwords are vague, fuzzy, open, polysemous, and sometimes verging on meaninglessness. On the other hand, buzzwords are compact, powerful, appealing, and packaged in a way that grants them a great deal of social efficacy, building bandwagons and "steering" fields.[113] In an increasingly crowded global communications environment, buzzwords are a way of shouting and being heard—they are terms that will capture attention and travel easily. Yet it is their unspecific and ambiguous character that promotes successful uptake in diverse social contexts. These characteristics apply especially well to sexual health, and they suggest how it is that sexual health may simultaneously be so potent an idea yet so flexible in its meanings across different domains of employment.

Among the research questions we might pose about sexual health, a number of interesting ones concern its trajectory and temporality as a buzzword. At what stage in its own history can a novel term most appropriately be called a buzzword? And at what point in our familiarity (or overfamiliarity) with them do buzzwords cease to be buzzwords? Do buzzwords "die" when they reach the limits of overextension? Or (as Michael Penkler and coauthors suggest, in a study of "diversity" in health care), do buzzwords more typically resolve into more crisply defined concepts as particular meanings and uses, by particular communities of practice, come to predominate as a practical necessity, and as "doable" tasks are articulated?[114] No doubt the answers vary depending on the buzzword.[115]

Specifically, in the case of sexual health, one might reasonably wonder about the likely fate of its current dispersion across semantic and social space. Can "sexual health" retain its attachment to multiple social problem arenas? Or, will the term gradually fall out of favor in particular frames while consolidating its hold in others? Or, alternatively, will it prove possible to construct bridges that connect some or all of the different islands of sexual health? I return to these questions in subsequent chapters and in the conclusion, where I consider different potential futures of sexual health.

But most immediately—in the next chapter—I turn attention away from the "centrifugal" tendencies of sexual health to examine the "centripetal" possibilities. What happens as key actors seek to connect the different social problem frames of sexual health—and to expand the definition of sexual health to include more and more of those frames under a sexual health umbrella? This chapter has emphasized what can be accomplished by means of ambiguity and diversification. The next looks at the work that gets done by generating new, hybrid objects that connect the worlds of sexual health and bring different problem domains into conversation with one another.

3 *New Projects of Health, Rights, and Pleasure*

RECOMBINING SEXUAL HEALTH

My badge for the Twenty-First Congress of the World Association for Sexual Health (WAS), held in Porto Alegre, Brazil, identifies me as a "Non-Prescriber." Though prompted by an arcane rule of the Brazilian Health Surveillance Agency,[1] the badge designation inscribes a visible distinction among the roughly one thousand attendees, between those authorized to write medical prescriptions and those not authorized—or as one conference-goer tells me, it immediately separates the sheep from the goats. (I neglect to ask who is which.) Indeed, across dozens of presentations that I hear over the course of three days, I encounter striking differences between conceptions of sexuality—for instance, between biomedical and neurological approaches and psychosocial and social-structural ones. "They think that sex is all right here [points to her head] or here [points to her groin]," a sociologist complains to me, over breakfast: "But there's no person, no relationship."

Yet what stands out overall is how the conference creates a "big tent" for a sprawling array of understandings of sexuality and sexual health—as if all the concerns and constituencies referenced in chapter 2 were assembled in one place. Listening to presentations, I learn about the positive correlation between activation in the left anterior cingulate gyrus and the level of perceived sexual arousal; how the launch of Viagra fueled a "biologization of the psychological"; the benefits and risks of aesthetic vaginal procedures; the notion of sexual rights as fundamental and universal; plant-based supplements for sexual pleasure; clitoral therapy devices; and how "recognition theory suggests that human sexual pleasure can be progressively harnessed and expanded by a reciprocally relating couple as a special form of intersubjective engagement." Mariela Castro Espín—daughter of Raúl, niece of Fidel, and director of the Cuban National Center for Sex Education in Havana—describes how capitalist crisis and neoliberalism lead to social disintegration; and having gotten that out of the way, she proceeds to speak passionately about the harms of discrimination against transgender people.

At a lunchtime symposium organized by the condom manufacturer Durex and the MTV Staying Alive Foundation, a crowd of several hundred people—younger and hipper looking than the conference attendees overall—turn out for free sandwiches and a panel discussion, conducted on a white leather couch, on the topic "Your Love. Your Life. Sex Education for a New Generation." The creative director from MTV International then previews a short film in which a diverse group of young people from around the world, speaking in English, answer questions about their sex lives and HIV risk and show us their bedrooms. Afterward, the host solicits feedback in the style of a television talk show with audience participation.

The conference attendees themselves are diverse in many respects. Medical doctors and academic researchers mingle with sex therapists, educators, counselors, policy makers, and members of nongovernmental organizations. The organizers report proudly that program speakers come from thirty different countries, while the book of abstracts includes presentations from eighty-eight countries. North Americans and Europeans appear to make up a majority of those present, but the Congress has a substantial number of attendees from Latin America and the Caribbean, and also many from Asia and a few from Africa. Quite a number this year are from Brazil itself, and in a nod to the local culture, the opening ceremony begins with a samba presentation that is enthusiastically received.

Is this another story of the dramatic and seemingly uncontained diversification of sexual health projects? Certainly, the WAS conference offered a grab bag of sexual health possibilities, but in fact, I want to argue something different. While the previous chapter emphasized "fuzz" and "buzz"—and the resulting blossoming of semantic and practical possibilities—the work of the WAS, together with the WHO, demonstrates concerted efforts to gather many of those disparate activities together under a single, big umbrella. Congresses of the WAS are more than just conventions of adherents of different approaches to what they all call sexual health, briefly united under a single banner. The important point is that the WAS has enjoyed success in building conceptual and practical bridges that connect the sexual health frames—stitching together some of the distinct meanings, activities, and forms of expertise that run across the different social problem domains. In this regard, the WAS exerts more organizational energy than the National Sexual Health Conference that I described in the introduction, which also functioned as a meeting point for people from different social worlds but had less of a distinct agenda of its own.

The WAS has come a long way from its founding in 1978 as the World Association for Sexology. Initially designed to revive the dormant field of sexology, the organization was reborn as the World Association for Sexual Health, having formally changed its name (while keeping the acronym) in 2005. At that same moment, the World Congress of Sexology became the World Congress for Sexual Health.[2] "Sexual Health represents a common goal and reflects in a more direct way our vision and mission," announced the organization's president at the time, the Mexican sexologist Eusebio Rubio-Aurioles.[3] As Eli Coleman, a leader in the organization and a past president, recalled, the name change prompted concern and some resistance on the part of some of the clinicians and researchers within the WAS, who were skeptical about a move into the domains of public health and advocacy.[4] But in the intervening years, the broadening of emphasis signified by the name change has succeeded in placing the organization at the center of wide-ranging concerns related to sexuality and health.[5] On World Sexual Health Day, inaugurated by the WAS in 2010 and celebrated each year on September 4, the WAS coordinates a global advocacy and awareness campaign marked by events in a growing number of countries—forty-six as of 2019, including Argentina, Australia, Austria, Bahrain, Brazil, Chile, Colombia, Croatia, Cuba, Indonesia, Israel, Italy, Japan, Lebanon, Mexico, Pakistan, Spain, Sweden, Turkey, and Venezuela.[6]

Through its construction of a federation of international, regional, and national member organizations; its avowedly transdisciplinary emphases and embrace of multiple professional constituencies; and its sponsorship of the *International Journal of Sexual Health*, the WAS has sought to enact a broad and ambitious agenda. As expressed in the association's "Sexual Health for the Millennium" declaration from 2008, that agenda includes recognizing and protecting sexual rights; advancing gender equality; condemning and combating sexuality-related violence; providing universal access to comprehensive sexuality education; emphasizing the centrality of sexual health within reproductive health programs; halting and reversing the spread of HIV and other STIs; treating sexual concerns, dysfunctions, and disorders; and achieving "recognition of sexual pleasure as a component of holistic health and well-being."[7] Certainly, many of these ambitions go far beyond any narrowly medical or professional conception of sexological research and practice—though, to be sure, since its founding days, sexology has always had broad foundations and aspirations.[8] Notably, the organization has linked its identity closely to the idea of human rights, or "sexual rights for all."[9]

In pursuit of these goals, the WAS has allied itself with the WHO, seeking its support while also working to influence its statements and activities in the domain of sexual health. Just as sexologists were central to the defining of sexual health at the WHO-sponsored meeting in 1974, so the WAS—both before and since its renaming—has sought both to put sexuality on the agenda of the international agency and to piggyback on its credibility and imprimatur. And without a doubt, the WHO has itself become more and more invested in the term. While the 329-page report issued by the agency to summarize its annual activities in 1975 devoted only the briefest mention to the publication of the report that contained the original working definition,[10] over time, as I will describe, the agency has come to claim sexual health as a significant focus of its activities and concerns.

The synergistic activities of the WAS and the WHO hold important implications for the proliferation of sexual health and its possible futures. This chapter looks at what happens when organizations seek to establish new connections across sexual health projects and locate them under a broader sexual health umbrella. These organizations treat the hybridity of sexual health as an opportunity: they seek to construct more complex hybrid objects that join different dimensions of sexual health. In so doing, they seek to locate sexual health as a more general framework (or boundary object) that can unite scientific and humanitarian goals.[11]

In effect, institutional actors like the WAS and the WHO have sought to treat the different ways of framing sexual health described in the previous chapter as modular components that can be assembled into a larger architecture. Of course, it is not obvious that such efforts will necessarily succeed. The question of whether the different agendas (and value commitments, and ontologies) of the different social problem frames of sexual health will ultimately collide, combine, or merely coexist is mirrored by the question of whether the centripetal force within the worlds of sexual health will prove more powerful than their centrifugal tendencies.

To assess the attempts to develop new connections, new projects, and new hybrid objects, I first consider the twists and turns in the story of WHO attention to sexual health and its meanings in the years following the promulgation of a definition in 1974. While the capacious nature of the early WHO working definition helped create possibilities for the term to travel, the successful spread of the term prompted, in turn, efforts to revisit the definition and expand it to encompass more of the domains and issues that the term by then had begun to reference.

Thus, the mutually reinforcing relationship between definitional development and the spread of the term has presented possibilities for forging conceptual unity across diversity. At the same time, the challenges in coming to consensus on definitions has further demonstrated how yoking sexuality to health inevitably frames sexual questions from the standpoint of normative judgments—that is, claims about who or what should be considered healthy or not—and that such judgments are often highly controversial. Similarly, the growth of a transnational sexual health industry has inevitably raised questions about whether sexual health can be defined in universal terms—or whether attempts to do so inevitably privilege the perspectives of wealthier and more powerful countries.

After analyzing the evolution of definitions over time and the role of the WHO and the WAS in the process, I proceed to examine the broader influence of the current WHO working definition as a touchstone in discussions of sexuality and health. The cultural authority of the WHO and its status as one of the largest and most important agencies of the United Nations has caused the term and the definition to travel far and be taken up, though sometime in altered form, by many groups interested in promoting sexual health.[12] However, the very success of the definition may occlude attention to alternative histories and to other groups that have also been influential in shaping thinking about sexuality and health.

The latter part of the chapter examines recent extensions of the sexual health umbrella through the assembly of new, hybrid objects: it explores the organizing work pursued under the rubric of "sexual and reproductive health and rights," as well as attempts to strengthen the "triangle" of sexual health, rights, and pleasure. These initiatives undergird many recent projects designed to promote justice, equity, and fulfillment, but they also raise questions. While the fuzzy nature of the concept of sexual health creates openings for such extensions, it remains unclear whether the disparate visions of sexuality and health implied by these and other projects can be brought together into a coherent picture. In addition, the increased emphasis on goals such as sexual rights adds, to the prior debate over whether sexuality can be conceived of in universal terms, the similar question of whether "rights" can be specified in universal ways. Finally, the very breadth of the new connections being forged "inside of" sexual health demands consideration of sexual health's "outside." I argue that it is important to consider who is left out—which issues and groups fail to obtain shelter under the sexual health umbrella.

Defining, Refining, and Redefining: The WHO Revisits Sexual Health

I have argued that the buzzwording of sexual health reveals the potency—and exploitability—of conceptual ambiguity, fuzziness, and flexibility. Yet this does not mean that those invested in defining sexual health have abandoned the effort to say just what it is. Indeed, one striking development is the repeated willingness of the WHO to revisit the working definition—not to narrow the usage of the term or corral its possible meanings but, rather, to reach out and encompass more of the extant shades of meaning within the organization's embrace. In other words, while the 1974 definition granted legitimacy and visibility to the concept of sexual health and launched it on the path of differentiation, the more the meanings of sexual health have multiplied since then, the more the WHO has seen fit to rethink the definition and expand its scope—which, in turn, has given license to those around the world who have sought to use the term in ever more diverse ways. Thus, the relationship between definitional clarity and conceptual fuzziness is more complicated than might be supposed—perhaps less one of opposition than a powerful feedback loop.

NORMATIVE JUDGMENT AND THE PROBLEM OF CULTURAL VARIATION

The WHO's process of definitional work has been less than entirely linear. Indeed, when the agency convened a working group of experts in

Copenhagen in 1987 "to clarify the concepts of sexual health" and discuss how to promote it, the group repudiated its mandate and declared, flat out, that "sexual health is not a scientific concept." What's more, given that "concepts of sexual health are related to culture and time and express value and norms of the society from which they come," it followed that definitional specificity was impossible and the attempt to achieve it was dangerous. As the committee report explained: "Clearly a definition of sexual health would be normative, and restrictive; it would also not be feasible. People in different age groups, those living in their own home, or in their parents' home or in institutions, prisons, hospitals, residential homes, people with physical or mental or sensory impairments, or people with different sexual preferences, people in different social classes, from different cultures or countries, religions or ethnic groups, people who are single, in a relationship or married, all are likely to experience their sexuality differently and to have different perceptions as to what is healthy."[13]

According to Eli Coleman, a WAS president and key long-term supporter of the definitional process, the German sexologist Gunter Schmidt "was particularly critical of this effort. He said that sexual health implied certain norms for 'proper' sex that can be termed 'healthy.' Attempting to define sexual health risked propagating sexual norms disguised as medical truths."[14] In the end, the committee members, who came from thirteen different countries, pointed not only to the enormous cultural variation in beliefs about proper sexual conduct but also to what they called the "power element" that inheres in definitional work. They therefore declined to grant a stamp of scientific legitimacy to projects of symbolic power (and, potentially, symbolic violence)—that is, attempts to say what constitutes sexual "normalcy."[15] In place of an effort to specify "objective measures of sexual health"—a proposition deemed "impossible"[16]—the authors of the 1987 report instead put their emphasis on "the variety and uniqueness of individual sexual experiences and sexual needs, and . . . the rights of individuals to be free from sexual exploitation, oppression, and abuse."[17] Thus, while professing and preaching value neutrality, the group in fact strongly endorsed its own preferred values, specifically those of individual choice and self-determination.

In one sense, the emphasis on variability in the meanings attached to sexuality resonated with the "fuzzy" and "buzzy" processes that I described in the previous chapter, as "sexual health" increasingly came to mean different things in different contexts: perhaps the WHO "non-definition" of 1987 effectively gave license to the polysemous and proliferative phase of sexual health speak that began just a few years later. But this expert body's refusal of its own cultural authority—its renunciation of a presumed ability to state how things are in the world, or should be[18]—proved to be an anomalous moment in the history of sexual health. Still, it introduced a thirteen-year gap in the WHO's formal consideration of the concept.

Then, at the start of the new millennium, the WHO (by then working closely with the WAS) returned to the definitional project, with no tremendous concern expressed about the dangers that had been identified earlier. But making sense of the new thinking that then took shape around sexual health requires that we first examine an intertwined development: the coincident emergence of political investments in promoting sexual rights. The rise of concern with sexual rights would prove central to a redefinition of sexual health.

SEXUAL RIGHTS?

There is nothing obvious about the idea of a kinds of rights called sexual. As the sociologist Ken Plummer has observed of rights in general and sexual rights in particular, rights are "part of the day-to-day world of lived meaning [rather than the] theoretical and philosophical or even legal heavens." Those, according to Plummer, "who suggest that rights are straightforward, inalienable, uncontested—and many do—work from a shallow and culturally limited idea of rights."[19] Therefore, it is important to reconstruct the pathways by which, in particular places at particular times, the existence of specific rights has been asserted and established.

The concept of sexual rights as well as its complex intertwining with health concerns can be traced back to multiple origin points and reflect the convergence over time of several relatively distinct streams of political thought and action.[20] The historian Nancy Cott has described how early twentieth-century feminists in the United States spoke of what they termed "sex rights for women," which involved both a repudiation of the reigning sexual double standard for women and men and a call for the frank recognition "that sexual drives were as constitutive of women's nature as of men's."[21] More typically, scholars interested in constructing a genealogy of sexual rights have pointed to the second-wave feminists of the 1970s and their close attention to sexual issues—including those, like the authors of *Our Bodies, Ourselves*, who emphasized connections between empowerment, sexuality, health, bodily autonomy, and reproductive control.[22] These ideas influenced, and were influenced in turn, by the transnational feminist movement and its work in subsequent decades.

Meanwhile, the emergence of the gay liberation movement in the early 1970s and the development of global LGBTQ activism placed on the table not only the idea that sexual self-definition is a basic human right that should not be curtailed but also the important argument that pleasure itself, grounded in the embodied experience of sexuality, is at stake in political struggle.[23] Moreover, the global HIV epidemic has, from its earliest days and into the present, sparked the emergence of "sex-positive" strategies for confronting STIs.[24] Advocates have claimed not just that rights to sexual expression and pleasure need not be trampled in the name of public health but in fact that health promotion activities that defend sexual pleasure are more likely to be efficacious than those that oppose it or fear it.[25] As AIDS activism developed and became more multifaceted in its goals, more diverse in its social composition, and more evident around the globe, the idea of a crucial linkage between sexual health and sexual rights was powerfully reinforced.[26]

Thus, many advocates of sexual health have become interested in sexual rights precisely on the hope (as described by Richard Parker and colleagues) that it would "serve as the foundation for a transformed public health praxis with regard to sexuality and sexual health."[27] More generally, the political scientist Dennis Altman has stressed how global advocacy in relation to HIV "has coincided with a broader move to recognize gender and sexual issues as intrinsic to the development of international human rights," as reflected in a wide array of concerns, from sex trafficking to rape as a war crime.[28]

Over the course of several decades, the idea of sexual rights has gradually thickened and has taken on more substantive content, as a consequence of the international "maturation of a more sophisticated and diverse coalition of civil society groups advancing sexual rights."[29] At the same time, the discourse of sexual rights has been taken up by a broad range of individuals and groups in various occupations and professional domains, including public health, family planning, sex education, and academia.[30] This work has been undergirded by the development of legal standards that gradually have forged linkages between the domain of sexuality and the promotion of human rights on a global stage. As Alice Miller has emphasized, these standards have important precursors that arguably date back a century and that include UN measures and human rights treaties from the 1970s and 1980s.[31] However, the pivotal decade for the emergence of what we would now recognize as a notion of sexual rights is the same decade that saw the proliferation of sexual health: the 1990s.[32]

As I described in chapter 2, the defense of sexual rights was broached but not formally adopted at the International Conference on Population and Development (ICPD) in Cairo in 1994: at this early stage, sexual (and even more so, reproductive) health provided a cover of respectability to discussion of sexual rights, given the strong rejection of the latter by representatives from many participating countries.[33] However, the following year, at the Fourth World Conference on Women in Beijing, the adopted Platform for Action proclaimed: "The human rights of women include their right to have control over and decide freely and responsibly on matters related to their sexuality, including sexual and reproductive health, free of coercion, discrimination and violence."[34] Defenses of sexual rights increasingly have been undergirded by international treaties as well as case law in international courts.[35] In 2004, the UN Special Rapporteur on the Right to Health declared sexuality to be "a fundamental aspect of an individual's identity" and asserted that sexual rights (including "the right of all persons to express their sexual orientation") were human rights.[36] To be sure, these efforts have encountered resistance framed as political, cultural, and religious.[37] For example, attempts to insert a broader conception of sexual and reproductive rights into the United Nations' highly touted Millennium Development Goals, adopted in 2000, were whittled down to the narrower objective of promoting "improvement in maternal health"—in part as a result of objections from the Bush White House, where one official asked: "Isn't there a greater unmet need for eyeglasses than contraception?"[38]

Perhaps most centrally among transnational agencies, the WHO has played a key role in sponsoring discussions, involving academics, advocates, and foundations, that have sought explicitly to link the idea of sexual rights with that of sexual health.[39] This brings us back to the narrative of the WHO's shepherding of the process of clarifying the definition of sexual health, as well as the coincident promotional efforts of the WAS.

REDEFINING SEXUAL HEALTH: LINKING TO SEXUAL RIGHTS

Despite having supervised a meeting in 1987 that declared sexual health to be undefinable, the WHO got back in the definitional game thirteen years later. Acting jointly with the Pan American Health Organization and in collaboration with the WAS, the WHO organized another meeting, held in Antigua, Guatemala, in 2000, that resulted in a new report: *Promotion of Sexual Health: Recommendations for Action.*[40] According to Alain Giami, the meeting was undertaken "mostly on the initiative of sexologists from Central and South America," and Eli Coleman, then the president of WAS, "considerably contributed to the text."[41]

The meeting brought together participants from many Latin American countries, plus others countries including Canada, the United States, China, Spain, the Netherlands, and Nigeria. Attendees noted the important developments in the quarter century since the first WHO report that led to the defining of sexual health: advances in knowledge about human sexuality, the global spread of the HIV epidemic, the impact of feminist scholarship, the consolidation of the field of reproductive health, public attention to the problem of sexual violence, advocacy by sexual minorities, and the development of medications to treat sexual problems—in short, many or most of the topics encompassed by the social problems described in chapter 2.[42] To address such concerns, the participants concluded, "it [was] essential to have commonly agreed-upon, precise definitions of the terminology used in the fields of human sexuality and Sexual Health."[43] The report did not dwell on the questions of cultural variation, normative judgments, or the "power element" associated with universalizing definitions— indeed, while characterizing the report from the 1975 WHO meeting as "a historic document" and "a stimulus for the development of the field of Sexology," the new report mentioned the intervening document from 1987 only in passing.[44]

The new report then proceeded to lay out a whole series of definitions of basic terms, notably including an expansive definition of "sexuality" as "a core dimension of being human which includes sex, gender, sexual and gender identity, sexual orientation, eroticism, emotional attachment/love, and reproduction."[45] This established the parameters for a revised and expanded definition of sexual health: "*Sexual health is the experience of the ongoing process of physical, psychological, and sociocultural well being related to sexuality*. Sexual health is evidenced in the free and responsible expressions of sexual capabilities that foster harmonious personal and social wellness, enriching individual and social life. It is not merely the absence of dysfunction, disease and/or infirmity. For Sexual Health [*sic*] to be attained and maintained it is necessary that the sexual rights of all people be recognized and upheld."[46]

Compared to 1974, the wording of this definition of sexual health was a bit more jargon-laden, with the fostering of "harmonious personal and social wellness" replacing the goal of enhancing "personality, communication, and love." Yet many of the emphases were similar. As before, sexual health was imagined as a capacious and multidimensional state of generalized well-being in relation to sexuality, and it was understood to rest on both individual and societal underpinnings. Two differences are noteworthy, however. One is the new pairing of "freedom" with "responsibility": the latter term was absent from the 1974 definition, and its inclusion here presaged moral emphases that later became more pronounced. The other difference, of course, is the strong assertion of the central place of sexual rights—an emphasis that was consistent with the broader historical development of the concept of sexual rights that had taken place over the previous decade, as I have described. While the 1974 definition had referred, briefly and without elaboration, to "the right to sexual information and the right to pleasure,"[47] the working group report in 2000 was considerably more specific and detailed. It cited the World Association of Sexology's Declaration of Sexual Rights (first approved in 1997), which, it was noted, made reference to rights to sexual freedom, autonomy, integrity, safety, privacy, equity, and pleasure, as well as the rights to reproductive choice, sexual information, comprehensive sexuality education, and sexual health care.[48]

WHOSE RIGHTS?

The commitment to rights gave the new definition a more explicitly political edge, and it informed the working group's recommendation that sexual health education and services be offered as universal entitlements.[49] But the foregrounding of rights also provided an avenue for addressing and resolving the sorts of concerns about norms and values that had led the 1987 working group to abandon the definitional project. In 2000, the working group neither proposed that its various definitions of terms were value-free nor despaired of offering definitions because they would be value-laden. Instead, the working group observed that values always infuse science: because "scientific activity, and therefore science-based health care and promotion cannot be performed from a totally value-free stance," it followed that "value-defined propositions, definitions, and concepts are unavoidable." The group then laid its own cards on the table by declaring its value commitments: "establishing a definition of Sexual Health is both possible and desirable provided that the definition is derived from . . . and embodies the concept of sexual rights."[50]

The point here is that the working group members saw rights as providing a special grounding: rather than representing just one value commitment among many possible ones, rights were deemed uniquely unassailable. "Human rights are above cultural values," the working group asserted: "If a particular culture has a practice that contravenes a human right, the cultural value should be changed."[51] Thus, by treating human rights as inalienable and universalistic in character, the working group members presumed they could sidestep the concerns about cultural variability that had bedeviled the previous working group in 1987. Indeed, these experts did not shy away from articulating what they took to be the component "characteristics of a sexually healthy society," including preferred features of its politics, policies, laws, institutions, and culture.[52]

Yet these universalistic claims are controversial: many scholars have argued that conceptions of human rights are, in fact, derived from a fundamentally Western (or global North) perspective rooted in historically and culturally specific ideas about the modern liberal individual.[53] Even more specifically, scholars have argued that ideas about sexual rights and sexual democracy not only privilege a global North vantage point but also provide fuel for drawing dubious and harmful distinctions between "enlightened" and "backward" nations and regions.[54] As Stephen Seely has described it, an uncritical adoption of ideas about human rights and democracy not only "systematically encodes certain Euro-American sexual values as synonymous with the values of 'democracy' itself" but also, simultaneously, "[positions] other sexual value systems—particularly those of Africa and Islam—as inherently anti-democratic."[55] In this way, beliefs about rights and democracy become a linchpin of what Eric Fassin has termed the thesis of a "sexual class of civilizations"—and they may be put to invidious uses, for example in the treatment of immigrants deemed less "civilized" unless they adopt specific norms with regard to gender and sexuality.[56] At the same time, particular ideas about how sexuality should be lived and experienced—for example, ideas about authentic self-expression and the social visibility of sexual minorities—give rise, as Ghassan Moussawi has observed, to "linear narratives of progress and modernity" that are then imposed as universal pathways of proper development.[57]

This critique is compelling and deserves more attention than proponents of sexual health and rights have sometimes given it. But at the same time, the genealogy of sexual rights may itself be more complicated than critics of the concept acknowledge. Visions of sexual rights in international forums—at the ICPD, at the Beijing Conference, and in subsequent venues organized by the United Nations—have often been put forward by representatives of countries in the global South, and as Sonia Corrêa has argued, the genealogy of sexual rights also includes the development in the global South of indigenous ideas of sexual self-determination.[58] In addition, one influential and oft-cited articulation of sexual rights, the "Yogyakarta Principles on the Application of International Law in Relation to Issues of Sexual Orientation and Gender Identity," is broadly understood to represent a global South perspective as much as one from the global North. Crafted by a diverse group of activists and experts who convened in Indonesia in 2006, half of whom came from the global South or non-Western countries, the Yogyakarta Principles declare that "sexual orientation and gender identity are integral to every person's dignity and humanity and must not be the basis for discrimination and abuse."[59] In short, while it may be problematic to take sexual (or other human) rights at face value as intrinsically universal, it may also be problematic to presuppose that their endorsement necessarily reflects the hegemony of Western or global North values.

Proponents of sexual rights seek to perform substantive political work. While borrowing legitimacy from the alignment with health, they also undertake a complicated political reframing and a new "articulation":[60] they seek to center sexuality-related social change within a distinctive vision of a freer and more just world.[61] The effort has been influential, and even organizations not specifically concerned with sexuality, such as the American Jewish World Service, have seen fit to take up "sexual health and rights" as a specific area of emphasis in global advocacy.[62] However, the efficacy of "sexual health and rights" as a political project depends not only on how much it attracts adherents; ultimately, it also hinges on the outcome of competition with political opponents. Indeed, some of those opponents have specifically targeted the very idea of sexual rights for political critique. Family Watch International, a nonprofit international organization that, in its words, "works at the United Nations and in countries around the world educating the public and policymakers regarding the central role of the family," has criticized organizations and countries that "aggressively promote radical sexual rights" and has bemoaned the "disturbing trend" of the appearance of the term within UN publications that have not been approved by all member states. The organization has also warned of the "potential damage that would result to societies, families, and individuals—especially children" if proposed conceptions of sexual rights were broadly adopted, including through the promotion of contraception, abortion, "transgenderism," pornography, adultery, prostitution, same-sex marriage, polygamy, and other practices, identities, and institutions it opposes.[63]

THE LATEST DEFINITION

On the heels of its collaboration with the Pan American Health Organization and the WAS, the WHO sponsored efforts that led to the current working definition of sexual health. In January 2002, the WHO convened a technical consultation that generated a report (finally published in 2006) entitled "Defining Sexual Health" (fig. 7).[64] Held at WHO headquarters in Geneva, Switzerland, and described as a joint effort with the WAS (with funding from the Ford Foundation), the consultation reflected a growing interest and commitment of resources: it followed a series of regional meetings and was overseen by "an interdepartmental working group within WHO headquarters as part of a collaborative consensus-building process."[65] These investments notwithstanding, the WHO not only took four year to publish the report but also, once again, disavowed any official responsibility for the working definitions of sex, sexuality, sexual health, and sexual rights that

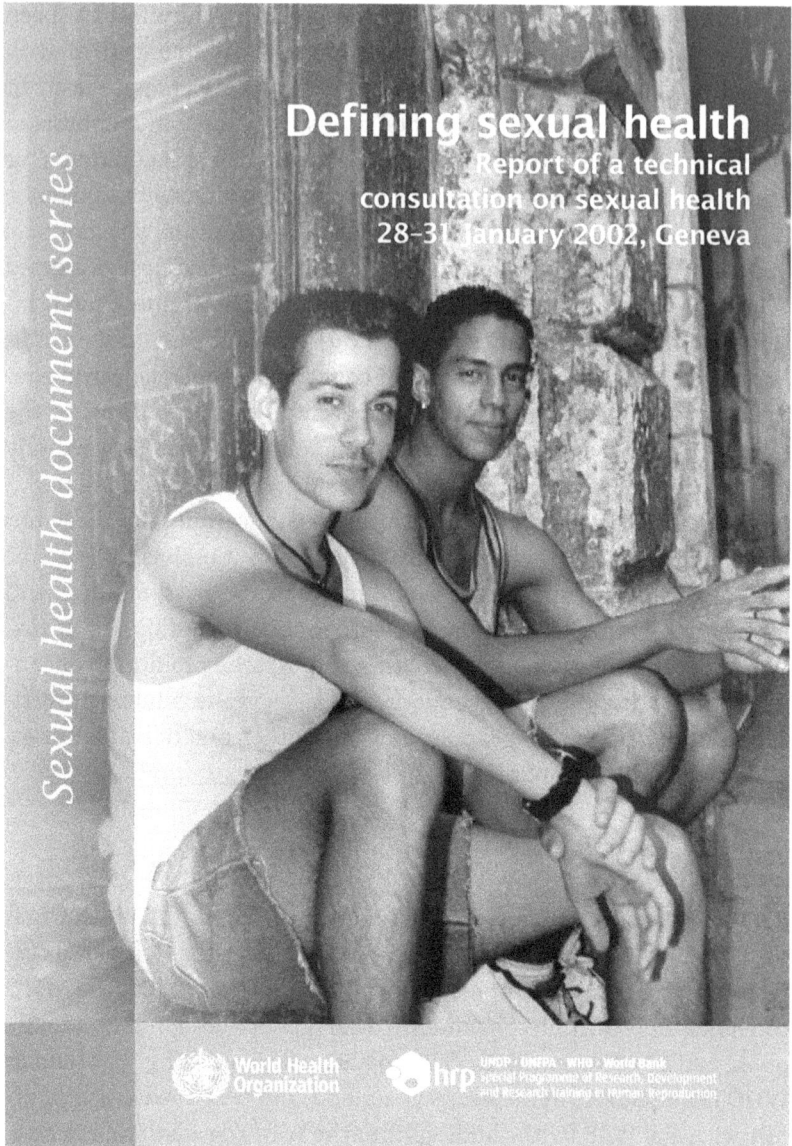

Figure 7: *Defining Sexual Health* (WHO, 2006)
Cover art reprinted with permission from *Defining Sexual Health: Report of a Technical Consultation on Sexual Health, 28–31 January 2002, Geneva* (Geneva: World Health Organization, 2006).

emerged. As described in a footnote, "these working definitions were developed through a consultative process with international experts [and] reflect an evolving understanding of the concepts." However, because they were never taken up and voted on by the World Health Assembly, "they do not represent an official position of WHO."[66]

Whatever their formal status, the new definitions borrowed heavily from the recent WHO-PAHO report—in fact, the definition of sexuality was nearly identical. In the case of sexual health, the end product was a mix of ideas from the 1974 definition and the WHO-PAHO report, combined with some important new emphases: "Sexual health is a state of physical, emotional, mental and social well-being in relation to sexuality; it is not merely the absence of disease, dysfunction or infirmity. Sexual health requires a positive and respectful approach to sexuality and sexual relationships, as well as the possibility of having pleasurable and safe sexual experiences, free of coercion, discrimination and violence. For sexual health to be attained and maintained, the sexual rights of all persons must be respected, protected and fulfilled."[67]

Thus, the definition encompassed several of the concerns of the social problem frames that had developed in the 1990s, including sexual rights as well as new attention to the problem of coercive or violent sex. Indeed, the same consultative process simultaneously generated a working definition of "sexual rights" themselves (borrowing on the work done on this topic at the earlier WHO-PAHO meeting, and reflecting the influence of the WAS).[68] This definition of sexual rights was multipronged and encompassed various subsidiary rights, including (somewhat circularly) a right to sexual health, but also rights to information and education; bodily integrity; partner choice; choice of whether to be sexually active; freedom from forced sex or marriage; reproductive choices; and, most abstractly, the right to "pursue a satisfying, safe and pleasurable sexual life."[69]

As Sandfort and Ehrhardt have noted, it is also evident that by this point the WHO conceived of sexual health within a broadly social framework that transcended individual health concerns.[70] "What does being sexual mean in the context of power differentials?" the report asked, in one of several mentions of issues of power dynamics and social inequalities.[71] The report also invoked the significance of diversity along various dimensions, including "sex, marital status, class and socioeconomic status, place of residence, age, ethnicity, sexual orientation, level or manner of sexual experience (voluntary or involuntary), motivations for sexual activity (affection, status, and needs) and health status"—all of which can affect how sexuality is experienced and understood.[72]

Yet respect for difference within the boundaries of the nation-state did not seem to translate into similar regard for cross-cultural variations in sexual beliefs and practices, and the hesitations about making normative judgments that were keenly felt by the experts in 1987 were little in evidence here. Indeed, one of the report's concluding proposals for future action by WHO was to "develop normative guidance documents on sexuality and healthy sexual development and maturation for developing countries."[73] Furthermore, the insistence in the very definition that sexual health requires one to hold "a positive and respectful approach to sexuality" suggested a willingness to entertain questions of moral judgment about how sexuality should be addressed and even thought about. It is also noteworthy that the language of "responsibility"—which surfaced in 2000—is much more present in this document (though not in the definition itself).[74] Variants of the word "responsible" appeared fourteen times in the twenty-one-page report in reference to sexual and reproductive behaviors. Indeed, the very first sentence of the report's introduction affirmed that "sexual and reproductive health and well-being are essential if people are to have responsible, safe, and satisfying sexual lives"—apparently placing responsibility and safety ahead of satisfaction as preferred dimensions of sexual experience.[75]

ELABORATIONS AT THE WHO: LINKING AND DISTINGUISHING SEXUAL HEALTH AND REPRODUCTIVE HEALTH

Since 2002, the WHO's working definition of sexual health has remained unchanged. Experts advising the WHO have continued to puzzle over issues of value judgments and cultural differences. For example, at a meeting convened in 2010, participants objected to the tendency to use "sexual health" and "healthy sexuality" as interchangeable terms. Participants deemed the latter term problematic and best avoided, "as it suggests that there is 'unhealthy sexuality,' which might be used to designate expressions of sexuality that are not considered acceptable in some societies, such as same-sex relationships."[76] Yet presumably "sexual health" similarly suggests the possibility of "sexual *ill* health," which by definition would be deemed undesirable—so it was not clear how the term "sexual health" would be any less conducive to the drawing of moral boundaries between favored and disapproved sexualities.[77]

Meanwhile, sexual health had gradually become institutionalized as a formal concern of the WHO's Department of Reproductive Health and Research—which, finally in 2020, became the Department of Sexual and Reproductive Health and Research (SRH), officially signaling the conjoined emphasis on reproduction and sexuality that was already the department's de facto mission.[78] Especially given global sensitivities around issues of sexuality, the department has had to tread carefully at times in addressing a topic that, until recently, was not formally signified in its name. However, the funding received in support of its activities from a range of cosponsoring governments and private foundations has enhanced its capacity to expand its remit.[79] Lianne Gonsalves, a technical officer working within SRH, characterized sexual health as an area "where there is interest in all six of our Regions," even while the topics of greatest concern vary across them.[80] In a series of reports, SRH has sought to unite sexual and reproductive health concerns while attempting not to conflate them.[81]

On September 4, 2017, the WHO took the occasion of World Sexual Health Day to announce the launch of "a new WHO framework for operationalizing sexual health and its linkages to reproductive health."[82] In a report, advertised by an editorial in the prominent medical journal the *Lancet*, the WHO sought to visualize and concretize the placement of sexual health and reproductive health on an equal footing: the report depicted a "rosette" of sexual health and reproductive health concerns that, like the petals of a rose, were to be considered "distinct yet inextricably linked."[83]

Part of the motivation for so carefully establishing this close relation between sexual and reproductive health was a particular organizational imperative: translating the United Nation's Sustainable Development Goals, or SDGs (which were announced in 2015) into concrete action plans in the domain of sexual health.[84] Of the 169 identified action targets associated with the SDGs, Target 3.7 calls for universal access to sexual and reproductive health care services by 2030.[85] As Gonsalves, the lead author on the report, described, "we saw that opportunity when the SDGs came out . . . to get a sexual health portfolio going."[86] In practice, however, the formal indicators associated with Target 3.7 all focus on reproductive health.[87] Yet the very fact that the wording of the target explicitly links reproductive health to sexual health presented the promoters of the latter with what the working group called "opportunities for enormous progress in sexual health in the SDG era."[88] Thus, the SRH attempted the delicate balancing act of, on the one hand, maintaining the strategically useful link between sexual health and its more visible cousin, while, on the other, avoiding having the former be overshadowed by the latter.

Alternative Pathways and Definitional Legacies

Genealogies are treacherous undertakings, because it is nearly impossible not to read the present back into the past. Having charted the proliferation of sexual health, and having traced the evolution of WHO working definitions, I feel confident in proposing that the latter has undergirded the former while the former has motivated the latter. The danger is to lose sight of the historically significant tributaries that have run somewhat independently of these larger streams.

Past contributions of grassroots social movements perhaps stand in particular risk of elision via historical amnesia. As Laura Carpenter has observed, the Boston Women's Health Book Collective, publishers of the influential *Our Bodies, Ourselves,* "glossed sexual health [early on, in its 1984 edition] as 'a physical and emotional state of well-being that allows us to enjoy and act on our sexual feelings.'"[89] This characterization did not just go "beyond" disease and dysfunction but seemed almost to leave those concerns behind. Most important, it built on an analysis of embodied female subjectivity and health politics that predated—and no doubt indirectly informed—the WHO's definitional work.[90]

Similarly, scholars have begun to unearth the story of efforts by gay men and lesbians in the United States in the 1970s and early 1980s—before the advent of the HIV/AIDS epidemic—to undertake health promotion in the spirit of sexual liberation. As the historian Katie Batza has chronicled, "a colorful cast of doctors and activists built a largely self-sufficient gay medical system that challenged, collaborated with, and educated mainstream health practitioners" in the United States in the 1970s and that addressed issues of sexual health squarely from the standpoint of gay liberation. "In short," according to Batza, "many men had a lot of sex with a lot of other men without the shame or harassment of previous decades, but they also got tested and treated for VD

regularly and saw that as a necessary part of being sexually active."[91]
The historian Jennifer Brier has likewise described how the insistence
that gay sexuality is itself healthy was the cornerstone of the foundation of gay community health care clinics in the 1970s, such as the
Fenway Clinic in Boston, the Howard Brown Health Center in Chicago,
and the Whitman-Walker Clinic in Washington, DC.[92]

The sensibilities that underlay these efforts fueled initiatives that
set the stage for responses to AIDS from the gay community. By 1980,
the National Coalition of Gay STD Services (NCGSTDS) was already on
its fourth revision of its "Guidelines & Recommendations for Healthful Sexual Activity," designed by gay health professionals and other gay
community members from around the United States, and suggesting
a variety of risk-reduction practices to avoid STIs.[93] Thomas Blair has
also excavated the roots of what would later become known as "safer
sex" not only in the work of the NCGSTDS and the Bay Area Physicians for Human Rights, but also in the more grassroots-based Sisters
of Perpetual Indulgence—a political, cultural, and philanthropic organization of gay men who dressed in parodic fashion as nuns and could
often be seen roller-skating across San Francisco. In 1981, the Sisters
produced "Play Fair!," a pamphlet that advocated basic steps to prevent
the spread of sexually transmissible infections, for distribution at the
San Francisco gay pride parade.[94]

Such stances and activities suggest complicated pathways to subsequent understandings of sexual health. In particular, and mostly as a
consequence of the global HIV/AIDS epidemic, the unabashedly sex-
positive sensibilities of gay liberation have filtered into much more
widespread discussions of sexual health promotion—just as the feminist inclinations reflected in *Our Bodies, Ourselves* have added texture
to a huge swath of contemporary thinking regarding sexual and reproductive health. These nuances in the recent historical record of how
"health" and "sexuality" have been brought together deserve careful
attention.

Yet it remains indisputable that the WHO, because of its global
prominence and authority, has played a pivotal role in conferring credibility on the concept of sexual health as a medical topic. As the former
WAS president Eli Coleman observed, "Having the WHO imprimatur
gave an amazing legitimacy to talk about this, to have programs in
academic institutions, and to promote professional organization."[95] At
the same time, because the WHO's definition of sexual health, like the

WHO's definition of health in general, insists on a "positive" conception of health that exceeds the absence of disease, the WHO's definitional authority can—and has been—invoked to justify sexual health
projects that extend well beyond the terrain of the biomedical.

Still, there is little direct evidence that the WHO's definition was
influential in the 1970s and 1980s. Only when sexual health entered
the proliferation phase, in the 1990s, did the WHO working definition
acquire broad cultural authority. One clear indicator comes from medical dictionaries: When my research assistant examined successive
editions, we learned that as prominent dictionaries began to include
entries on sexual health—as *Taber's Cyclopedic Medical Dictionary* first
did in its sixteenth edition in 1989 and *Mosby's Medical Dictionary* did in
its fourth edition in 1994—the WHO working definition from the time
was the explicit point of reference. For example, the entry in Taber's
began, "The World Health Organization has defined three elements of
sexual health," while Mosby's entry read: "A condition defined by the
World Health Organization as freedom from sexual diseases or disorders and a capacity to enjoy and control sexual behavior without fear,
shame, or guilt."[96]

Nowadays, the WHO working definition from 2002 is the simple
fallback for health agencies (and others) seeking to invoke the term. As
opposed to the situation in 1994, when (as described in chapter 2), attendees of the ICPD found themselves wondering whether a definition
existed and had to contact WHO officials in Geneva to find out, today
enough other organizations cite the WHO working definition for it to
be widely available and accessible.

Moreover, many of the organizations invested in sexual health that
do not reproduce the WHO working definition nonetheless offer alternatives that are, to a certain degree, variations on the same themes. Out
of many possible examples, a useful one to consider is the American
Sexual Health Association (ASHA). Not only does the group include the
term "sexual health" as part of its name, but also, much like the WAS,
it has sought an expansive definition of sexual health in order to bring
various concerns under that umbrella.

As I described in chapter 1, ASHA began life in 1914 as the American
Social Hygiene Association and, after various transmutations, adopted
its current name in 2012. According to ASHA, "the change reflected
a shift from ASHA's traditional focus on sexually transmitted infections to a broader emphasis on sexual health."[97] ASHA disseminates

educational materials on sexual and reproductive health to patients, parents, and physicians; seeks to destigmatize portrayals of sexuality in the mass media; works in alliance with other advocacy groups; and from its policy office in Washington, DC, works to influence policy formation on prevention, diagnosis, and treatment of STIs.[98] According to ASHA, sexual health is "the ability to embrace and enjoy our sexuality throughout our lives. It is an important part of our physical and emotional health." The ASHA statement goes on to say that being sexually healthy means "understanding that sexuality is a natural part of life and involves more than sexual behavior"; "recognizing and respecting the sexual rights we all share"; "having access to sexual health information, education, and care"; "making an effort to prevent unintended pregnancies and STDs and seek care and treatment when needed"; "being able to experience sexual pleasure, satisfaction, and intimacy when desired"; and "being able to communicate about sexual health with others including sexual partners and healthcare providers."[99] Thus, ASHA's definition, like the WHO's, includes but extends beyond issues of disease and dysfunction, encompasses both sexual and reproductive concerns, and references both pleasure and sexual rights.

New Assemblages of Sexuality, Health, Rights, and Pleasure

As variants of the WHO working definition have become disseminated (and have absorbed other currents of discourse linking sexuality with health), many different organizations have also become involved in activities that expand the coverage of the sexual health umbrella. Two important assemblages have been developed through "mergers" of the disparate ideas connoted by sexual health: a complex conjunction that has become known as "sexual and reproductive health and rights," or SRHR; and a renewed emphasis on "pleasure" as the crucial third term linking "health" with "rights."

THE ASSEMBLING OF "SEXUAL AND REPRODUCTIVE HEALTH AND RIGHTS"

Especially in the past two decades, advocacy groups, academics, and the WHO have collaborated to generate a new and complex object within the sexual health umbrella: "sexual and reproductive health and rights." The phrase itself has traveled widely: it appears in commentaries published by WHO officials, in a program of the Dutch Research Council, and in a "plan of action" of the African Union Commission.[100] It has its own Wikipedia page, and it has even merited its own acronym, SRHR.[101] In 2018, the WHO's Department of Reproductive Health and Research began its annual report by asking, "Why sexual and reproductive health and rights?"—demonstrating how salient this assemblage has become to that office within the WHO and how well it functions as a unifying frame for its many activities.[102]

The potency, visibility, and transnational circulation of SRHR reflect the growth of a transnational advocacy network,[103] but also the combined salience of its component buzzwords, notably including the resonant concept of rights. This new concept therefore reflects a deliberate blurring of the boundaries between two of the social problem frames that I described in chapter 2: containing population growth and promoting procreative autonomy, and also solving injustices linked to the absence of sexual rights. Put another way, SRHR involves a conjunction of two different bridging enterprises, both of them described above. On the one hand, "health" is linked to "rights" with the claim of a necessary connection. On the other hand, "sexual" is conjoined with "reproductive"—acknowledging their close links in practice but without subsuming sexual rights under reproductive rights.

Drawing on the conceptual and practical work of transnational agencies such as the WHO, liberal international foundations have been important financial backers of SRHR. The Ford Foundation sponsored an initiative called Promoting Reproductive Rights and the Right to Sexual Health, which offered grants to local advocacy groups in support of "reproductive and sexual health policies and laws that protect the rights of the most marginalized" in the United States, Mexico and Central America, and Indonesia.[104] The Open Society Foundation created the Sexual Health and Rights Project that took up a number of concerns, including funding advocacy work in countries of the global South to defend the rights of sex workers in the face of punitive legislation and policies threatening their health.[105]

Progressive civil society organizations have also been important contributors to the construction of SRHR. The International Planned Parenthood Federation (IPPF), which currently has member associations in more than 170 countries around the world, drew up the Charter on Reproductive and Sexual Rights in 1994.[106] By 2008, in a collaboration that involved the Ford Foundation, the IPPF had expanded its discussion of sexual rights into a "declaration" that described ten basic sexual rights that member associations were expected to defend and promote.[107] The Guttmacher Institute, a research and policy organization, describes its mission as the advancement of "sexual and reproductive health and rights in the United States and globally."[108] In 2018, together with the *Lancet*, Guttmacher announced a new SRHR agenda to address a host of global social problems including inadequate access to contraception, unsafe abortions, gender-based violence, homophobia, and the spread of HIV and cervical cancer.[109] The Guttmacher-Lancet Commission report declared that "sexual and reproductive health and rights (SRHR) are fundamental to people's health and survival, to economic development, and to the wellbeing of humanity."[110]

The intertwining of academic and activist investment in SRHR is apparent in the pages of the journal *Sexual and Reproductive Health Matters*, which "explores themes across the field of sexual and reproductive health and rights."[111] Founded in 1993 and known for many years as *Reproductive Health Matters*, the journal changed its name in 2019 to reflect "enormous strides forward" in the recognition of the intertwining of sexual and reproductive health.[112]

In short, the careful bridging work that nowadays connects the four component terms of "SRHR"—sexuality, reproductivity, health, and rights—draws on the efforts of a diverse assortment of people and institutions: activists, scholars, professionals, foundations, and international agencies, operating variously at local, national, and transnational levels. Through their intellectual and practical work as well as monetary expenditures, "sexual health" has frequently become aligned with an expansive set of political goals. In recent years, however, some of its promoters began to argue that an important piece was missing: "pleasure" needed to be drawn into the equation in order to tether health and rights more profoundly to sexuality.

THE PLEASURE PRINCIPLE

"This week, Mexico City was abuzz with sexual pleasure," declared one commentator, characterizing the Twenty-Fourth Congress of the World Association for Sexual Health, held in that city in October 2019.[113] But in their featured lecture, Anne Philpott and Arushi Singh, directors of the Pleasure Project in the United Kingdom and India, highlighted the fundamental dilemma. On the one hand, "pleasure is one of the key motivators of sex globally." On the other hand, "the framing of sex education and sexual health programmes continues to be one of avoiding danger, avoiding death, and avoiding disease rather than seeking pleasure, enjoying and affirming our bodies, and articulating desires." Calling for "pleasure audits" of organizations purporting to advance sexual health, Philpott and Singh acknowledged that the "two worlds of pleasure and prevention are strange bedfellows." But they argued they the two worlds have "much to learn from each other" as we revise the "tired narratives" of sexual health promotion.[114]

The conference closed with the announcement of WAS's approval of a new "Declaration on Sexual Pleasure" that had been drafted, behind the scenes, in recent months.[115] Of course, at least nominally, pleasure had been part of the discourse around sexual health for some time, mentioned at least in passing since the WHO's first working definition in 1975, and referenced directly in the enduring working definition from 2002. Moreover, alternative approaches to joining sexuality with health, with origins in gay communities (as I have described) and other alternative sexuality communities, had long insisted on valorizing pleasure, rather than fear, when seeking to protect people from unwanted consequences of sexual activity. Now the goal was to move pleasure to center stage in mainstream sexual health discourse.

Once again, the first step was a definition of terms. The WAS borrowed text from the Global Advisory Board for Sexual Health and Wellbeing, an independent group based in the United Kingdom. Importantly, that organization sought to build on the prior work undertaken under the banner of SRHR: it identified sexual pleasure as "the forgotten link in sexual and reproductive health and rights" and promoted what it described as "the triangle of sexual health, sexual rights and sexual pleasure" in order to advance a "positive approach" to sexuality.[116]

According to the WAS declaration, sexual pleasure is "the physical and/or psychological satisfaction and enjoyment derived from shared or solitary erotic experiences, including thoughts, fantasies, dreams, emotions, and feelings." However, the ability to experience such pleasure depends on various "enabling factors," including "self-determination, consent, safety, privacy, confidence and the ability to communicate and negotiate sexual relations."[117] As Eli Coleman, an insider to the discussions, described, "wrestling with the definition" was a complicated business, given that "sexual pleasure is something different to everybody." Yet contemporary political considerations, such as those reflecting an era of #MeToo feminism, clearly helped shape the process and the outcome: pleasure was not just "something that feels good"; and "in this social historical context there needs to be some language . . . on consent, mutuality, equity."[118]

Notably (and not surprisingly), the WAS emphasized the tight connection between the safeguarding of sexual pleasure and the defense of sexual rights, and the WAS urged governments as well as nonstate actors to "promote sexual pleasure in law and policy as a fundamental part of sexual health and well-being, grounded in the principles of sexual rights as human rights, including self-determination, nondiscrimination, privacy, bodily integrity, and equality." More concretely, the WAS called for a reform of such domains as sexual health education, which ought to incorporate sexual pleasure "in an inclusive, evidence-informed and rights-based manner."[119]

In advocating the turn to pleasure while linking it to health and rights, the WAS and its associated circle of academics and sexual health advocates focused their attention on weighty issues of politics and policy. However, others who hailed the WAS's promotion of sexual pleasure were located more directly in the social problem domain that approaches sexual pleasure, well-being, and self-actualization more from the standpoint of commerce and consumption. For example, Gerda Larsson, the commentator who described Mexico City during the WAS Congress as being "abuzz with sexual pleasure," is the cofounder and managing director of the Case for Her, described as "a philanthropic investment portfolio for menstrual health and women's sexual pleasure and wellness." According to Larsson, the Case for Her was "leading [the] charge" to implement the pleasure agenda through investment in various projects, including a sex product company and an initiative to promote pleasure-oriented sex education in El Salvador.[120] Thus, an emphasis on pleasure seemed to hold open possibilities for building quite diverse kinds of connections across the worlds of sexual health.

Synthesis and Its Limits

In chapter 2, I described the various social problem frames that characterize the practical activities unleashed in the name of achieving something called sexual health. These activities are unfolding in a wide range of professional and nonprofessional contexts in many locations around the world. By contrast, in the current chapter, I have analyzed attempts to build a sexual health umbrella that extends over much of the range of sexual health activities. I have also shown how that process of extension rests on the elaboration of new compound objects, such as "sexual and reproductive health and rights" and the "triangle of sexual health, sexual rights and sexual pleasure."

Proponents aspire to link the concerns of multiple professional groups and constituencies within the various social problem frames—or assemble them in modular fashion into new combinations. I have argued that the evolution of the WHO working definition of sexual health is central to this story—that WHO expert advisory bodies have sought to keep pace with the expansion of meanings and incorporate them into revisions of the definition, and conversely that changes in the scope of the definition have facilitated the proliferation and diffusion of meanings.

The various expert committees that have debated and promulgated definitions have struggled with many questions, crucially including the normative stakes and global reach of their own recommendations: Who is to say what constitutes healthy sex? Is it the same thing everywhere? And if we cannot easily say, then what grounds the very concept of sexual health? Despite such difficulties, they have succeeded in forging a definition that has become broadly influential, fueling new sexual health activities, and subsuming (and perhaps sometimes obscuring) alternative approaches to questions of health and sexuality.

The elaborations of WHO-sponsored definitions of sexual health since 1974 are replete with references to real-world developments: AIDS; the ICPD conference in Cairo; the advent of new approaches to the treatment of sexual dysfunction; and the growing concern with rights (and more recently, pleasure) in relation to gender, reproduction, and sexuality as promoted by nongovernmental organizations and particularly by social movements, including feminist, LGBTQ, and AIDS activist movements. By this route, at least four of the six social problem frames came to be referenced squarely by the WHO working definition: containing the threat of sexually transmissible infections, addressing failures of sexual functioning, controlling population growth and promoting procreative autonomy, and solving injustices linked to the absence of sexual rights. The frame concerned with promoting sexual self-expression is also clearly implicated in the definition: it is reflected in much of the accompanying psychological language as well as the frequent references to "wellness"; and it is also referenced in recent work by the WAS on pleasure. Finally, the social problem frame associated with the goal of containing threats of irresponsible sexual behavior, while not specifically incorporated in the working definition, makes periodic appearances nonetheless, particularly in the 2002 report. Importantly, the discourse of responsibility is generally consistent with the tendency—questioned in 1987 but tolerated, if not always welcomed, since then—to identify a normative sexuality whose proper functioning serves the paramount goal of health.

Yet the consensus statements of expert committees cannot fully reconcile the distinct and sometimes competing meanings associated with the different social problem frames—any more than a conference that functions as a big tent can truly forge a lasting sense of common purpose. To conceive of sexuality as a bundle of risk practices, or in terms of physiological and neurological mechanisms, is ultimately rather different from viewing it as self-actualizing practice or an integral component of social identity. And to imagine health in terms of risk reduction, or performance enhancement, is to stand some distance from conceptions of health that emphasize autonomous decision making, or freedom from unwarranted coercion, or social betterment, or generalized wellness. No definition, however synthetic, can completely paper over the tensions among these competing goals, priorities, and visions of the self and the world. Therefore, the WHO definition-making process has proved influential but also has left open the possibility that other actors might pick and choose among the different threads of meaning of sexual health or leverage some against others.

Left Out in the Rain?

I have considered the forging of connections to extend the remit of sexual health to encompass various rights and pleasures—but any project of extension encounters limiting cases, and these can be revealing. Before concluding this analysis, therefore, it is worth considering what we might call sexual health's "outside." What is *not* covered by the sexual health umbrella? Who is denied the shelter it offers?

There are different ways of approaching this question. One relevant group includes all those who are "othered" by sexual health programs—those deemed intrinsically incapable of achieving sexual health. The list might include physically and intellectually disabled people, who are often treated as lacking the agency needed to manage their sexuality, as well as asexual people, who are often seen as sexually unhealthy by definition.[121] Then, there are those who are treated not so much as "other" but as invisible. For example, mainstream approaches to sexual health often presume a cisgender subject and fail to focus on the specificity of transgender, intersex, and gender nonbinary people. Participants in one study of trans and nonbinary people's past experiences with sexual health education described feeling "lost" and "confused" by what they had learned, as well as being left to their own devices in determining how to pursue sexual and reproductive health in the context of their diverse anatomies, identities, and processes of transitioning.[122] Another assumption embedded in many approaches to sexual health is that sexual relationships necessarily involve couples. This renders invisible people who reject "mononormativity" and engage in relationships involving more than two participants.[123]

A different way of thinking about the "outside" of sexual health is suggested by considering alternative mechanisms for the social management of sexuality aside from "healthicizing" it. Just as "illness" and "badness" have long functioned as contrasting approaches by which social issues might be construed and managed,[124] so a chief alternative to a sexual health approach is sexual criminalization. The sociologist Trevor Hoppe has made this point through his analysis of the criminalization of HIV transmission, or what he terms "punishing disease": in many jurisdictions of the United States, laws have been passed that make it a crime for HIV-positive people to have sex without informing their partners of their HIV status. Such legislation takes a carceral approach to matters of health, in the process positioning the offender (often presumptively nonwhite) as impervious to the benefits of sexual health education.[125] Other cases in which sexuality is criminalized rather than healthicized include the institutional management of sex offenders, who may be legally subject to indefinite confinement,[126] and the prosecution of women (particularly, women of color) who are deemed to have endangered their fetuses by failing to avoid health risks during pregnancy.[127]

In the above situations, the possibilities of sexual citizenship are denied to some, who instead become positioned as carceral subjects.[128] In other cases, however, while sexuality is not explicitly criminalized, sexual citizenship is effectively withheld from those who are considered incapable of exercising sexual agency. For example, the history of forced sterilization, practiced in the United States for more than half a century—driven, as the historian Alexandra Stern has described, "by a shifting mix of anxieties about sexual deviance, the promiscuity of teenage girls, fear of biological deterioration, and a discourse of institutional cost savings"—demonstrates a clear failure to extend the rights, protections, and presumptions of agency that we now associate with the sexual health umbrella.[129] Such concerns are not merely of a historical nature. Some scholars have found worrisome echoes of this egregious practice in the present-day promotion of long-acting reversible contraception (LARC) for young Black and Latina women: according to Chris Barcelos, "the strategy of promoting LARC as a magic bullet to lower teen pregnancy rates restricts user agency by minimizing the interpersonal complexities of contraceptive use and eclipses the history of LARC in reproductive coercion."[130]

As opposed to cases of outright criminalization or absolute coercion, the case of long-acting contraception would seem to lie within the boundaries of sexual health's jurisdiction, if somewhat closer to the hazy frontier between the "inside" and "outside" of sexual health. Yet what connects it to more extreme cases, as Dorothy Roberts has observed, are the dynamics of race and racism that prove so fundamental to the determination of whose sexuality is administered in what way.[131] While race is not the only relevant consideration, it does offer tangible clues in helping us locate the borders of sexual health terrains.

The question of who falls within or beyond the protective shelter of the sexual health umbrella is one to keep firmly in mind while analyzing the wide range of projects that promote sexual health. The remainder of this book takes up these projects and assesses the consequences of the investments in sexual health—consequences for the pursuit of knowledge, for practices of governing, for self-improvement, and for political work to bring about social change. That is, previous chapters of this book have emphasized the changing meanings of sexuality and health and the effect of each on the other. Now, I shift the analysis to ask a somewhat different question: once sexuality and health have become coupled in the ways I have explored, what else gets done?

Part 2: Operationalizing Sexual Health

ENABLING SCIENCE, MEDICINE, AND HEALTH CARE

If sexual health is so hard to "catch hold of," how does it ever get pinned down? How is it stabilized and made an object of knowledge and a focus of medical care? As we have seen, at times sexual health need not be imagined very precisely in order for work to proceed: even a vague idea can be put to powerful uses, and that very vagueness can itself be enabling. But in certain contexts—especially scientific, medical, and technical ones—before they can work with the concept of sexual health, people first need to operationalize it: they must develop techniques to recognize, measure, and employ it with relative ease and confidence. Such efforts to impose order and rationality are central to the production of new truths of sex.

The chapters that comprise part 2 consider how sexual health has been made a workable object of knowledge in ways that matter for people's everyday lives. They trace the efforts to improve patient-provider encounters through a focus on sexual health. They examine how a reform effort is transforming the global diagnostic categories for sexual problems. They investigate how knowledge about the sexual health of a population is generated by survey research. And they consider how experts of many sorts produce knowledge and give advice under the banner of sexual health. Each of the four chapters describes a distinct mode of operationalizing sexual health: standardizing, in the case of the clinical encounter; classifying, for diagnostic reform; enumerating, when taking surveys; and evaluating, in the case of expert advice giving.

The various projects that operationalize sexual health reflect an imperative to impose order on a disorderly domain with the goal of generating knowledge and providing care. In all these domains, people's sexuality is scrutinized, assessed, measured, and considered. Here, the "health" in sexual health serves not just to legitimize attention to sexuality but also to "scientize" it, by making sexuality the province of experts performing knowledge-intensive work. The stakes are high: people often seek the benefits that expert knowledge and health care can bring, but operationalization also has potential costs. As I describe, these processes make it possible to better address the full subjectivity of patients or reduce them to "risk factors," to identify sexual problems in ways that either bring desired treatment or medicalize people's identities, and to produce knowledge about the sexual practices of the population that may either challenge existing prejudices or reinforce them.

Operationalization may also have complex effects on understandings of differences and inequalities within the broader population. At times, it may serve to standardize the population in ways that render invisible those who differ from the majority in various ways, such as according to their race, ethnicity, nationality, age category, gender identity, or sexual identity. But at other times, it may make certain forms of difference "hypervisible," shining a spotlight on the particular health risks believed to be associated with those groups.

In these ways, techniques of knowing and ordering sexual health can propel—or challenge—processes of normative judgment that matter for people's lives. By virtue of the practices described in these chapters, experts and professionals claim the ability to say who is healthy or ill, normal or abnormal, responsible or problematic, behaviorally typical or a statistical outlier. Yet the ability of "operationalizers" to do these things does not go unchallenged, and at times, the experts and professionals may find themselves to be the ones under scrutiny.

4 Sexuality in the Medical Encounter

STANDARDIZING SEXUAL HEALTH

Significant percentages of people around the world experience what they perceive to be sexuality-related medical problems, including sexual dysfunction, pain during intercourse, sexually transmitted infections, and issues related to contraception.[1] Yet an international study conducted in 2005 with 27,500 participants, in which half of those who were sexually active reported at least one "sexual problem," found that only 19 percent had sought medical care, and only 9 percent had been asked about their sexual health by a doctor in routine visit over the previous three years.[2] Especially in the years since then, as interest in sexual health has flourished, advocates have pursued what I have termed a sexualization of medicine and health care: the incorporation of sexual matters into the very heart of medical concerns.[3]

This chapter shows how the sexualization of health care practice has gone hand in hand with the operationalization of sexuality. It emphasizes the development of new ways by which sexuality can be managed and made an object of knowledge and practice—in particular, by *standardizing* it. But the chapter also reveals the many obstacles that surface. Medical practice is not so easily transformed to accommodate the charged topic of sexuality, one that many professionals resist engaging. Advocates of reform also struggle to accommodate the tensions between simple, standardized approaches and the complex and differentiated character of patients' sexual health issues. While standardized techniques and tools may make it easier to bring sexual health issues to medical attention, they may also occlude the complexity of patients' subjective experiences, reducing lives to identifiable risk behaviors and performance scores.

Sexualization and Its Discontents

The growth of specialty areas such as sexual medicine has provided new niches within the medical profession in which physicians are prepared and trained to tackle sexual topics, particularly sexual dysfunction. But what about other arenas of modern medicine? In a growing number of domains both likely and unlikely, physicians are encouraged to take sexual health seriously as an integral component of their work, and patients are likewise enjoined to embrace sexual health as part of broader processes of recovery. Medical journal articles now urge physicians to discuss sexual matters directly with patients in settings—such as spinal care—where sexuality is more typically ignored.[4] The Sexual Medicine Society of North America has a standing committee that focuses on the sexual health needs of cancer survivors, including problems resulting from chemotherapy and surgery, and has declared cancer a "relationship disease."[5] At the same time, patients of all sorts are encouraged to embrace their sexual health as part of a broader return from illness to health. As STS scholar Judy Segal has described, this emphasis can at times feel overwhelming: "The woman with cancer, especially, is exhorted on countless Web sites and in articles, films, and on television shows to discover, or rediscover, her sexual self. In fact, she is told she must do so, or she will not be returned from the land of the sick."[6]

However, for most patients, the entry point into the medical system remains the primary care physician, and these generalists may have little experience with sexual health issues or inclination to engage with their patients on such topics. This lack of knowledge and motivation was the original impetus for the WHO-sponsored meeting in 1974 that first led to a working definition of sexual health—but the problem has persisted. A key barrier has been the relatively limited success in educating physicians about sexuality during their formal training in medical schools. As the sociologist Marie Murphy discovered through ethnographic observation at one major US medical school, sexuality had "an 'absent presence' within the formal curriculum"—not so much ignored as addressed occasionally, inconsistently, and often haphazardly in ways that "reinforced sexuality's ambiguity and unknowability."[7] Moreover, Murphy discovered "a hidden curriculum of heteronormativity" by which "a certain set of sexual possibilities (i.e., heterosexual ones) were repeatedly rendered natural, knowable, and unremarkable, while other sexual possibilities were largely excluded from the realm of the obvious, the normal, and the intelligible."[8] In recent years, promoters of sexual health have sought to reform the medical curriculum: one petition, promoted by the Multidisciplinary Joint Committee of Sexual Medicine, has called for establishing sexual medicine "as an integral and obligatory part of the core curriculum for students in all medical schools."[9] Others have sought to require course work or training in sexual health as a component of continuing medical education for practicing physicians.[10] But change has been a gradual process at best.

Once out in practice, doctors' squeamishness about sexual matters may subtly but significantly influence medical care in a wide variety of ways. For example, the sociologist Anny Fenton has studied physicians' greater reluctance to challenge parental suspicion of vaccines in the case of vaccination to prevent infection with the (sexually transmitted) human papillomavirus: apparently, doctors are far quicker to set aside their steadfast commitment to promoting vaccination when sexual matters come into play, sometimes preferring just to keep quiet.[11]

Taking a Sexual Health History: Beyond the "Five Ps"?

Perhaps the greatest impact of inadequate training with regard to sexual matters is a simple tendency not to want to ask patients direct, relevant questions, even when these might reveal significant health problems or risk factors. The reasons for this failure to engage are multiple and may include "negative attitudes regarding sexual problems, time constraints, unrealistic fears of offending the patient, deficits in communication skills, reimbursement concerns, the lack of available or approved treatments, and a growing knowledge gap between developments in sexual medicine and the clinical skills of practicing physicians."[12]

Studies indicate that the disinclination to inquire into sexual matters is widespread but may extend especially to certain categories of patients, including older adults, homeless people, and transgender people.[13] One study found that male physicians were especially uncomfortable asking female patients about sexual matters, and vice versa.[14] Entrenched gender biases may compound the tendency to shy away from asking patients about their sexual behaviors, desires, and identities. As one female OB/GYN described it: "we often find that some

non-OB/GYN physicians emerge [from medical school] uncomfortable taking a sexual and reproductive history. Some physicians express
these uncomfortable biases when they consult us . . . as if there's an
ick factor around the [female] patient's reproductive system."[15] While
general practitioners may be especially at fault in the failure to engage
with sexual matters, apparently even OB/GYN specialists are not immune from this problem. One survey of more than one thousand OB/
GYN's in the United States in 2012 found that only 40 percent routinely asked patients about sexual problems. Even fewer asked questions about sexual satisfaction (29 percent) or pleasure (14 percent),
and nearly three-quarters failed to inquire about sexual orientation or
identity.[16]

　While calls for improved sexual history taking date back at least to
the 1980s,[17] serious efforts to take corrective action are more recent. In
2008, citing a range of motivating concerns including the spread of
HIV/AIDS and the need to respect LGBT patients, the American Medical Association released an online video that advised doctors on how
better to conduct a "sexual health history."[18] The AMA construed the
barriers to be overcome as largely of a communicational nature: hesi-
tancy on the part of patients to speak openly, combined with a tendency on the part of physicians to be judgmental or make assumptions
(for example, that patients are heterosexual) that deter them from asking the right questions. The video devoted attention to such issues as
how to phrase questions in a nonjudgmental way and the kind of language physicians ideally should use. The video also proposed an im-
pressively expansive agenda for the issues doctors should explore as
part of sexual history taking. Physicians were advised to think beyond
a narrow focus on STIs and inquire into such matters as the gender of
partners, the number of partners, the type and frequency of sexual behavior, alcohol or drug use, sexual practices and fetishes, the exchange
of sex for money or drugs, forms of protection used to prevent STIs,
timing of first sexual activity, cultural influences on sexual behaviors,
psychological or physical problems, and histories of sexual abuse or
nonconsensual sexual activity.

　That the AMA would back such an effort is noteworthy and reflects
social change within the organization—especially with regard to LGBT
issues, toward which the association had been hostile or indifferent until the 1990s.[19] However, the AMA's endorsement of a wide-ranging conversation between doctors and patients about sexual concerns bucked

other trends in modern health care. Most doctor-patient encounters are notoriously brief and driven by practical exigencies; and many doctors prefer a simple algorithmic logic of risk assessment and diagnosis. From medical school onward, physicians are also enamored of mnemonic devices that help them learn and recall the innumerable details of health and disease.[20] Such features of modern medicine explain the appeal of simpler, standardized, and easily memorized approaches to sexual health history taking. Hence the tendency, in many instructional guides on taking a sexual health history, to lay out "standard operating procedures"[21]—or to boil it down to what the CDC has dubbed the "Five Ps": partners, practices, protection from STDs, past history of STDs, and pregnancy prevention.[22]

The CDC's brochure "A Guide to Taking a Sexual History" exemplifies the tension between a recognition of complexity and a desire for simplification and standardization. On the one hand, the document offers disclaimers early on: the brochure "is not meant to be a standard for diagnosis or a complete reference for sexual history taking," and the information contained therein "may need to be modified to be culturally appropriate for some patients." On the other hand, the material in the brochure is organized straightforwardly around the Five Ps and proceeds through them sequentially.[23] The Five Ps surface repeatedly in discussions of taking a sexual health history, and not just in government documents.[24] Even the thorough, thirty-four-page "tool kit" called "Taking Routine Histories of Sexual Health," put out by the National LGBT Health Education Center at the community-based Fenway Institute in Boston, offers an "algorithm" for conducting a sexual history that leads directly into a risk assessment organized around the CDC's "simple categorization of sexual history questions that may help providers . . . remember which topics to cover."[25]

The Fenway Institute's tool kit explicitly acknowledges another exemplar and driver of medical standardization in recent years: the need to efficiently and systematically capture patient information in the form of electronic medical records. The tool kit includes several pages of screenshots of sample sexual health risk assessment forms, as well as a list of relevant diagnostic codes that can be used in record keeping "as part of your overall business strategy."[26] Certain other countries where health care delivery is highly bureaucratized have developed even more formalized and systematic guidelines on sexual health. For example, in the United Kingdom, the Clinical Standards Committee of the Faculty of Sexual and Reproductive Healthcare of the Royal College of Obstetricians and Gynaecologists has published a 142-page report that identifies eleven general service standards for sexual health, all based on current evidence of best practice, which are recommended for use by all providers working with the National Health Service.[27]

Meanwhile, advocates of social change continue to press for more inclusive forms of sexual history taking that inevitably pose challenges for standardization. In 2018, the *American Journal of Public Health* published a commentary entitled "Venturing beyond the Binary Sexual Health Interview." Reminding readers that "sexuality and gender issues are a perfect example of multidimensional, nonbinary experiences," the author encouraged health providers to take sexual histories that "assess which parts go where instead of who is having sexual contact with whom." At the same time, the author called for giving patients the opportunity to present their own self-descriptions of their identities: "We find that people self-describe beyond lesbian, gay, bisexual, transgender, questioning, intersex, and asexual and use words such as agender, androgyne, demigender, gender fluid, gender nonconforming, demisexual, polysexual, or pansexual. Allowing for self-description shows the profound need to change the sexual health interview."[28]

The proliferation of gender and sexuality identity labels—combined with some people's resistance to providing any category at all—are indeed striking features of the contemporary social landscape, prompting adjustment from a growing number of institutions. (The sociologist Arlene Stein has noted that Facebook recognizes fifty-six custom gender options, while New York City now recognizes thirty-one genders.[29]) Yet attempts to acknowledge this profusion of diversity inevitably run up against challenges—for example, when providers confront software that encodes a delimited set of response categories.

The Standard Way to Sexual Health?

Standardizing—that is, constructing uniformities across time and space through the generation of agreed-upon rules for the production of objects—is a pivotal background feature of the modern world.[30] Scientific inquiry depends on the availability of standardized instruments, tests, and protocols, and modern governance is likewise impossible without standardized forms, procedures, and measures.[31] The perceived desirability of standardizing reflects, in part, the variety of things that it can accomplish: standardization specifies how procedures should be carried out, how objects should be named, how tools should be designed, and which outcomes should be expected.[32] In modern medicine, standardization is a driving force—a key feature of the evidence-based medicine movement that employs protocols, guidelines, decision tools, and algorithms in order to align professional practice with the best available evidence and solve the problem of "practice variation." Yet the pushback against medical standardization is also powerful at times. People don't always fit the categories; the "standard human" is no one in particular.[33] Indeed, the resistance against standardization in medicine invokes cherished professional values such as the uniqueness of the individual patient and the irreplaceability of clinical judgment, while also embracing the movement to offer "culturally competent care"; and it takes aim at little-liked features of modern medical practice such as "cookbook medicine" and the surveillance exerted by managed-care "bean counters."[34]

In practice, standardization is often painfully difficult to bring about, at least in the form that designers may have envisioned.[35] In the case of efforts to standardize sexual health history taking or define service standards for delivery of sexual health care, one would need to conduct ethnographic research in medical clinics or analyze recordings or transcripts of patient-provider encounters to obtain a realistic sense of just how successful those efforts may be. But even my introduction to the topic above suggests the tension between recognizing the sheer complexity of human sexuality and streamlining providers' engagement with it. Thus, for example, the CDC has laid out the Five Ps within a document that, they maintain, "is not meant to be a standard." On the one hand, physicians need mnemonics and toolkits; on the other hand, much of the discussion of taking a sexual health history imagines a strikingly complex and very human patient: a communicatively rational individual who is deserving of respect, whose cultural circumstances matter, whose sexuality may be multidimensional in character, and who may possess a hidden diversity of experience (perhaps shaped by race, ethnicity, sexual identity, disability, and so on) that needs to be revealed through open and unbiased questioning.

Yet standardization projects are worthy of study even when their accomplishments are uneven or incomplete: "Even the standards that do not obtain anything materially may have an important signaling function."[36] What do standards of sexual health history taking signal? First, this standardizing effort and its limits tell us something about the discomfort that sexual topics provoke among medical professionals, who often feel unprepared to discuss them with their patients. Second, the discourse around taking a sexual health history reveals a particular idea about what sexuality itself might be, or how it should be known. In essence, sexuality in this case is imagined as a multifaceted bundle of risk behaviors, which patients must be induced to divulge, and whose implications for health must then be formally assessed. As we will see in the next example, this conception of the truth of sexuality differs even from that presupposed by other sexual health standardization projects.

Performance Standards: Measuring Sexual Dysfunction

A second group of standardizing projects—inventories and questionnaires to diagnose sexual function and dysfunction—have been offered, in part, as a solution to the limits of the sexual health history. As Giovanni Corona and colleagues observed in the *International Journal of Impotence Research*: "Finding the correct way to ask questions and to decode answers on sexual health and illnesses might be difficult and, in some way, embarrassing. Hence, expert-guided, validated and standardized sexual inventories (i.e. structured interviews and self-report questionnaires) might help naive and more experienced physicians alike to address sexual health and diseases." That is, the hope is that the introduction of these tools—which "have the advantage of being standardized [and] easy to administer and score," and which are "relatively unobtrusive and substantially inexpensive"—will obviate the need for the physician to engage in potentially awkward and extended dialogue with patients about sensitive topics. Yet as Corona and colleagues acknowledge, these tools "carry a risk of oversimplification and are sensitive to language differences . . . , semantic perception, and . . . ethnic, religious, education and cultural factors."[37]

As opposed to the sexuality-related risk factors that are emphasized in most discussion of the sexual health history, the literature on inventories and questionnaires is concerned almost exclusively with sexual function and dysfunction. That is, the focus here is not on disease transmission, infection, or pregnancy but rather on the mechanics of sexual performance and the various difficulties that may impair it: erectile dysfunction, low sexual desire, premature or delayed ejaculation, pain during intercourse, and so on. Therefore, the purposes of the tools are to identify individuals in need of treatment, to measure outcomes in clinical trials of such treatments, and to establish the prevalence of dysfunction in epidemiological surveys. These interview guides and self-report questionnaires typically consist of anywhere between four and twenty-five closed-ended questions, the responses from which are then scored and, typically, summed up. For example, the nineteen-item Female Sexual Function Index (FSFI) asks questions like "Over the past 4 weeks, when you had sexual stimulation or intercourse, how *often* did you reach orgasm (climax)?" and requests responses on a scale ranging from "Almost always or always" to "Almost never or never."

The variety of such instruments in circulation yield an alphabet soup of abbreviations and acronyms: the SHIM (Sexual Health Inventory for Men), the CHEES (Checklist for Early Evaluation Symptoms), the PEP (Premature Ejaculation Profile), the MSHQ (Male Sexual Health Questionnaire), the FIEI (Female Intervention Efficacy Index), the IIEF (International Index of Erectile Function), and various others. Reflecting a neatly binary conception of human gender and sexuality, nearly all of the instruments are intended for use either only with men or only with women.

A significant scholarly literature concerns itself with the evaluation of these instruments to determine their sensitivity, specificity, reliability, and construct validity.[38] A key concern is to show that this means of producing sexual truth legitimately aspires to being universally applicable. Researchers have sought to overcome insularity and demonstrate that these tools may be used successfully and without modification on people of different ethnicities, ages, socioeconomic status levels, and education levels.[39] In some case, proponents tout the benefit that the tool in question "does not assume heterosexual intercourse as the primary or sole form of sexual activity."[40] Researchers have also claimed the ability of these instruments to bridge national and cultural—or at least, linguistic—boundaries successfully. For example, the MSHQ (first developed in 2004) has been translated into Arabic, Bulgarian, Chinese, Czech, Dutch, French, German, Greek, Hungarian, Italian, Latvian, Lithuanian, Polish, Portuguese, Romanian, Russian, Spanish, Swedish, Tagalog, Thai, Turkish, and Ukrainian.[41]

The investment in these tools is also driven substantially, in some cases, by the interests of pharmaceutical companies, who have sponsored research validating the instruments. For example, the IIEF was developed hand in hand with clinical trials for Viagra, and the SHIM (also known as the IIEF-5 because it is a shortened, five-item version of the IIEF) is used routinely to assess patients' suitability for treatment with erectile dysfunction drugs.[42] A striking demonstration of the "healthist" impulse in consumer-oriented medicine is that potential end users are sometimes urged to take these simple tests themselves and perform their own assessments. Notably, the pharmaceutical company Pfizer has called on potential patients to compute their own SHIM scores and then, on the basis of the results, consult a physician about whether Viagra is right for them.[43] Indeed, the SHIM has spread well beyond the confines of professional health care domains. My own web browsing turned up a "wellness" website at which visitors were invited to take an online SHIM while also booking a dinner reservation and shopping for wellness products.[44] An important implication is that these various scales and inventories are more than just "tools" for assessment: they come along with implicit "scripts" that guide and coordinate the actions not only of health providers but also of current and potential patients.[45]

Such developments suggest the potent links between standardization and selfhood. In an article on the medical standardization of transgender experience, Demetrios Psihopaidas has called attention to how standardization also affects intimate life and everyday understandings of selfhood and identity—sometimes in unexpected ways as people creatively adopt and adapt the standards that are applied to them by professionals and experts.[46] Somewhat similarly, certain standardization projects related to sexual health appear capable of stitching together the domains of prominent organizations—medical clinics, research labs, schools—with inner worlds of intimate, embodied experience. These effects of standardization are important because of the classificatory work that the tools perform—not simply assigning a numerical value but, in the end, sorting individuals into diagnostic "boxes" and thereby declaring them to be "healthy" or "dysfunctional."

The tools are also important because of their capacity to group individuals and provide statistical measures of disease conditions. As Ayo Wahlberg and Nikolas Rose have argued about health-related rating scales more generally, they can be understood, somewhat paradoxically, "as efforts to quantify the 'patient perspective' in order to enable aggregation and comparison across different diseases and populations." By this path, "the existential condition of living with disease is rendered calculable, subjected to expertise and thereby amenable to novel forms of health intervention."[47]

Here, too, the standardizing project throws open the question of what sexuality "really is" by casting light on what a group of doctors and researchers imagine sexuality to be. Unlike the sexual health history, where sexuality is construed as a package of risk behaviors, in this domain sexuality is conceived of as a set of *capacities* inferred from patient ratings of their behavioral and performative histories and their assessments of satisfaction or dissatisfaction.

My point is not to question the scientific legitimacy of these projects nor to doubt their ability to help bring benefit to many people who are suffering. Yet the potential limits of standardization and simplification surface and raise questions. How much of the profound complexity of sexuality can be materialized by these simple scales? What happens to the goal of sexualizing medicine and health care—transforming them to take sexuality fully into account—when sexuality is rendered as a simplified scientific object? What happens to people, such as those who are intersex or gender nonbinary, who don't fit the presumed categories of users of this technology?

Finally, we should consider how encounters between patients and providers in the clinic play out against the backdrop of broader debates about how sexual issues should be diagnosed and classified. What is a sexual health "condition," and how does our classification of health and illness change over time? The next chapter takes up diagnosis as a global concern—and as the focal point of controversies that are simultaneously scientific, ethical, and political.

5 *Diagnostic Reform and Human Rights in the ICD*

CLASSIFYING SEXUAL HEALTH

On May 25, 2019, the World Health Assembly, the decision-making body composed of delegates from all 194 member states of the World Health Organization, voted to ratify the first major revision in more than a quarter century to the world's most widely used medical classification system. Formally called the International Statistical Classification of Diseases and Related Health Problems, but better known as the International Classification of Diseases or, more simply still, the ICD, this tool will undergo the transition from the tenth to the eleventh version on January 1, 2022.[1] According to the WHO, which has been responsible for managing this instrument as part of its core mission ever since the creation of the agency, the ICD is "the foundation for the identification of health trends and statistics globally, and the international standard for reporting diseases and health conditions."[2] Within the tree-like structure of the ICD, every disease and health condition is designated by an alphanumeric code. These codes are aggregated into "chapters," which constitute major disease categories, such as neoplasms, diseases of the immune system, and diseases of the skin.

Member states are committed, by international treaty, to using the ICD as their standard for collecting and reporting health data for a variety of purposes. The goal is to promote comparability and standardization across national borders, as the ICD (in the words of the WHO) "provides a common language that allows health professionals to share health information around the globe."[3] Just as important, within countries, the ICD is also the backbone of national health programs and insurance reimbursement systems. Typically, every patient must be assigned a diagnostic code, from A00.0 ("Cholera due to Vibrio cholera 01, biovar cholera") to Z99.9 ("Dependence on unspecified enabling machine and device").[4] For example, in the United States, a version of the tenth edition is the only official coding system permitted under the Health Insurance Portability and Accountability Act of 1996 (HIPAA), and its use is required for government programs such as Medicare, as well as by most private insurance companies.[5] As scholars of the "sociology of diagnosis" such as Annemarie Jutel have observed, all diagnoses are in the business of doing work.[6] But as Geof Bowker and Susan Leigh Star emphasized in their influential study of the politics of classification, a *system* of diagnoses like the ICD performs an enormous amount of "infrastructural work," undergirding many other systems and processes, and "facilitat[ing] the coordination of work among multiple agencies."[7]

For these reasons, the transition from one edition of the ICD to another is a substantial undertaking. My focus in this chapter is on the process leading to the adoption of the latest revision, ICD-11. Specifically, I examine the noteworthy fact that among the handful of chapters that appear in ICD-11 for the first time, one is a chapter devoted to "conditions related to sexual health." This is a remarkable achievement considering that the total number of chapters is fairly small—there were only twenty-two in ICD-10, and there are only twenty-six in ICD-11—and especially considering that the phrase "sexual health" did not even appear anywhere in ICD-10.[8]

Indeed, the adoption of ICD-11 marks a milestone in the long march of the idea of sexual health from its first promulgation under the auspices of the WHO forty-five years earlier. "Sexual health has come of age," commented Eli Coleman in his remarks at an award ceremony marking his own lifetime contributions to the field, two months after the World Health Assembly ratification vote. "We have a complete chapter called 'Conditions Related to Sexual Health,'" he explained to the audience, grinning widely.[9] This is proof positive of what I have called the "sexualization of health"—the transformation of global health institutions as they encounter and grapple with the domain of sexuality. Of course, it simultaneously demonstrates the "healthicization of sex"—the conversion of sexual matters into problems on which health institutions may do their work.

The Politics of Classification

While the previous chapter called attention to standardization as a way of operationalizing sexual health, this one focuses on the closely related process of *classification*—a kind of scientific and social labor with profound consequences. Diagnostic reform is something that matters because classification is a form of power: systems of classification reflect prevailing hierarchies and dominant beliefs, and they serve to shape both moral and social order.[10] In their canonical work on the topic, Bowker and Star treated the previous (tenth) edition of the ICD as a quintessential example in an extended case study that occupied three chapters of their book.[11] For Bowker and Star, who emphasized the pragmatic character of the decisions that shaped the ICD's internal logic, the ICD's organization and wording encapsulate—but also hide from view—"a series of technical, social, political, and economic decisions taken at different moments."[12] Indeed, the ICD "can . . . be read as a kind of treaty, a bloodless set of numbers obscuring the behind-the-scenes battles informing its creation. This dryness itself contains an implicit authority, appearing to rise above uncertainty, power struggles, and the impermanence of the compromises."[13]

The shift from ICD-10 to ICD-11 demonstrates the continued relevance of Bowker and Star's analysis.[14] The new chapter on "conditions related to sexual health" does the important work of bringing together, under one rubric, health concerns that previously had been spread throughout the ICD. More subtly, the classifications and descriptions of specific sexual issues in ICD-11 reflect significant changes not only in "what goes where" but also in the medical (and, in effect, social) consensus on what actually constitutes a problem meriting medical intervention. ICD-11 destigmatizes, in some cases "de-psychiatrizes," and in other cases demedicalizes, a range of sexual and gender-related social practices in ways that reflect broad social changes and specific advocacy work undertaken over the course of recent decades.

Tracing the pathway to ICD-11 sheds light on the larger politics of classification, but it also calls attention to specific features of contemporary debates about sexuality and health. Two such features are central to the analysis that follows. First, this is a story about norms and universals. The specifics of the new diagnostic categories will have powerful downstream consequences in terms of choice of treatment modalities, insurance coverage, and other practical concerns that affect patients, providers, and governments. But the sexual health chapter also holds important implications at the level of cultural beliefs, both reflecting and shaping how normality and pathology are understood.[15] What makes the "politics of normality" even more complicated and contentious is the attempt to articulate a formal classificatory regime at the global level, in a world where gender, sexuality, and health care are hot-button issues, and where both practices and opinions vary significantly across national borders.

Second, diagnostic change in this case came about through a conscious and deliberate attempt at progressive reform. As we will see, the experts who debated the details of sexual health in the ICD brought medical evidence together with ethical arguments in order to justify the fine details of classificatory change—the recodings, delistings, and redescriptions. In the process, experts found themselves engaging with a wide range of interlocutors, importantly including advocates representing transnational social movement organizations. This aspect of the process guaranteed that, in this case of diagnostic reform, some of "the diagnosed" would have the opportunity to "speak back."

Collaboration and the Politics of Transgender Health

Although its precursors extend back into the nineteenth century, the first edition of the ICD was adopted in 1893 (well before the birth of the WHO), and subsequent editions have been approved about once a decade ever since.[16] However, the time lag between ICD-10 and ICD-11 is the longest gap between revisions in the history of the tool. ICD-10 was approved in 1990 and took effect in 1993. (After much delay, the United States adopted a modified version of it in 2015.) ICD-11 (which, among other things, is the first fully electronic version) has been long in the making: work began in 2007; the "Beta Draft" was made public in 2012; and a (temporarily) finalized list of fifty-five thousand unique codes and descriptions was released in June 2018.[17] As noted above, ICD-11 was then ratified the following year and will first take effect in 2022.

One implication of the timing is especially significant for my purposes: ICD-10 was issued right at the start of what I have described as the "proliferation phrase" of sexual health. Thus the designers of ICD-11 have grappled not only with many changes in cultural and medical understandings of sexuality in the intervening years but also with the successful spread of the very idea of sexual health as a label for understanding sexual issues.

But in addition, what proved unexpectedly crucial to the origins of the chapter on sexual health was a specific set of debates about transgender health. These debates arose because individuals desiring medical services relating to gender transitioning, including gender-affirming hormone therapies and surgeries, have long found themselves caught on the horns of a dilemma. On the one hand, they have fought against a stigmatizing portrayal of transgender people as suffering from a mental illness or delusion—a belief that was routinely espoused by many physicians and mental health professionals in the twentieth century.[18] On the other hand, transgender people are deeply dependent on medical and mental health professionals, who, in many or most legal jurisdictions, stand as gatekeepers between them and desired services and statuses both medical and nonmedical.[19]

Specifically, transgender people may need to be assigned a diagnosis in order to qualify for gender-affirming procedures (or be reimbursed for them, in cases where health insurance covers such procedures) or in order to amend birth certificates and passports or defend legal rights.[20] A diagnosis, as one sympathetic expert described it, amounts to "the difference between a necessary medical procedure and something that can be perceived as cosmetic surgery that insurance won't cover."[21] Therefore, transgender people have had to engage strategically with medical categorization—often acquiescing to, yet also resenting, a characterization of themselves as having a medical or mental health condition.[22] The unfairness of this predicament has been widely remarked upon. As the sociologist Arlene Stein has observed: "People make major decisions about their lives—they reshape their noses, undergo grueling exercise regimens, and join demanding religious communities—all the time without having to justify their decisions to others. Most adults are capable of making their own decisions regarding their bodies. We have a right, we increasingly believe, to be happy. But although such ideas are beginning to influence the world of transgender care, in order for patients to gain access to surgery and hormones they must still use the language of suffering, pathology, and cure."[23]

Under ICD-10, this characterization took the specific form of a grouping within the chapter on mental and behavioral disorders called "gender identity disorders," and within it a category called "transsexualism." This was defined as "a desire to live and be accepted as a member of the opposite sex, usually accompanied by a sense of discomfort with, or inappropriateness of, one's anatomic sex, and a wish to have surgery and hormonal treatment to make one's body as congruent as possible with one's preferred sex."[24]

Yet with the rise of a global grassroots movement for "trans depathol-ogization," advocacy groups increasingly took aim at stigmatizing med-ical diagnoses, as well as at the presupposition that a diagnosis should be required as a prerequisite for obtaining needed health services.[25] In 2012, in response to many years of lobbying by transgender activists, the American Psychiatric Association announced that it would remove "gender identity disorder" from the DSM, and that DSM-5 would in-stead include "gender dysphoria" as a diagnosis available for those dis-playing "a marked incongruence between one's experienced/expressed gender and assigned gender."[26] While activists welcomed the departure of the formal designation of trans identities as "disordered," many con-sidered it a "pyrrhic victory":[27] the new diagnosis not only continued to view transgender people as meriting a psychiatric designation but also located the "problem" as being within them, as reflected in their "dys-phoric" response to their gender assignment.[28] Still, as Cal Garrett has argued, the change in terminology in DSM-5 indicated an important if incomplete shift among medical experts, away from viewing gender in strictly binary and categorical terms and toward an appreciation of gender as a domain of natural variation.[29]

These complicated developments placed squarely on the table the issue of how "gender identity disorders" would be handled in the ICD. One question, clearly, was what terminology to use. But whatever this category might be called, a second question immediately arose: Could the category be moved out of the mental and behavioral disor-ders chapter—and if so, where might it happily live? What would be a medically appropriate home, and what would be the least stigmatizing association possible? Although transgender experiences have come to be understood principally as a question of gender identity, not sexual-ity, the growth of an infrastructure around sexual health within the WHO afforded a specific opportunity. At the same time, the perceived need to find a place to locate a transgender category provided an im-petus to think about other categories that might be housed alongside it. Eli Coleman, a close observer of the process, goes so far as to claim that "the [sexual health] chapter came about because of the dilemma of 'transsexualism,'" and that, "knowing that they can't just have one diagnosis in [the chapter], the brilliant idea was to really start to put [in] all the various conditions to protect this whole chapter."[30]

My own research suggests that Coleman's claim is a bit overstated, but that, in essence, the desire to "de-psychiatrize" transgender health issues converged nicely with a simultaneous commitment to further solidifying sexual health as a distinct area of concern within the WHO. That is, as described in earlier chapters, the WHO had become increasingly invested in defining, measuring, and promoting sexual health, and this effort had been taken up explicitly by the Department of Reproductive Health and Research. As WHO staff members later described: "Taking into account the definition of sexual health and the need to measure sexual health, experts proposed the creation and inclusion of a new chapter on sexual health within ICD-11. Presenting the concepts within one chapter helps to better define the realm of sexual health and facilitates related specialized tabulation of data."[31] Thus sexual health concerns would no longer be scattered across different domains of the ICD but would be gathered together into one easily referenced chapter.

TRANSNATIONAL PARTICIPATORY POLITICS AND THE FOCUS ON HUMAN RIGHTS

In preparing for the ICD-11 revision, the WHO created "topic advisory groups" within different agencies of the WHO. In part for the reasons described above, two of those advisory groups—reporting to the Department of Mental Health and Substance Abuse and the Department of Reproductive Health and Research, respectively—found themselves considering an overlapping set of issues involving gender, sexuality, and reproduction. These two groups therefore collaborated in appointing the joint Working Group on Sexual Disorders and Sexual Health. In the ICD development process, working groups are intended to bring together internationally recognized experts and incorporate the perspectives of relevant stakeholders.

According to Doris Chou, a medical officer in the Department of Reproductive Health and Research who served as a liaison to the working group, this particular group functioned as a "meeting point" for professionals with mental health backgrounds and those with expertise in genitourinary medicine.[32] Thus, in addition to what Chou described as the usual emphasis on diversity by gender and geography in WHO working groups, the Working Group on Sexual Disorders and Sexual Health spanned multiple specialty areas. Functioning as an example of what the historian of science Peter Galison has called a "trading zone" for scientific communication,[33] the working group promoted "mutual teaching and collaborative learning" across domains of professional expertise.[34]

The participation of mental health experts meant that working group discussions inevitably tacked back and forth between categories found in ICD-10 and those appearing in recent editions of the DSM.[35] However, research shows that the ICD is the classification system most used by psychiatrists around the world, with the DSM (a commercial product of the American Psychiatric Association) lagging far behind.[36] Moreover, the revision of the ICD presented pathways for depathologization that are absent from the DSM revision process. After all, any condition listed in the *Diagnostic and Statistical Manual of Mental Disorders* is presumptively a mental disorder, and therefore the only clear way to depathologize a diagnosis is to remove it from the DSM altogether. By contrast, because the ICD includes all varieties of medical conditions, it is possible to "de-psychiatrize" a condition without demedicalizing it, simply by moving it out of the mental disorders chapter. And, because the ICD is intended to cover the full gamut of patients' engagement with the health care system—again, the full name is the "International Statistical Classification of Diseases *and Related Health Problems*"—the fact that a category is included in the ICD certainly implies a medicalized status but does not necessarily tag it as a disease as such. Indeed, the ICD contains many codes for health-related issues that are well understood not to be diseases, including "contact with health services for concerns about pregnancy" and "contact with health services for immunizations."

Transgender health issues seemed in this respect similar, as Chou explained: "The transgender concern largely allowed us to say, 'This is an example of where we need to put things in a classification that are not necessarily what we call or consider, from a clinical standpoint, . . . a disease.'"[37] However, others disagreed and argued that simply locating any identity within the ICD was in effect to spoil that identity by medicalizing it. "[The] ICD will destroy any good name that you put there," was the pithy assessment offered by Mauro Cabral Grinspan, the executive director of Global Action for Trans* Equality (GATE) and a longtime activist on transgender and intersex issues.[38]

Alongside the encounters across expert professional communities, certainly one of the most distinctive features of the working group process was the presumption of a public voice in the revision process, at least in the form of "active input from multiple global stakeholders":[39]

"Submission of proposals for revisions to ICD-10 had been encouraged by WHO beginning in 2008 and could be submitted in three languages. Proposals . . . were received from a variety of scientific societies, professional associations, and advocacy organizations, as well as from several individual experts."[40] To be sure, working group meetings themselves were essentially closed to the public, and the opening of the process to public comment was carefully managed; Cabral Grinspan of GATE described being invited to one meeting in Geneva in 2012 to give a short presentation and then being ushered out before the ensuing discussion.[41]

However constrained, the inclusion of voices such as Cabral Grinspan's reflected larger shifts in the worlds of medicine and public health, away from paternalism and toward a relatively recent emphasis on incorporating the perspectives of patients and of stakeholder communities.[42] Véronique Mottier and Robbie Duschinsky's reflections on revision of the DSM apply equally well to the ICD: "The DSM-5 is very much a product of the twenty-first century: while the DSM still constitutes an authoritative source . . . for medical practitioners . . . , patients and advocacy groups nowadays talk back and voice criticism of the labels that are being applied to them. Indeed, such views were solicited as part of the process . . . , something which would have been unthinkable in the 1950s."[43]

The inclusion of research and opinions offered by members of trans communities and advocacy groups is a clear illustration of these trends. As Zowie Davy and coauthors have described, in reference to both DSM-5 and ICD-11: "Including research and opinions from medical stakeholders, members of trans communities and political advocacy groups seems to be a novel method of creating diagnoses for trans people. . . . Internal workgroups from the APA and WHO were tasked with developing diagnoses that reflect trans people's medical, economic and social lives."[44]

In the case of the ICD, regional networks of activists working on transgender issues—including GATE (registered in the United States), Iranti and Gender Dynamix (based in South Africa), Akahatá (a Latin American network), the Asia Pacific Transgender Network (based in Thailand), and Transgender Europe (TGEU, based in Germany)—took advantage of any openings provided them to make the case for depathologization.[45] Cabral Grinspan recalled sitting down with WHO employees as early as 2011, at an international meeting convened by the Dutch government, "to start the conversation about what we wanted or what was possible in the ICD."⁴⁶ Two years later, GATE organized a follow-up meeting that WHO officials attended, though only informally and without representing the agency. In these conversations, activists for transgender rights were able not only to press for specific changes in the ICD but also to emphasize, as Cabral Grinspan put it, "the power that classifications have to frame our world [and shape] the way in which people understand us."⁴⁷ As an Argentinian, Cabral Grinspan was also well situated to emphasize the lessons of that country's progressive Gender Identity Law, adopted in 2012: by eliminating the need for a diagnosis in order for transgender people to receive access to legal recognition, surgeries, and hormones, the law "allowed us to tell WHO that depathologization was possible."⁴⁸

In addition to opening the process to a range of viewpoints, working group members also emphasized that their classificatory work was "undertaken with awareness of the human rights standards endorsed by the United Nations."⁴⁹ In their published commentary on the revision process, these experts made frequent allusions to the recent history of social change in relation to gender and sexuality as well as ethical considerations in that domain, though always in ways that aligned the social and ethical concerns with the scientific character of the project. From Eli Coleman's perspective, the formal endorsement of human rights as a criterion for assessing recommendations reflected the ascendancy of the compound concept of "sexual and reproductive health and rights" (see chapter 3) and of the idea that sexual health and sexual rights go hand in hand, as the World Association for Sexual Health (WAS) had long insisted—and the percolation of that idea through the WHO's Department of Reproductive Health and Research: "By then the [department] had really embraced the concept that the only way they could promote reproductive health was through human rights. There was a clear understanding that they were going to examine these diagnoses, not just from a mental health or scientific perspective, but from a rights perspective."⁵⁰

Here, the WHO's point of view was ostensibly global but as perceived from the vantage point of dominant institutions that valorized human rights, such as the United Nations. Yet at least one report of the working group simultaneously referenced both the UN High Commissioner for Human Rights and the "Yogyakarta Principles on the Application of International Law in Relation to Issues of Sexual Orientation and

Gender Identity" as having codified the "emerging human rights standards" that the group invoked as necessitating diagnostic reform.[51] This reference to the Yogyakarta Principles is significant because of their specific focus on gender and sexuality, which are deemed "integral to every person's dignity and humanity."[52] In addition, the Yogyakarta Principles were produced by a diverse group of activists and experts who convened in Indonesia in 2006, half of whom came from the global South or non-Western countries, and therefore the document is less susceptible to the suggestion that it hegemonically construes "human rights" from a global North perspective.[53] The Yogyakarta Principles are often invoked by advocates of depathologization in relation to gender and sexuality because they include the insistence that "a person's sexual orientation and gender identity are not, in and of themselves, medical conditions and are not to be treated, cured or suppressed."[54]

Sexual Health in ICD-11

Drawing, therefore, on what they termed "current scientific evidence, best clinical practices, and human rights considerations," the working group, in effect, appropriated and repositioned—but in some cases also redefined or even eliminated—conditions that had been listed elsewhere in ICD-10, so as to build a new chapter of conditions related to sexual health.[55] Upon completing its work, the group reported back to the two topic advisory groups, which in turn made recommendations to the ICD Secretariat at the WHO.

In its final form as approved by the World Health Assembly, the new chapter (which is slight in comparison with most others in the ICD) contains five general groupings of sexual health concerns: sexual dysfunctions, sexual pain disorders, gender incongruence, changes in female genital anatomy, and changes in male genital anatomy. Several additional groupings housed in other chapters of the ICD are also cross-listed in the sexual health chapter—or in the lingo of the ICD, for these categories, "conditions related to sexual health" serves as a "secondary parent." For example, the various sexually transmitted infections have a primary home in the chapter on "certain infectious or parasitic diseases," but sexual health is a secondary parent. Similarly, the category of paraphilic disorders (which involve "persistent and intense patterns of atypical sexual arousal") finds its primary home in the chapter on "mental, behavioural or neurodevelopmental disorders" (hereafter, the "mental disorders" chapter) but secondarily appears under sexual health. The sexual health chapter is also a secondary parent for "contact with health services for contraceptive management." Thus, the kinds of conditions or issues that either are located directly in the sexual health chapter or that cross-reference it from elsewhere in the ICD are quite varied—just as we would anticipate given the proliferative and polysemous character of sexual health that I described in previous chapters. However, in the hopeful view of Coleman and coauthors, in an article published before the ratification of ICD-11, the new chapter recognizes "the interrelatedness of these issues—and [will] help promote integrated sexual health care."[56] If true, this would be a significant step forward in the development of what I have called the sexual health umbrella.

A noteworthy feature of the ICD revision is that the entire grouping of sexual dysfunctions has been moved from the mental disorders chapter to that on sexual health, where it has been joined with other conditions previously found in the chapter on diseases of the genitourinary system. The various dysfunctions have also been reorganized into new categories that locate each dysfunction as a problem of either desire, arousal, orgasm, ejaculation, or pelvic organ prolapse.[57] The effect is to create an "integrated classification"[58]—one that, as Coleman and coauthors point out, "[bridges] the mind/body divide, which has long been a prominent feature of medical care related to sexual dysfunction."[59] (Of course, the WHO's working definition of sexual health, with its unusual inclusion of both physical and psychological components, paved the way for such bridging.) "They're finally catching up to the recognition that sexual dysfunctions are not all in people's heads," Coleman commented.[60] It is also worth observing that this "depsychiatrization" of sexual dysfunctions is consistent with the general move to destigmatize them that undergirds the phenomenal success of new "sexuopharmaceutical" therapies such as Viagra.

Three additional aspects of the differences between ICD-10 and ICD-11 are especially significant indicators of medical reform (and its limits): the details of the changes in the medical management of transgender people, a reworking of the paraphilic disorders, and the placement of compulsive sexual behavior. I take up these issues in turn.

DEPATHOLOGIZING TRANSGENDER EXPERIENCES

Rather than following the path of DSM-5 and replacing "gender identity disorder" with "gender dysphoria," the working group for ICD-11 instead invented the new category of "gender incongruence."[61] Notably, gender incongruence is not a "disorder," and instead of being located in the chapter on mental disorders, it is placed in the chapter on conditions related to sexual health. (However, gender incongruence is "secondarily parented" by the mental disorders chapter, as well as by the chapter on "factors influencing contact with the health system.") The idea, according to the working group, was to "preserve access to health services" while mitigating the "doubly burdensome" stigma that has resulted from the combination of hostility toward transgender people combined with negative attitudes toward the mentally ill: "Stigma associated with the intersection of transgender status and mental disorders appears to have contributed to precarious legal status, human rights violations, and barriers to appropriate health care in this population."[62]

However, this category was one that attracted significant public input—the working group received 190 comments and proposals specifically related to gender incongruence[63]—and trans activists did not necessarily embrace the details of this change. A communiqué issued by the activist campaign Stop Trans Pathologization in 2013 criticized the language of "gender incongruence," which appeared to pathologize those transgender people who had not fully transitioned, and which also seemed to imply the existence of "a normative state of 'congruence.'"[64] Of course, the simple fact that the institutional and medical constraints facing transgender people are not uniform around the world guarantees that no classificatory solution is ideal in all cases. Going further, there is good reason to be skeptical of the very idea that a single social identity and corresponding term—"transgender"—can adequately and fairly capture the diverse embodied experiences of those non-cisgender and gender nonconforming people around the world who may seek medical intervention.[65]

From Doris Chou's perspective, the phrase "gender incongruence" was "maybe the least problematic" option available in English, as well as the choice that best lent itself to nonstigmatizing translations into other languages.[66] The working group also took the opportunity to modernize the language for describing gender issues, dispensing with terms such as "opposite sex" and "anatomic sex" and "using more contemporary and less binary terms such as 'experienced gender' and 'assigned sex.'"[67] All these modifications reflected, in the words of the working group, "rapid change in social attitudes in some countries, and . . . controversy"; and the group noted having received commentary on transgender issues "from a wide range of civil societies, professional organizations, and other interested parties."[68]

To be sure, the placement of "gender incongruence" in the chapter on sexual health was an imperfect choice and clearly a compromise: it folded questions of gender into the domain of sexuality, and it "depsychiatrized" trans issues while retaining a medical diagnosis as the gateway to care. From Cabral Grinspan's perspective, the problem was that "the ICD doesn't have a lot of rooms," and the question was which "room" might be least inhospitable. While many trans activists would have preferred a primary home in the chapter on "factors influencing contact with the health system," this placement would not have guaranteed health insurance coverage for gender-affirming treatments—not a concern in Cabral Grinspan's home county of Argentina, thanks to the Gender Identity Law, but a powerful barrier in much of the rest of the world.[69]

The placement of gender incongruence in the sexual health chapter also suggested that it fell under the rubric of sexuality rather than that of gender identity and gender expression. "It's not necessarily the most ideal for everybody" was Chou's summary of reactions to the placement: "You end up having to ask: 'What is something that is okay for everybody to live with?'"[70] Eli Coleman had no problems with locating gender incongruence in the sexual health chapter, on the logic that "if you go back to the definition of sexual health, it includes gender. . . . Gender identity is in the definition of sexual health."[71] Others disagreed. In 2013, at a "consensus meeting" on ICD-11 organized by the World Professional Association for Transgender Health, an influential interdisciplinary professional and educational organization supporting those providing services to transgender people, participants expressed a preference for locating the diagnosis within a "sex and gender health" chapter or, perhaps, a "gender health" chapter.[72] However, trans activists who were more thoroughly opposed to diagnostic categorization rejected the idea of locating gender incongruence in a gender chapter precisely because doing so would "contaminate" gender identity by medicalizing it.[73] At an early stage, the working group considered the possibility of moving gender incongruence to a chapter all its own, arguing that "the revised categories for gender incongruence represent highly unique clinical challenges and merit placement in an entirely separate ICD chapter that would contain no other entities."[74] But at the level of the WHO, there was no mandate for a chapter consisting of a single code, and ultimately, to the working group, the new sexual health chapter seemed the most viable option.

When the finalized version of ICD-11 was announced in June 2018, and again when the World Health Assembly voted to accept ICD-11 in May 2019, the de-psychiatrization of transgender people was among the most widely noted specific changes in the ICD as a whole. "Being Transgender No Longer Classified as Mental Illness" was the headline of a USA Today article that called the development "a key sign of progress for an often-marginalized community."[75] CNN quoted Lale Say, coordinator of WHO's Adolescents and At-Risk Populations team, who explained that the category "was taken out from the mental health disorders because we had a better understanding that this wasn't actually a mental health condition, and leaving it there was causing stigma. . . . So, in order to reduce the stigma while also ensuring access to necessary health interventions, this was placed in a different chapter."[76]

Transgender advocacy groups by and large have treated the ICD-11 changes as a limited step in the right direction. But they have retained concerns about various issues of classification, including the vexed question of whether and how to diagnose gender-variant children.[77] Earlier, in 2014, the activist group GATE had commented: "Despite the challenges of both the new categories and the new chapter, we can celebrate this small step in the long struggle for depathologization."[78] Yet in 2018, Nua Fuentes, a Mexican activist with the Trans Pride World Platform, called the WHO action "positive" but "incomplete" and "nothing new"; while the group Stop Trans Pathologization pointed out that if medical gatekeeping were eliminated and trans-specific health care were provided freely, then the medical category would be rendered unnecessary.[79] Thus, the root problem, as Cabral Grinspan observed, was that "in some countries the right to health has been expropriated and [privatized] by insurance companies."[80] A joint statement issued by nine organizations in 2019 concluded: "We consider the ICD-11 to be a *transitional* version, *acceptable only as a step towards depathologization.*" The statement described "gender incongruence" as "a *temporary and imperfect solution* to the needs of those trans and gender diverse people who require access to specific health care (e.g., surgeries and hormones) under health systems that otherwise will exclude them"; and they characterized their acceptance of the compromise as one that "was very difficult to make and ultimately was made based on international solidarity and a strong shared commitment to continue to make submissions to WHO on alternative wording and criteria."[81]

The reference to international solidarity in the statement highlighted the dilemmas that arise from the simple fact that the experiences of being "transgender," and the institutional and medical constraints facing transgender people, vary considerably around the world, as do the gender and sexual identities and labels that people adopt for themselves.[82] And this point, in turn, underscores a broader critique made by trans studies scholars: that a key consequence of the maintenance of diagnostic categories for transgender health experiences has been precisely the reinforcement of rigid, monotonic, and stereotypical conceptions of what it means to be trans.[83]

ATYPICAL SEXUALITIES AND THE CRITERION OF CONSENT

An additional set of changes aimed at destigmatization concerns the "paraphilic disorders"—referring to so-called atypical sexual preferences—which are "secondarily parented" in the sexual health chapter. While the working group concluded that, for practical reasons, the paraphilias ought to retain a primary location in the mental disorders chapter, it recommended that several of the paraphilias be eliminated or redefined.[84] Notably disappearing is a vestige of an earlier era: an ICD-10 diagnosis called "ego-dystonic sexual orientation." The term originally marked a compromise following the contentious process by which homosexuality was removed from the DSM in 1973—a consequence of social change within the psychiatric community propelled by disruptive activism by gay liberationists who targeted the American Psychiatric Association's annual meetings.[85] The idea had been that while homosexuality per se was no longer to be considered an illness, people distressed by their unwanted same-sex desires could be diagnosed with ego-dystonic homosexuality and "treated" for that condition.[86] The term did not survive in the DSM past 1987, but it remained in ICD-10 and consequently the diagnosis lingered for decades.[87] But the working group took exception to the idea that mental distress resulting from societal discrimination should be classified as a mental illness: "There are several socially stigmatized conditions, such as physical illness or poverty, that are also likely to lead to distress. These conditions could be labelled 'ego-dystonic' to the extent that they are unwanted but the ICD does not treat such distress as constituting a mental disorder."[88]

Ultimately, the working group concluded that not just "ego-dystonic sexual orientation" but the entire grouping of "psychological and behavioural disorders associated with sexual development and orientation" to which it belonged should be deleted from the ICD. The working group argued that these categories lacked clinical utility, had not generated scientific publications, and failed to contribute to public health surveillance; moreover, retaining them threatened to bring "suboptimal care" to people with a same-sex orientation and could "also be construed as supporting ineffective and unethical treatment that aims to encourage people with a same-sex orientation to adopt a heterosexual orientation or heterosexual behaviour."[89] Finally, "from a human rights perspective, the . . . categories selectively target individuals with gender nonconformity or a same-sex orientation without apparent justification."[90] That is, the working group's argumentation proceeded seamlessly from the scientific, to the practical, to the ethical, stitching these concerns together.

Certain sexual practices, such as pedophilia, exhibitionism, and voyeurism, also remained in ICD-11 as paraphilias, although only if the individual either acted on the impulse or was distressed by its presence. But as a general rule, the working group took a dim view of treating sexual predilections as diseases unless they involved coercion, harmed others, or risked significant injury or death. Consensual sadomasochism was therefore eliminated, but a new category called "coercive sexual sadism disorder" was added to describe the "infliction of physical or psychological suffering on a non-consenting person." Cross-dressing ("fetishistic transvestism" in ICD-10) was likewise removed, as was fetishism.

"I think the [question] of 'what is normal sexual behavior?' was a bit of a minefield," Doris Chou observed: "So I think this is where the colleagues who were working in mental health made a bit of a distinction. If somebody was doing something of their own free will, with consent and without harm to anyone else, on the spectrum of things, it's probably okay."[91]

The emphasis on consent nicely signals the working group's clear investment in normative and ethical concerns. The sexologist and sexualities scholar Alain Giami has highlighted the historical significance of the emphasis on the criterion of consent in ICD-11. For Giami, the emergence of new understandings of sexual health and sexual rights has coincided with the triumph of a "democratic normative model of sexual activity grounded in individual responsibility, communication, love, well-being, and respect for others." This perspective displaced an older conception of sexual "normality" linked to reproduction and replaced it with "a framework based on communication, individual freedom, well-being, and equality." In this context, it became self-evident that "consent" should serve as "the key criterion for distinguishing normal sexual activity and its variations from pathological and criminal forms."[92]

Giami's observations suggest, yet again, how the rise of the framework represented by sexual health signifies broad shifts in contemporary understandings of gender and sexuality. As we will see especially in later chapters of this book, the consenting subjects of sexual health discourses are conceived as those who make healthy choices that enhance the self while respecting the rights and prerogatives of others. Indeed, Giami may understate the significance of the selection of consent as demarking normal sexuality and gender in the ICD (and well beyond). Certainly from the vantage point of the United States, it is difficult to read this shift without reference to the charged critiques of sexual assault advanced by #MeToo feminists as well as the debates on college campuses about the adoption of policies of "affirmative consent."[93] Nowadays, the focus on consent is overdetermined.

Yet it is interesting, in that regard, to point to pushback against the triumph of consent. As Sam Winter, a member of the working group complained, the WHO "retreated somewhat from the Working Group's original recommendations" by adding an unwieldy grab-bag diagnostic category called "paraphilic disorder involving solitary behaviour or consenting individuals."[94] This designation was to be reserved for cases in which "the person is markedly distressed by the nature of the arousal pattern and the distress is not simply a consequence of rejection or feared rejection of the arousal pattern by others" or in which "the nature of the paraphilic behaviour involves significant risk of injury or death either to the individual or to the partner (e.g., asphyxophilia)."[95]

Still, in Winter's view, "this diagnosis re-pathologises behaviour patterns the Working Group sought to depathologise."[96] Arguably, this
overruling of the working group suggests a degree of instability in the
historical changes to which Giami has pointed and indicates the contemporaneous presence of multiple understandings of how to locate
the dividing line between normal and pathological sexuality.

SEX AS COMPULSION?

An interesting case of classificatory politics concerns the controversial
category known generally as sexual compulsivity or, more colloqui-
ally, sex addiction. According to a critical analysis by the sociologist
Janice Irvine in the 1990s, the category of sex addiction was invented
in the 1970s by various professionals in the United States who used
the addiction metaphor to repurpose older ideas about nymphomania
or out-of-control sexual urges. In the view of Irvine and many critics
since, the category of sex addiction is an example of how the process
of medicalization takes social problems and recharacterizes them as
defects within individuals. The discourses of sex addiction, she argued, problematically "site deviance in the individual physical body,
reinscribe stereotypic ideas of gendered sexuality, and expose deep cultural anxieties about sex."[97]

The idea of sex addiction has continued to be controversial, especially as social and scholarly attention to the issue has climbed in
recent decades. Drawing on data from the National Survey of Sexual
Health and Behavior, researchers have suggested that "10.3% of men
and 7.0% of women [experience] clinically relevant levels of distress
and/or impairment associated with difficulty controlling sexual feelings, urges, and behaviors."[98] Alarm about sexual compulsivity has also
coincided with rising concerns about the effects of viewing pornography, especially online. As we saw in chapter 2, at least one group, the
Society for the Advancement of Sexual Health, has sought to bring the
treatment of sexual addiction within the domain of sexual health—
indeed, to position the overcoming of sex addiction as the essence of
sexual health. But other, more representative organizations, including some specifically concerned with sexual health, have opposed the
use of the diagnosis. A proposal to include a mental illness category
called "hypersexuality" was rejected by the US psychiatric community
when the fifth revision to the DSM was issued in 2013, in part out of

objections to dictating what constituted the "right amount" of sex.[99] And in November 2016, the American Association of Sex Educators, Counselors and Therapists, a large and well-established interdisciplinary professional organization, issued a position statement that declared there was not "sufficient empirical evidence to support the classification of sex addiction or porn addiction as a mental health disorder." Citing issues of both evidence and rights, one of the statement's authors observed: "These are real problems, but sex therapy counseling and education requires a higher standard of sexual science to ensure sexual rights and sexual health. The sex addiction concept is an oversimplification of a complex area of human sexual behavior and is not substantiated by sexual science and sex therapy."[100]

In ICD-10, sexual compulsivity was called "excessive sexual drive" and appeared within the sexual dysfunction grouping in the chapter on mental disorders. But in ICD-11, the excessive sexual drive category was eliminated in name, and no remnant of it is to be found among the set of sexual dysfunctions that were relocated to the new sexual health chapter. However, this does not mean that the condition has ceased to be medicalized. Instead, a new category called "compulsive sexual behavior disorder" has been added to the grouping of "impulse control disorders" found within the mental disorders chapter—and the new sexual health chapter does not serve as a secondary parent. That is, rather than being grouped with sexual dysfunctions, paraphilias, or any other conditions related to sexual health, compulsive sexual behavior now sits alongside three nonsexual conditions—pyromania, kleptomania, and "intermittent explosive disorder"—that are understood to involve "the repeated failure to resist an impulse, drive, or urge."[101] Notably, the other three kinds of impulse control disorders involve a substantial risk of harm to others, while compulsive sexual behavior disorder is defined solely in terms of harmful consequences to oneself.

This classification came about through a settlement of sorts between ICD working groups: while orphaned by the Working Group on Sexual Disorders and Sexual Health (whose members do not even mention sexual compulsivity in two key publications describing differences between ICD-10 and ICD-11[102]), the condition was adopted by a different ICD working group that focused on "obsessive-compulsive and related disorders." The latter group found it "more clinically useful," from the standpoint of both diagnosis and treatment, to view sexual compulsivity through the lens of failed impulse control, "rather than placing the primary focus on the fact that the behaviour involved is sexual in nature."[103] This relocation has numerous potential consequences for those so diagnosed, especially in light of interest in the use of medications, often in combination with talk therapy, to treat disorders of impulse control.[104] That it was controversial is suggested by the fact that the working group received forty-seven comments from stakeholders specifically on this diagnostic category.[105]

The new definition of compulsive sexual behavior disorder is suggestive of the tensions and contradictions that follow from a concerted attempt to define sexual "excess" as a scientific, rather than moral, category. The ICD text clarifies that simply being above the norm in wanting sex doesn't merit the diagnosis. For an individual to qualify, engaging in repetitive sexual activities has become "a central focus of the person's life to the point of neglecting health and personal care or other interests, activities and responsibilities," or the person has made "numerous unsuccessful efforts to significantly reduce repetitive sexual behaviour," or the person continues to engage in repetitive sexual behavior "despite adverse consequences or deriving little or no satisfaction from it." Moreover, the behavior must continue over at least six months and must cause "marked distress or significant impairment" in personal or social functioning.[106] Clearly, the authors of the definition sought to provide a diagnostic opportunity for patients and clinicians while inoculating themselves against the charge that they were acting merely as enforcers of cultural norms—indeed, they state explicitly that "distress that is entirely related to moral judgments and disapproval about sexual impulses, urges, or behaviours is not sufficient" for diagnostic purposes. Yet while the inclusion of such a disclaimer is noteworthy and important, it is not clear how individuals are expected to fully separate their own sense of whether their behavior brings them "satisfaction" from their distress about being on the receiving end of negative social judgments.

In short, despite the careful phrasing, the retention of the category of compulsive sexual behavior disorder raises important concerns about the moral policing of sexuality—even though, or perhaps especially because, in this case, the behavior has been separated from other sexual practices and housed alongside noxious, nonsexual neighbors. While ICD-11's conception of sexual health has resulted in the declassification of a number of conditions, compulsive sexual behavior disorder stands as an example of how a controversial sexual diagnosis can remain in the ICD by means of being—oddly enough—desexualized. That precisely the condition associated with sexual excess should be the one subject to categorical desexing is a curious irony in the story of ICD-11.

Consequences

There is a risk of exaggerating the significance of adding a sexual health chapter to the ICD. At the level of innovation, ICD-11 mostly does not come up with new classifications of sexuality but rather redefines, relocates, or eliminates old ones. Moreover, a number of specific changes with regard to sexual terms and definitions were prefigured in the earlier move from DSM-4 to DSM-5. Yet the creation of a sexual health chapter (even a short one) clearly signifies the rise into prominence of the concept of sexual health—and therefore, the increasing "sexualization" of global health institutions. And it reveals how its proponents, in deliberate fashion and with an eye to recent social change, have sought to stitch together scientific and normative concerns in the hope of taking a medical and ethical agenda in relation to gender and sexuality and making it workable on a global scale. To the extent this effort succeeds, the result is a redefinition of what we take to be knowledge about the sexual and knowledge about the human. As I argue throughout the book, conjoining "sexual" with "health" is not trivial: it changes the meanings of both terms, and establishes new truths of sex.

Inevitably, such work has multiple and complex effects. From the standpoint of proponents of a strong concept of sexual health, the advent of the chapter promises unity, visibility, and greater capacities for data collection and aggregation. According to a statement issued by the WAS: "By using a sexual health approach, these guidelines will improve the way that public health practitioners approach, record, and report diagnoses, moving away from a persistent emphasis on negative outcomes toward an approach based in integrated, holistic care."[107] More broadly, this package of diagnoses will serve as an "obligatory passage point" on the way to satisfaction of a diverse set of institutional imperatives and personal aspirations:[108] it will permit patients to get treated, medical providers to get paid, researchers to conduct studies, and governments to organize the delivery of health care services.[109]

Of course, it is hard to know exactly how or to what degree the changes reflected in ICD-11 will affect everyday encounters between patients and providers. As the STS scholar Andrew Lakoff has observed about diagnostic systems, it is no simple matter to take the diverse life experiences of particular patients and render them "liquid"—capable of conversion into a generalizable format that can travel around the world.[110] In particular, it is hard to gauge what health providers will do with the diagnostic labels made available to them. One might assume that clinicians necessarily take their cues from formal nosologies, but studies have shown that clinicians often resist their logics or nego- tiate their use of them.[111] My point, though, is that well outside the micropolitics of encounters between providers and patients, ICD-11's destigmatization of many conditions sends powerful messages that potentially reverberate much more broadly. This signaling effect of the ICD, which speaks to the cultural authority of the tool and of the WHO itself, may prove more enduring and significant than its impact on the diagnosing of individual patients.

SEXUAL BOUNDARY DRAWING AND THE RENEGOTIATION OF THE NORMAL

Perhaps most consequentially of all, the repositioning of sexual mat- ters within ICD-11 marks the renegotiation of various boundaries. When asked about the lasting impact of the sexual health chapter, the WHO's Doris Chou emphasized the disembedding of the sexual from the domain of the reproductive: "it separates the notion of sexual health [and] sexual activity from reproductive health and reproductive activity."[112] This motivation, of course, has been a key driver of the de- velopment of the concept of sexual health since its inception, and (as I described in chapter 3), Chou's department has been at the center of efforts to insist both on the intrinsic connections between sexual and reproductive health and rights and on the relative autonomy of the sexual from the reproductive. But this is only one boundary at stake in the debates around sexuality and gender in the ICD. Others include that between mental disorders and other health conditions, and of course, most fundamentally of all, the ever-shifting boundary between the normal and the pathological. This last point is hardly surprising, given the historical salience of sexuality to the very idea of the normal in Western societies;[113] but it bears close attention all the same.

In her classic and still widely read polemical essay from the 1980s, the anthropologist, sexualities scholar, and activist Gayle Rubin bemoaned the widespread cultural practice of condemning, medicalizing, or criminalizing nonnormative sexual practices simply because they differed from mainstream sexual tastes. "One need not like or perform a particular sex act in order to recognize that someone else will, and that this difference does not indicate a lack of good taste, mental health, or intelligence in either party," argued Rubin, criticizing the typical ways of drawing boundaries between "acceptable" and "unacceptable" sexualities: "Most people mistake their sexual preferences for a universal system that will or should work for everyone."[114]

Certainly to some degree, the reorganization of sexual diagnoses in ICD-11 represents a triumph of Rubin's critique within the bureaucracy of modern global medicine. Even if depathologization, in the end, is just one step along the path to substantive social change,[115] nonetheless the working group's efforts reflect an impressive move away from a previously well-ingrained assumption that being sexually different is, ipso facto, a symptom of illness.

But two points are worth noting in this regard. First, while depathologization is a fascinating outcome, the impetus to destigmatize and depathologize at least certain sexual and gender behaviors and identities in ICD-11 wars against the desire to use classifications to say what is normal—and to do so in universalist ways that aspire to global relevance. It could be argued, for example, that the retention of categories such as exhibitionism and voyeurism in the chapter on mental disorders, along with the relocation of sexual compulsivity, as well as the creation of the new diagnostic category of "paraphilic disorder involving solitary behaviour or consenting individuals," all reflect an unproven assumption that certain activities that sometimes (but not always) are socially problematic are best understood as psychological defects and best remedied through psychological or pharmacological intervention. Moreover, it seems predictable that the various qualifications and potentially ambiguous terms in the definitions of specific conditions—What exactly is "consent"? How marked is "marked distress"? What qualifies as an "adverse consequence"?—not only will be interpreted in varying ways in different contexts and cultures but also will leave sufficient wiggle room for those who are so inclined to capture many sexual nonconformists in the diagnostic web. Given the historical links between sexual classification and the exercise of power over sexual deviance, it seems likely that the opposing tugs of two goals—upholding sexual normality, and destigmatizing sexual differences—will continue their face-off in the new era of ICD-11.

The second point is an analytical one, and it revolves around the questions raised by my use of various overlapping "de-" terms in this discussion: Are behaviors and identities related to gender and sexuality being demedicalized? Depathologized? Destigmatized? "De-psychiatrized"? The case of ICD-11 indicates that the various implied oppositions—between the medicalized and the nonmedicalized, the stigmatized, and the nonstigmatized, and so on—just don't all neatly line up.[116] Conditions may be de-psychiatrized without being demedicalized, destigmatized without being de-psychiatrized, demedicalized while still being treated as "health-related," and so on. This observation reinforces my suspicion, highlighted in the early pages of this book, that broad-brush concepts such as medicalization tell us little in the end about the meanings of the rise of sexual health, and that we are sorely in need of a more differentiated conceptual vocabulary. At the very same time, the complex relations among these non-overlapping sets of opposing terms should give us pause before we attribute theoretical solidity to the construct known as "the normal." The implication, also suggested by recent critical work on the history of normality, is that the normal and the pathological are complex and unstable concoctions, derived from multiple sources, whose apparent coherence at a given moment is a crucial dimension of their hold on our minds and deeds.[117]

STATISTICS AND THE MEASUREMENT OF SEXUALLY HEALTHY SOCIETIES

The diagnostic categories of ICD-11 matter for health providers and patients but also hold significance for practices of measurement and monitoring at the scale of the nation, the region, and the globe. (It is worth recalling yet again the full name of the ICD: the International *Statistical* Classification of Diseases and Related Health Problems.) From the standpoint of the WHO, aspirations for the ICD (and for measuring sexual health more generally) are tightly intertwined with the goal of documenting progress toward broader institutional imperatives laid down by the United Nations. Once the United Nations had established the target of "achieving universal access to reproductive health by 2015" as a component of Millennium Development Goal 5

("Improve maternal health"),[118] WHO officials were keen to find ways to measure progress toward global sexual health. Later, but similarly, once the UN had established the target of ensuring "universal access to sexual and reproductive health-care services" as a component of Sustainable Development Goal 3 ("Ensure healthy lives and promote well-being for all at all ages by 2030"),[119] then finding ways to operationalize and measure sexual health took on added importance.

Indeed, the WHO for some time has sought means to express, quantitatively, the sexual health of populations. In March 2007, at a technical consultation meeting organized by the WHO and the United Nations Population Fund, participants were tasked with recommending an array of nation-level indicators that could be used to monitor progress toward the goal of universal access to sexual and reproductive health.[120] While there appeared to be many indicators available to document reproductive health conditions around the world, sexual health indicators were deemed lacking. Therefore, in September 2007, a working group of experts on sexual health indicators met to propose steps forward.[121] After much discussion of potentially measurable features of different aspects of sexual health, the working group proposed a matrix of indicators.[122]

In 2015, WHO officials returned to the agenda of "expanding the measurement of indicators related to all aspects of sexual health, both positive and negative." They noted one obvious obstacle standing in the way: "Unfortunately, many countries, particularly low and middle-income countries, struggle to produce meaningful data on sexual health due to lack of resources and sometimes the commitment required."[123] But a partial solution, in their view, was provided by the ICD, and particularly the ratification of ICD-11. Because the ICD provides a standardized format for collecting and reporting health statistics; because its use is obligatory within the 194 member states of the WHO; and—crucially—because ICD-11 would contain a new chapter on conditions related to sexual health, the advent of ICD-11 was expected to facilitate measurement of a variety of concepts at the nation level. Specifically, the officials proposed to use ICD-11 categories to measure and report statistics on sexual dysfunctions, female genital mutilation, gender incongruence, sexually transmitted infections, violence against women, unwanted pregnancy, and induced abortion.[124]

Measuring progress toward national sexual health by collecting a full array of indicators is largely aspirational at this stage. Standing in the way are many practical obstacles and political considerations. These include the limitations involved in capturing complex social phenomena using simple quantitative measures,[125] but also the complication that measures designed for one set of purposes—say, health promotion and epidemiological tracking—do not always lend themselves to smooth employment for other purposes, such as propelling policy changes or political action.[126]

Moreover, it is not obvious that discrete measures of sexual health conditions in a given country retain their meanings when divorced from the social contexts that give sexuality its distinctive features.[127] And the risk is that decontextualized numbers may lend themselves to facile assessments of which countries are "ahead" or "behind"—perhaps privileging the taken-for-granted background characteristics of wealthier, Western societies and inadvertently using those countries as the standard to which others are compared and by which they are judged. Thus, if it is tricky and problematic to classify, diagnose, rate, and rank *individuals* with regard to their sexual health and measure their deviation from sexual norms, then the complications may be amplified considerably when we seek to classify, diagnose, and rank entire countries. Undoubtedly, any future advance of this measurement project will give rise to new debates and prompt pushback of various sorts from governments, policy advocates, and activists.

PARTICIPATION AND THE "HEALTHICIZATION" OF GLOBAL GOVERNANCE

As Bowker and Star put it previously in their analysis of ICD-10, the ICD serves to "stabilize" the natural and social worlds by "describing disease in a way that folds the socially and legally contingent into the classification system itself," whereby the contingency becomes invisible.[128] In the move from ICD-10 to ICD-11, this normally hidden work of stabilization has been brought into public view—quite evidently so, in the creation of a new chapter on sexual health. As made apparent by the working group's frequent references to "civil society organizations," the need to counter "stigma," "human rights violations," and "harm to individuals so labeled," classificatory changes in the ICD reflect not just scientific concerns but also (as they noted) "major changes in social attitudes and in relevant policies, laws, and human rights standards."[129] Similarly, the substantial emphasis on consent as a criterion of normality indexes a complex negotiation among evolving medical, ethical, and political judgments.[130] While upholders of a purist conception of the autonomy of science might lament what they view as the "politicization" of global health, it seems more useful to understand cases such as these, conversely, as instance of the contemporary global "healthicization" of politics and governance. That is, public health and medicine are increasingly understood to be domains in which a host of political problems can be worked out, including the nature of social justice, the boundaries of belonging, and the definitions of normality and abnormality.[131]

Moreover, the changes encapsulated in the sexual health chapter reveal the substantial incursions made into biomedical worlds by commentators from beyond its immediate bounds. They testify both to new emphases on deference to so-called stakeholders and to the growing power of knowledgeable advocacy groups—uncredentialed "lay experts"—to offer guidance that draws on hybrid mixes of experiential and official knowledge.[132] Here, again, transgender politics emerges as central to the story of the sexual health chapter as a whole: as Damien Riggs and coauthors have emphasized, it is precisely "the traffic between clinicians, guidelines, and transgender communities"—and not any monolithic definitional authority wielded by medical or psychological professionals—that nowadays defines the production of knowledge, classifications, guidelines, and standards governing transgender health care.[133] Thus, global transgender health advocacy is an exemplary case of the new models of confrontation and collaboration between experts and laypeople found cropping up, in varying forms, across the landscape of medicine and health care today. And therefore, while the revision of the ICD might appear as a totalizing project of global medical standardization, it has been fueled by the delicate interplay of a diverse set of actors, whose intricate negotiations leave openings for flexibility of interpretation and also seem to guarantee future contestation.[134]

This includes debates about the very meaning of sexual health. Recently, some transgender health activists have pointed to the inclusion of "gender incongruence" within the ICD's sexual health chapter as grounds for demanding that practitioners in the broad field of sexual health revisit some fundamental assumptions: they should not only attend more systematically to transgender people's sexuality but also reject a binary gender logic when considering sexuality generally.[135]

It remains to be seen whether actors in the many domains of sexual health will be motivated to act in response to such interventions. But one of the ramifications of a participatory process of diagnostic reform is the opening up of new discussions about how sexuality and health should be conceived in the first place.

CLASSIFICATORY POLITICS

Finally, the story of ICD-11 raises familiar and complex issues in the history and politics of classification. Chou, for example, referred to the tension between the "purists" and the "pragmatists" in debates over matters such as "gender incongruence"—debates that, inevitably, cut differently for those who actually had to "live" the category. She noted, as well, the familiar problem that diagnostic nosologies tend to be "one size fits all": "And I say this many times. 'One size fits all' will do, but it might not fit everyone perfectly."[136]

A related set of issues concerns what Bowker and Star have described as the "permanent tension between attempts at universal standard-ization of lists and the local circumstances of those using them."[137] By maintaining that sexual classifications are universally applicable, ICD-11 reaffirms the tendency of its predecessors to assume that the process of arriving at a diagnosis can take place in ways that are essentially inde-pendent of particular social contexts of doctor-patient interaction. Yet, not only, as I have said, will clinicians and patients negotiate their uses of nosologies, but they likely will do so differently in different places. To suggest otherwise is to flatten social distinctions and homogenize cultures (medical, sexual, and otherwise) around the world.[138] As the an-thropologist Didier Fassin has warned, medical diagnoses aim for uni-versalism in both a geographical and a moral sense; and the spread of diagnoses therefore "functions simultaneously as spatial expansion and moral normalization."[139] Claims to universality—even when backed by "field studies being implemented in multiple languages"[140]—inevitably collide with the "consistent finding of the history of science" described by Bowker and Star: that "there is no such thing as a natural or univer-sal classification system," and "classifications that appear natural, elo-quent, and homogeneous within a given human context appear forced and heterogeneous outside of that context."[141]

Yet while many aspects of the ICD-11 story may be familiar from other studies of classification debates, the case is distinctive, precisely because of the explosive politics of gender and sexuality. No doubt it can also be difficult to come to a global consensus about how to define measles, malaria, or meningitis. But diagnoses related to gender and sexuality pose special challenges, and not just because (though certainly partly because) many of these diagnoses cross the borders between so-called physical and mental disorders. In addition, questions related to sexuality and gender are among those that the 194 member states of the World Health Assembly are most likely to disagree about in general. In a world of nation-states marked by sharp divisions (and conflicting laws) around issues such as homosexuality, abortion, contraception, premarital sex, gender equality, and transgender rights, coming to agreement on classifying sexual health conditions is fraught with complexity. (While media coverage of the ratification of ICD-11 zeroed in on the transgender health issue, it is perhaps not surprising that the WHO's 10-page memo introducing ICD-11 as an agenda item for voting bypassed the transgender health categorization issue entirely and made only a passing mention of the new chapter on sexual health.[142]) Moreover, sexual and gender matters have been the occasion for a significant degree of global activism and advocacy that has questioned biomedical orthodoxies. Thus, the voices at the table seeking to influence the process of classification are exceptionally diverse, further complicating the business of standardization.

"We cannot escape classifications and categorizations," writes Jeffrey Weeks, a foremost historian of sexuality who has traced the history of sexological thinking: "Without them, the world is a formless mass. What matters is who makes the definitions and how they are lived."[143] Indeed, as the past history of activism in the face of diagnoses around homosexuality and transgender experience well suggests, the publication of ICD-11 is likely to spark a new round of debates about sexual and gender subjectivity. At the same time, it may engender its own "looping effects," to use the term offered by philosopher of science Ian Hacking:[144] Disease nosologies may sort people into categories but, given time, those who inhabit the categories may "talk back" in ways that lead, ultimately, to classificatory reform.

6 *Surveys and the Quantification of Normality*

ENUMERATING SEXUAL HEALTH

People are captivated by results from sex surveys—anxious to imagine what others are "getting up to," and to locate themselves, their fantasies, and their fears, in relation to the statistical means and the standard deviations. The conduct of such surveys invites many questions. How do such projects come about? How have they connected the topic of sexuality with that of health? How do they operationalize sexual health and transform it into the scientifically discernable attributes of a population? What questions are asked, and which topics are left unexplored? And what are the effects of the circulation of findings from sexual health surveys? What knowledge do they produce about the practices, identities, and beliefs of different groups in society? How does their uptake affect ideas about what it means to be a responsible sexual subject, or a normal and healthy sexual person?

This chapter takes up a distinctive way of knowing, shifting our attention in two key respects from the two previous chapters: from the biomedical and health sciences to the social sciences, and from scrutinizing the individual to measuring the whole population. It also focuses on a distinctive mode of operationalizing sexual health: *enumeration*, and specifically the counting and tallying of bodies and behaviors.[1] Enumerating practices and identities is consequential because it contributes to our understanding of what constitutes statistical "normality" and, by extension, who lies on the statistical margins. Enumeration via survey research also constructs quantitative knowledge about subgroups of the population: drawing on presuppositions about which identities should be studied, it measures how they differ from the "mainstream" and what the consequences of such difference might be. To the degree that findings from surveys circulate—and sex survey results prove particularly mobile—they may reverberate well beyond the domain of academic social science.

Between the "Will to Know" and the "Will to Not Know"

Compared to survey research generally, sex surveys are distinctive not only because of the special fascination they invite but also in light of the powerful challenges confronted by those who attempt them. The history of these surveys reveals the social, cultural, political, and financial roadblocks put in the way of acquiring clear knowledge of sexual practice. We can therefore think of sex surveys as facing agnotological barriers. If "epistemology" refers to how we know, then "agnotology"— its opposite and shadow—describes what remains unknown and why we don't come to know it. As Robert Proctor, a historian of science who uses the term, has put it: "If the politics of science consists (among other things) in the structure of research priorities, then it is important to understand what gets studied and why, but also what does *not* get studied and why not."[2] In the case of sex surveys, researchers confront not only the stigma that seems to cling to the topic of sexuality even as a research matter,[3] but also the preference in some quarters to simply not learn the truths of sexual behavior. Thus what Michel Foucault characterized as the modern "will to knowledge" about sexuality wars against a simultaneous will to not know.[4]

The history of sex surveys in the United States demonstrates that conducting such surveys is indeed an activity fraught with peril. Alfred Kinsey's pioneering research in the 1940s and 1950s, which resulted in two large volumes, based on interviews with 5,300 White men and 5,940 White women, respectively, was famously controversial, to the degree that some referred to his "blockbuster" volumes as the "K-bomb."[5] Widespread dissemination of his findings, which revealed his participants to be considerably more diverse in their sexual pursuits than Americans generally were deemed to be in that conservative era, prompted attacks from those who decried, in the words of the popular evangelist Billy Graham, "the damage this book will do to the already deteriorating morals of America." The *New York Times* did not review Kinsey's book on men and refused to let it be advertised in its pages, despite the volume's high position on the *Times*'s own bestseller list. Public outrage led to a congressional investigation and prompted the Rockefeller Foundation to terminate Kinsey's funding.[6]

The moral panic over Kinsey's research bears out historian Sarah Igo's contention, in her cultural history of modern survey methods, that "struggles over what we might call 'statistical citizenship' [are] often proxy wars for representation in other realms of U.S. society."[7] More specifically, conservatives have feared—with good reason—that surveys that tabulate the great variety of things that people do sexually inevitably challenge and, perhaps, shift broader social norms about what is considered acceptable and, in fact, "normal." This, indeed, had been a consequence of the Kinsey Reports, in Igo's view: "For Kinsey himself, but perhaps also for his readers, there was a certain strain simply in attempting to fix a singular container like 'normal sexual behavior' around the statistical abundance of the Reports. Kinsey's research, after all, virtually exploded the idea of a national 'average.'"[8]

Similar dynamics ensued when, in 1987, a group of sociologists that included Edward Laumann, Robert Michael, and Stuart Michaels at the University of Chicago and John Gagnon at SUNY–Stony Brook, responded to a request by the National Institutes of Health (NIH) for research proposals on the (euphemistically named) topic "Social and Behavioral Aspects of Health and Fertility-Related Behaviors." The investigators won a contract to design what they called the National Health and Social Life Survey (of course, the emphasis on "health" and avoidance of "sexuality" in the title is noteworthy)—a comprehensive national survey of adults on sexual attitudes and behaviors related to reproductive health and sexually transmitted infections, including HIV/AIDS. At a time when the AIDS epidemic was spreading rapidly and was finally being recognized as a substantial threat to the US population, the study proposed use of sophisticated techniques of data collection and analysis to fill in the yawning gaps in knowledge about sexual beliefs and practices and their relation to the risk of HIV transmission. The investigators also sought to correct the methodological limitations of Kinsey's research by conducting a nationwide survey using probability sampling to insure that it would be representative of the US population. In 1989, after extensive pretesting of their survey instrument, the researchers submitted it to the federal Office of Management and Budget (OMB) for review—normally a formality for federally funded research of this kind.[9]

This time, however, a furor ensued after word got out that the OMB was reviewing a "sex questionnaire." Conservatives in Congress denounced the study as an unwarranted intrusion into private matters as well as an attempt to promote the "agenda" of the gay movement. In response to mobilization by a Christian radio station, the OMB was bombarded with phone calls from opponents of the research.[10] The arch-conservative and staunchly anti-gay senator Jesse Helms (who took the opportunity to raise questions on the Senate floor about the "normality" of one of the researchers, John Gagnon, and falsely portrayed him as an advocate of sex between children and adults[11]) proposed a measure that permanently banned federal funding of this and another study related to sexuality, and the restriction ultimately was passed by Congress and signed into law in 1993.[12]

In the view of conservatives in Congress, when it came to sexuality, it was better not to know. After all, knowing—especially scientific enumeration—has consequences, as one of the opponents of the National Health and Social Life Survey, Rep. William Dannemeyer, made clear in a letter of protest sent to the assistant secretary for health. According to Dannemeyer, one problem with tabulating sexual behavior was that doing so might grant legitimacy to groups such as gay and lesbian Americans. "Imagine the political landscape if any one demographic grouping were to increase their rank from 10% of the population to 15% or 20%," wrote Dannemeyer: "This is the exact reason why the purveyors of laissez-faire sexual attitudes want to use tax dollars and the federal cloak of scientific legitimacy to produce this work."[13]

Meanwhile, the researchers had managed to piece together partial funding from a number of major private foundations and were then able to proceed with a scaled-down version of their original proposal. The results from the study were published in 1994 in book form as *The Social Organization of Sexuality*. Working with a journalist, the researchers also put out a thinner companion volume oriented toward a popular audience and called *Sex in America*.[14] Ironically, given the fuss, the study's well-publicized findings ran somewhat in the opposite direction of Kinsey's, portraying American sexuality as relatively conventional and suggesting that many people wrongly imagined that others must be having more sex than they themselves were.

The NSSHB as a Sexual Health "Snapshot": Identities and Differences

It is perhaps not surprising that no one again attempted a large-scale study of sexuality using a national probability sample for some years afterward in the United States,[15] until an interdisciplinary group at the Center for Sexual Health Promotion at Indiana University (the campus that is also home to the Kinsey Institute) took up the charge in the late 2000s. By this time, of course, the phrase "sexual health" was much more in vogue, and both the center's name and that of the research project—the National Survey of Sexual Health and Behavior (NSSHB)—put sexual health up front as the preferred and, perhaps, intellectually respectable and politically defensible way to frame a large-scale study of sexuality.[16] Indeed, the first write-up from the study, by public health researcher Debby Herbenick and coauthors, cited the WHO's 2002 revised working definition of sexual health in its opening paragraph.[17]

Rather than seek public funds or approach foundations, as previous sex survey researchers had attempted with mixed results, the designers of the NSSHB obtained all financing for the study from a single source in the private sector that was more sheltered from public disapproval: the company Church & Dwight Co., Inc., "maker of Trojan® brand sexual health products"—that is, condoms.[18] This partnership, according to the investigators, was designed "to better bridge public health research with the sexual health promotion activities and products to which American consumers are exposed daily."[19] The allocated funds were sufficient to collect survey responses, using the internet, from a representative sample of 5,865 women and men during a three-month period in 2009. This first wave of the study has been followed by six subsequent waves of data collection through 2018, providing a series of "snapshots" of the sexual lives of Americans.[20] The rich data thereby generated have yielded a slew of publications, beginning with a special issue of the *Journal of Sexual Medicine* in 2010 and continuing into the present. Perhaps not surprisingly, many of the articles have addressed condom use.

As noted previously, certain kinds of operationalizing projects—like the tools to assess sexual dysfunction, discussed earlier—seek to establish that social difference doesn't matter: the researchers are at pains to demonstrate that their instruments are neutral with respect to race, ethnicity, age, education, social class, and even language (once translated). By contrast, the NSSHB's "snapshot" sought to tease out and shine a light on difference—to make at least certain forms of difference hypervisible. While the earlier National Health and Social Life Survey had limited its respondents to those between age eighteen and sixty, the NSSHB expanded the age range to between fourteen and ninety-four.[21] Age therefore emerged as an important variable in the study, yielding publications specifically about the sex practices of groups such as adolescents and the elderly. The researchers have also reported results for women and men; for Whites, Blacks, and Hispanics; and for gay and lesbian participants. In this regard, Herbenick has described the approach of the NSSHB as the pursuit of "epistemic justice": representing the knowledge of diverse individuals and honoring voices and views that have been ignored or suppressed.[22]

Interestingly, this attention to difference has in some cases produced results that run contrary to the usual rendering of sexual health "risk groups." In particular, while much sexual health discourse generally portrays racial and ethnic minorities as "problematic" subjects who are more inclined to engage in sexual health risks,[23] the researchers found that African Americans and Hispanics reported higher condom use than did Whites.[24] More recent waves of the study have also challenged stereotypes about bisexuals by revealing huge variability in sexual behavior within the group of people who identity with the category.[25]

Surveying Pleasure and Danger

Was the NSSHB—dubbed a "sexual health and behavior" study and funded by a condom manufacturer—a "sex study," or was it a "health study"? The center's website juxtaposes quotes from the researchers that together express the two rationales. According to the public health researcher Michael Reece, the director of the center at the time of the study, "these data about sexual behaviors and condom use in contemporary America are critically needed by medical and public health professionals who are on the front lines addressing issues such as HIV, sexually transmissible infections, and unintended pregnancy." But Herbenick, the associate director, pointed to a less instrumental and more straightforward—and very human—interest: "People are often curious about others' sex lives. . . . They want to know how often men and women in different age groups have sex, the types of sex they engage in, and whether they are enjoying it or experiencing sexual difficulties. Our data provide answers to these common sex questions and demonstrate how sex has changed in the nearly 20 years since the last study of its kind."[26]

In fact, the NSSHB spoke to both of these perceived social needs. On the one hand, by asking participants whether they had engaged in various forms of sexual behavior, the investigators sought to provide a comprehensive picture of the kinds of sex Americans of different sorts were currently experiencing. On the other hand, such data about who was doing what with whom could be used to "inform clinicians about the proportions of patients who are likely to have engaged in various sexual behaviors since their last clinical exam and who may benefit from annual, detailed sexual history taking."[27]

The tight coupling of these two goals—describing sexual practice and assessing the nation's sexual health risk—provided both opportunities and constraints for the discussion of sexual matters in the NSSHB. This issue is best considered in light of findings about sexual topics in survey research more generally. Several scholars have observed that when survey researchers take up sexual matters as one component in large, multitopic surveys, sex tends to be cast in a negative light. Laurel Westbrook, Jamie Budnick, and Aliya Saperstein examined a number of important national surveys that address diverse topics, and found that when the surveys asked questions about sexuality, the tendency was to consider sexuality from the standpoint of "danger" rather than "pleasure"—the problems it may cause rather than the satisfactions it may bring.[28] Somewhat similarly, Megan Ivankovich and colleagues identified eighteen US-focused, nationally representative surveys that (to varying degrees) touch on matters of sexual health, and one of their findings was that issues of pleasure and sexual satisfaction were quite infrequently included, despite their relevance to sexual health.[29] What, then, about a large survey like the NSSHB that was entirely devoted to sexuality? Was the focus on "pleasure," "danger," or both?

We might expect that the healthicization of sexuality—the conversion of sexuality into a matter of health—might incline sex surveys away from pleasure and toward emphasizing various risks associated with sexual practice. Indeed, research by the sociologist Angela Jones suggests that this outcome characterizes sexual science research in general. Applying discourse analysis to three hundred articles in the *Journal of Sex Research*, Jones found an overall "erasure of pleasure" and a consistent emphasis on risk, disease, and dysfunction, and she speculated that this result might reflect the influence of the NIH, a leading funder of research by sexual scientists in the United States.[30] Yet it is important to note that the very expansiveness of the definition of sexual health can also cut in the other direction. The experience of a corresponding survey conducted in the United Kingdom, the British National Survey of Sexual Attitudes and Lifestyles, is instructive. The third wave of the study (called Natsal-3), conducted in 2010–12, explicitly "used WHO's definition of sexual health to frame the design, analysis, and interpretation of the study."[31] As the investigators observed, "this approach views sexual health as not merely the absence of disease but recognises the importance of having pleasurable and safe sexual experiences that are free of coercion, discrimination, and violence." In this case, therefore, the WHO's working definition of sexual health provided the warrants for the argument that "sexual violence, pleasure, and satisfaction should be routinely incorporated in sexual health datasets, as both explanatory variables and outcomes."[32]

How were these tensions between pleasure and danger negotiated in the case of the NSSHB? On the one hand, pleasure was clearly present as a theme in the questionnaire and in reporting of its findings. For example, among the key discoveries noted by the study team were that many older adults continue to have active and pleasurable sex lives and that adults having sex with a condom were just as likely to rate the sex positively in terms of arousal and pleasure. On the other hand, the finding about the enjoyable sexuality of older adults was linked to concern about their lesser use of condoms and was taken as evidence of the need for increased attention to the risk of STIs among this cohort, while the fact that adults apparently were not discouraged from using condoms by fears of diminished sensation implied that condoms could be an effective public health intervention to prevent unwanted pregnancy, HIV infection, and other undesirable outcomes.[33] Similarly, in a public presentation in 2019, Herbenick elicited much support from the audience for her straightforward endorsement of the pleasure and validation that come from sex, while also describing the survey's emphasis, in its most recent wave, on the social problems of the moment, such as coercive sex and the exposure of teens to hardcore pornography online.[34]

In other words, the billing of the NSSHB as a sexual health survey did more than simply insulate the study from attack and help make sexuality research seem more "respectable" (important as these legitimating functions no doubt were for the conduct of the study, even when it was publicly financed): it also reflected, and perhaps shaped, the study's methods and interpretations by welding sex to health and pleasure to risk in such a way that these pairings seemed both natural and inevitable. In effect, this way of grappling with sexual matters and making them legitimate for research purposes can be read as a means of managing the tensions in the broader society between the "will to know" and the "will to not know" sexuality.

Sex Surveys in the Public Domain

The various emphases of the NSSHB no doubt reflect the training and interests of the investigators—indeed, they call to mind Julia Ericksen's contention, in her book-length study of earlier sex surveys of the twentieth century, that "sex surveys tell us about survey researchers and their world views as well as about respondents."[35] But in addition to looking "upstream" at the knowledge producers, we might also wonder about the "downstream" effects of these ways of studying sexuality on members of the public who encounter the results. As several scholars have noted, surveys—certainly including sex surveys—do not simply describe the social world but may also help to shape it.[36] Indeed, as Igo has documented, the twentieth-century invention of national polls and surveys brought about, in the United States, "a little-noticed transformation: one whereby statistical majorities, bell curves, and impersonal data points came to structure Americans' social imagination."[37]

That is, not only do individuals and groups take up the results of surveys and use them to advance various agendas, but also people who encounter the findings of surveys—for example in media reports or via online social networks—learn lessons about what is normal, typical, or desirable. In response, they may reassess their own behaviors and beliefs accordingly—much as conservative opponents of sex surveys have feared. Of course, we should not exaggerate the influence of sex surveys in shaping opinions about sexual matters: nowadays, influential ideas about sexuality make their way to people from a multitude of sources, from popular literature to online pornography to the many experts who offer sex advice. Yet the authoritative character of sex surveys gives their findings a certain cachet.

In this case, announcements of findings from the NSSHB have sparked significant media coverage—not surprisingly, given what Lenore Tiefer has described as "the growth of mass media insatiability for sexual material." Tiefer has noted: "As many news outlets make a profit-seeking shift from information to infotainment, media fill their pages and websites with exciting sexuality 'news.'"[38] It is therefore interesting to see what people make of sex survey coverage—whether by embracing, evaluating, or rejecting survey findings. As Igo has described more generally, the popular uptake of survey research in the twentieth century helped bring into being a new kind of public: "at once highly intrusive and completely anonymous, self-scrutinizing and other-directed, familiar and impersonal."[39] Arguably, present-day combinations of traditional media with newer, alternative, online variants only accentuate this development.[40]

Public discussions of the first wave of the NSSHB fell generally into three categories. First, beginning with the publication of the study's initial nine articles in the *Journal of Sexual Medicine* on October 4, 2010, the survey drew attention as a historical event in itself. *Time* magazine heralded "the largest nationally representative survey of the sexual behavior of Americans ever undertaken," and the *New York Times* called it "a wide-ranging study of Americans' sexual behavior, based on the largest nationally representative survey since 1992." Another burst of publicity came two years later, when the Discovery Channel used the NSSHB to anchor an episode, "Sex in America," of its *Curiosity* series. The cable television program took the viewer inside the study—"Five thousand people. Hundreds of questions. No holds barred"—and cut back and forth between voice-over narration of its findings and the comments offered by a diverse set of individuals and couples who answered questions before the camera about their sex practices, almost as if they were actual respondents in the survey.[41] A review in the *Chicago Tribune* (one of many) announced that "Discovery Channel's 'Curiosity' this Sunday delves into two things most people enjoy: sex and numbers," and advised: "It's all extremely illuminating, but definitely not something to watch with your parents, or children."[42] Thus, much of the coverage of the survey (or the coverage of the coverage, in the case of the *Tribune* review) emphasized the scientific character of the enterprise while simultaneously playing to a presumed universal fascination with the details of the sexuality of others.

Beyond the reporting on the survey as such, a second category of discussion of the NSSHB in the public sphere has consisted of selective references to particular findings, by which the study is invoked to provide authoritative backing for claims related to sexuality. For example, in 2012 Dr. Logan Levkoff, a blogger on the *Huffington Post* website, cited the NSSHB in support of "pleasurable protected sex": "In fact, in the largest nationally representative study of sexual health and behaviors . . . , adults wearing condoms for intercourse were just as likely to rate the sex positively with respect to arousal, pleasure and orgasm as having intercourse without a condom. Don't believe me? Check it out for yourself (www.nationalsexstudy.indiana.edu)."[43] Alternatively, commentators have sought to pick apart the study's methodology to discredit specific claims—such as when the right-wing and anti-gay Family Research Institute turned a skeptical eye on the study's methods in order to cast doubt on the reported percentages of American men and women who are gay or bisexual.[44]

At a more substantive level, a third variety of public engagement with results from the NSSHB takes the form of preoccupation with salient cultural concerns. One example is generational experiences and differences.[45] *Time* magazine sounded this theme in an article headlined "Study of American Sex Habits Suggests Boomers Need Sex Ed." The article began: "As far as sexual behavior goes, we may be worrying about the wrong people. The kids, it turns out, may be all right. It's the boomers who are being all, like, irresponsible and stuff."[46] Similarly, a pair of articles in the *New York Times* juxtaposed two of the study's findings: while condom use was highest among teens, fiftysomething singles—"Grown-Up, but Still Irresponsible"—were having lots of sex but rarely using condoms or getting tested for STIs.[47] Such coverage simultaneously subverted expectations about young people (suggesting that concern about them is misplaced) while playing into stereotypes about self-indulgent baby boomers.

Another area of concern is gender equity.[48] Many commentators have invoked the NSSHB to discuss what is sometimes referred to as the "orgasm gap"—the problem that, in the worlds of an *MTV News* commentator, "statistically, men are occupying O-Town significantly more than women."[49] The cited source was the NSSHB's well-circulated finding that men reported reaching orgasm in 91 percent of their sexual encounters, whereas women said they had an orgasm in only 64 percent of theirs. The gender gap with regard to orgasm was also debated in venues including the statistical analysis website FiveThirty Eight.com; the *Daily Beast*, where a writer claimed the orgasm gap is "just as wide as the wage gap"; and the British newspaper the *Guardian*, which adapted the well-known recorded warning voiced on the

London Underground to urge its readers to "mind the orgasm gap."[50] Coming at a time of generalized concern about the character of heterosexual relationships and shortly before the #MeToo movement focused widespread attention on power imbalances between men and women and the sexual hazards that women regularly confront, the orgasm gap drew attention for appearing to demonstrate that inequalities between heterosexual men and women are embedded in the most intimate aspects of their interactions.[51]

An additional general topic of substantive interest is what David Rosen, writing on the website *Counterpunch*, described as "America's changing sexual appetites." Marshaling statistics from the NSSHB and comparing them to earlier findings from Kinsey's studies and the National Health and Social Life Survey, Rosen declared that "Americans across all age groups, genders and race/ethnic groups are enjoying a wider sexual pallet [sic], including masturbation, oral sex, anal sex and homoeroticism, then anytime in the nation's history."[52] Rosen and others portrayed this embrace of greater sexual flexibility as a welcome historical development; and some invoked NSSHB statistics on behavioral prevalence to proselytize, as a columnist writing on the women's website *Bustle* did on behalf of anal sex.[53] That is, the very fact that many people were doing a particular thing seemed to legitimize and normalize the behavior. Of course, the exposure of current sexual practices to public view is precisely what prompts opposition to the conduct of sex surveys—the agnotological "will to not know." Conservative opponents of sex surveys would rather that those sinners who feel alone in their deviance not begin to imagine themselves as standing in good company.

The New Normal

However, another, perhaps more troubling, side of this appreciation for sexual expansiveness among many readers of sex surveys is a resulting preoccupation with determining what constitutes normality. This consequence was anticipated by the double-edged effects of Kinsey's surveys half a century earlier, as analyzed by Igo: "By exposing the range of sexual behavior, Kinsey and his team might have believed that they were liberating individuals from the tyranny of social codes. But their statistics, tirelessly repeated and argued over, encouraged a new understanding of what it meant to be normal. Out of thousands of personal, emotional conversations, the surveyors had manufactured an authoritative batch of medians and modes. The possibility of using these data to monitor or regulate was always just under the surface."[54]

Recent public discussion of masturbation—a topic with a long and vexed history of medical and popular concern[55]—provides an example of how sex surveys promote the close comparison of individuals to norms. The health and fitness website *Greatist* referenced data from the NSSHB to address the question "How much masturbation is too much?" While reassuring readers that masturbation is extremely common (as NSSHB results indeed made clear), and after cataloging the potential benefits of the practice in the eyes of various experts, the article then observed that masturbation "can become a problem if it interferes with your ability to function in your everyday life," and that in some cases it "can lead to disconnecting emotionally or sensually when it comes to your partner—or being overly reliant on fantasy."[56]

On FiveThirtyEight.com, Mona Chalabi addressed a similar query from "Brandon, 31, New York": "Dear Mona, I masturbate eight times per week. Am I normal?" As befitting the ethos of the website, Chalabi's response treated "normal" as purely a statistical matter, and the graphic accompanying the article superimposed the text "Am I normal?" on a stylized frequency distribution curve. But despite Chalabi's general open-mindedness on the topic, this approach was bad news for Brandon in the end: while data from the NSSHB "suggest that self-petting is nothing out of the ordinary for a man of your age," Chalabi informed him, "your masturbation frequency means you're something of a statistical rarity."[57] Chalabi's response reveals how much the evaluative meaning of "normal" inevitably hovers around, and infects, the statistical sense of the term; and it is not hard to imagine that Brandon would have read the reply as a commentary on his moral worthiness as much as on his variance from a statistical mean.

More generally, these public investigations into the meanings of frequency distributions suggest the profound ability of enumeration exercises such as sex surveys to provide a space for the collective assessment of the normal and abnormal—permitting individuals to measure themselves against those norms and either receive validation or be found wanting. Of course, other sorts of surveys may have similar public effects. But sex surveys may be especially powerful in generating a screen onto which people project their aspirations and imaginings (for example, imagining that others are having more sex, or less sex, or sex that is better or worse). To be sure, survey researchers themselves may disavow such intentions and regret the uses to which sex surveys are put. "I can't stand it when journalists say to me, 'How often should people have sex?'" NSSHB researcher Herbenick confided at a plenary presentation at the National Sexual Health Conference in 2019. Not only may there not be a "right amount," Herbenick observed, but the question also presupposes that we are all in agreement about the definition of an act of sex and how to count it.[58] At the end of the day, however, the capacity of survey researchers to control the dissemination of their findings is limited at best.

The Consequences of Sex Surveys

Especially because sex surveys historically have attracted both voyeuristic attention and political opposition, the effects of such surveys on those who are exposed to their findings merits additional study. Sexual health surveys not only make manifest the societal tensions between the will to know and the desire not to know but also have multiple potential consequences as their findings circulate. They may document dramatic changes in sexual practices and beliefs and uncover serious public health needs affecting vulnerable groups in society. But by emphasizing certain categories and identities within the population while giving less attention to others, such surveys may also reinforce our assumptions about the categories that matter with regard to differences in sexual behavior. Indeed, by assuming the sufficiency of fixed categories of identity, such as "female" and "male"; "gay," "straight," and "bisexual"; and "Black," "White," "Asian," "Latino," and "Native American," surveys may further the process of making invisible all those who fail to conform to the categorical assumptions and who experience more fluid or mixed identities.[59] And to the extent they ignore pleasure or always pair it with danger, sex surveys may strengthen the everyday understanding of sex as a problematic and inherently risky endeavor.

Furthermore, I have suggested that sexual health surveys fuse statistical and moral conceptions of "the norm," thereby influencing contemporary understandings of sexual normality. By revealing what kinds and quantities of sexual behaviors are typical in the population, surveys may challenge existing norms by revealing the gap between official views and actual practice. But surveys may also quite potentially reinforce norms among those who worry whether their own sexual behavior matches up or falls outside the bounds—in effect, inviting them to conform. In both of these ways, sexual enumeration in the public sphere can play an important role in the forging of sexual subjectivity. Most generally, sexual health surveys can function informally to diagnose individuals, labeling them as either normal or pathological. Classificatory work of this kind is a consistent feature of the different modes of operationalizing sexual health: it is an obvious aspect of the sexual inventories and scales, and it is just as evident with the use of the ICD to diagnose sexual health conditions.

The wide circulation of potent findings from sexual health surveys and the diverse commentary about them also points to a broad question: When it comes to sexual health, who speaks with authority? The chapters in part 2 have focused attention on the *tools and techniques* of sexual health expertise: diagnostic codes, rating scales, surveys, and so on. Of course, behind those tools for operationalizing sexual health stand people who are trained to employ them. The next chapter—the last in part 2—moves the analysis more explicitly from instruments to persons: Who are the experts in the different worlds of sexual health? What makes someone an authoritative evaluator of sexual health matters, someone who can speak publicly and offer advice? As we will see, not only has sexual health expertise expanded significantly, but also the boundaries between expert and lay worlds have progressively eroded.

7 *The New Sexual Health Experts*

EVALUATING SEXUAL HEALTH

At a historical moment when the judgments issued by experts are omnipresent—yet when they face scrutiny and challenge as never before—experts strive to speak authoritatively about sexual health.[1] Whether engaging in one-on-one encounters with clients, performing professional and scientific duties, offering quotes to the media, or speaking or writing in other public forums, experts of many stripes claim the ability to say just what sexual health is, who best embodies it, and how it should be pursued. Their evaluative work proposes to pin down the free-floating meanings of sexual health.

Two implications follow from this observation. First, the expansive development of sexual health expertise proves an important marker, propeller, and consequence of what I have termed the "operationalizing" of sexual health. And second, alongside the other operationalizing processes I have already considered in part 2, such as standardizing, classifying, and enumerating, we should add to the list the process of *evaluating*. As Michèle Lamont has argued, activities of evaluation are omnipresent in contemporary societies, and experts are among the key players whose pronouncements are consequential in establishing what matters and who counts.[2] Especially in a domain like health, expert evaluative labor links the assessment of normality with the production, reinforcement, or contestation of norms.

While expert claims are often voiced in the name of science, what gives expertise its cultural authority and social significance is its important role in connecting "knowing" with "doing." As Reiner Grundmann has observed, "experts mediate between the production of knowledge and its application; they define and interpret situations; and they set priorities for action."[3] Therefore, expertise is best understood not as a possession—something one has, holds, or owns—but rather as a way of marshaling knowledge and skills to provide interpretive frames that will motivate action. Operating across the boundaries between the domains of science, politics, and culture, experts participate not only in making and validating knowledge claims but also in using those claims to evaluate the state of affairs and propose what should be done.[4] Of course, experts may prove more or less successful in carrying out such work, and as Gil Eyal has emphasized, our inescapable cultural dependence on expertise goes hand in hand with frequently voiced distrust of expert elites.[5]

How does "knowing" inform "doing" across the many world of sexual health? And how does the evaluative labor of experts create, reinforce, or challenge ideas about what sexuality and health are meant to be like? This chapter analyzes the development of sexual health expertise while emphasizing the wrinkles that complicate the understanding of expertise generally, as it operates in contemporary societies. The first complication is that experts *disagree*, and all the more so as the number and kinds of experts increase. In recent decades, sexual health expertise has become omnipresent, but it has also become just as varied as the diversification of sexual health would suggest. The many sexual health activities, responding to different social problems, all offer platforms from which a diverse assortment of experts now speak. The many components of the WHO working definition, and the various aspects of the sexual health "umbrella," likewise suggest very different groundings for expert claims and counterclaims. Among the cacophony of voices, which ones should be trusted?

The second complication is that, nowadays, not only are experts increasingly subject to challenge by the laity, but it also has become less clear, in many domains, who counts as part of which camp. Even as more and more professionals are involving themselves with matters of sexual health, and as expertise spills out beyond the boundaries of the medical profession to encompass many different understandings of "health," many of the speakers who claim authority to speak about sexual health transgress the boundaries between professional and lay worlds. The proliferation of expertise has coincided not only with its diversification but also with deprofessionalization—and with the emergence of new, hybrid "lay experts."[6] Along with all the platforms comes a seemingly infinite number of soapboxes. Thus, the complex dynamics between the "operationalizers" and their various clients and publics that we observed in the previous three chapters are even more sharply in evidence here, and it has therefore become much harder to say exactly what constitutes, or who embodies, sexual health expertise or to trace its ramifying effects.

I begin with an overview of the shifting boundaries of sexual health expertise, then focus on the social role of the purveyor of sexual health advice, and then consider various forms of challenge to expertise, including community-based expertise. Finally, the chapter takes up the question of norms and normality: I argue that the changing configurations of sexual health expertise have complicated our assessment of how experts contribute to defining normality.

Shifting Boundaries

SPECIALIZATION, PROFESSIONALIZATION, AND CREDENTIALING

Who gets to be called a sexual health expert? Against the backdrop of which social changes, and through which mechanisms, do people assemble the tools and techniques that allow them to intervene credibly and give voice to sexual health truths?[7] Some individuals stand out because of their foundational roles as field builders. Eli Coleman, whose name surfaces repeatedly in this book, has functioned not only as an innovator but also as a central node in transnational networks of sexual health expertise. When Coleman received a lifetime achievement award at the National Sexual Health Conference in 2019, the presenter, Dennis Fortenberry, commented plausibly: "You could easily say that without Eli's influence there wouldn't be sexual health as we know it in the United States." By that point, Coleman had served as president of the World Association of Sexology, the International Academy of Sex Research, the Society for the Scientific Study of Sexuality, the Society for Sex Therapy and Research, and the World Professional Association for Transgender Health, and he held the inaugural chair in sexual health at the University of Minnesota.[8]

Beyond the obvious cases, however, the criteria become more diffuse and harder to discern. Attention to specific professional domains helps clarify the nature of sexual health expertise, and the growth of fields such as sexual medicine is one prominent development. The International Society for Sexual Medicine reports having over two thousand members from eighty-nine countries across five continents, all of whom build and share expertise through the society's four official journals and its regular conferences.[9] While the practitioners of sexual medicine are known especially for their highly visible pharmaceutical solutions to sexual difficulties, the approaches within the field are broad enough to encompass various forms of expert knowledge and practice. At Northwestern University's Center for Sexual Medicine and Menopause, which opened in 2017 under the direction of Dr. Lauren Streicher, the emphasis is on addressing a range of sexual concerns experienced by women, including vulvar pain and painful intercourse. According to Streicher, "There's so many women who have a physical, hormonal or medical condition that has sabotaged her sex life." Her center promises to "develop a program that gets you back to your peak sexual health."[10]

However, clinicians practicing under the banner of sexual medicine stand as just one example of credentialed sexual health expertise. Increasingly, experts on sexual health can be found across a wide array of recognized professions. In 2007 the World Association for Sexual Health identified the following professional specialties as falling under the broad rubric of sexology, in a document endorsed by its general assembly: sexual counselor, sexual psychotherapist, sexual medicine practitioner, sexual health physician, sexual health surgeon, sexuality educator, sexological researcher, sexological anthropologist, and sexological sociologist. In defining each specialty, the WAS consistently emphasized the possession of proper credentials from the relevant discipline as well as the achievement of specialized training in sexual health—for example, a "sexual health surgeon" was defined as "a person with recognised medical qualification [who is] specifically trained in the practice of sexology as it applies to the provision of surgical services related to sexual health."[11] However, beyond the insistence on credentials and training, the looseness of the definitions and their somewhat tautological nature—a sexual health surgeon is a surgeon who does sexual health surgery—did little to bound or characterize these professional domains.

Other professional associations are even more capacious and inclusive. The American Association of Sexuality Educators, Counselors and Therapists (AASECT), a not-for-profit interdisciplinary professional organization, has described its membership as consisting not only of the aforementioned educators, counselors, and therapists but also of

"physicians, nurses, social workers, psychologists, allied health professionals, clergy members, lawyers, sociologists, marriage and family
counselors and therapists, family planning specialists and researchers,
as well as students in relevant professional disciplines." According to
the AASECT website, what all these kinds of members share is simply "an interest in promoting understanding of human sexuality and
healthy sexual behavior."[12]

Evidence from the worlds of scholarly research similarly demonstrates the substantial spread of sexual health expertise across recognized domains of scientific knowledge making. Using software that
traces the diffusion of a research topic in scientific journal articles, my
research assistant found that, in the early 1990s (just before what I
described as the proliferation period) sexual health was largely the
domain of researchers in general medicine, public health, psychology,
and a few other fields. Two decades later, the concern with sexual health
had spread to academics in pharmacology, geriatrics, computer science
information, sociology, women's studies, geography, economics, and a
host of other disciplines.[13]

Indeed, nowadays more and more categories of credentialed professionals are handing out their business cards, claiming to bring specialized expertise to bear on sexual health, if not to the general public
then for the benefit of other experts. For example, an article published
in 2014 in the journal *Sexually Transmitted Infections* asked in its title:
"What can geographic information science (GIS) offer sexual health
research?" and revealed a range of tools that geographers might provide to epidemiologists.[14] In another example, a roundtable discussion
in the journal *Games for Health* in 2015 examined the goal of enlisting
the expertise of game designers in order to develop "serious games" for
sexual health education—games that are "theory-driven," that invoke
"well established models," and that have been adequately tested using
"randomized controlled trials." As one participant noted, the success
of this work presumed the union of multiple forms of expertise, including not just "expertise in sexual health behavior change" but also
in programming skills, CGI animation techniques, and "end-user engagement."[15] Increasingly, then, the everyday business of sexual health
promotion requires, and provides the grounds for development of,
cross-fertilization across many existing and emergent expert domains.

Many of the new understandings of sexual health expertise invoke
and rely on the credentialing processes of established fields: the experts

are those who can brandish their medical degree, doctorate, or coun-seling degree and bring them to bear on sexual health. However, an increasing trend accompanying the expansion of expertise is the emer-gence of new credentials that are specific to sexual health. The Univer-sity of Michigan's School of Social Work, for example, offers a Sexual Health Certificate Program, intended "to provide comprehensive edu-cation and training to professionals about sexual health." Depending on their prior training and career interests, students may pursue a num-ber of different tracks, including sexuality education, sex therapy, and sexuality counseling.[16]

Other credentialing programs are based not in higher learning in-stitutions but out in the broader world of sexual health promotion and service provision. Options for Sexual Health, a sexual and reproductive health clinic in Vancouver, British Columbia, offers "sexual health edu-cator certification" (SHEC), attesting to the recipient's competence "to deliver comprehensive sexual health education sessions to a variety of audiences in the public and private sectors." After an investment of $3,600 and attendance at five three-day workshops, "graduates of the SHEC program will be eligible to say they are an Options for Sexual Health Certified Sexual Health Educator."[17] Credentialing programs such as these suggest how the field of sexual health has become sufficiently well established to generate its own pathways toward, and criteria for, the achievement of specialized expertise.

FROM MEDICINE TO HEALTH:
EXPERT, NONEXPERT, AND IN-BETWEEN

In 2013, an NIH-funded study conducted at Baylor University con-cluded that hypnotic relaxation therapy improves sexual health for post-menopausal women with hot flashes. The study's findings indicated that women's sexual comfort, sexual satisfaction, and sexual pleasure all benefited from the therapy, which therefore should be considered as a safe and effective alternative to hormone replacement therapy. While the study was led by a doctoral student in psychology and neurosci-ence, the treatment sessions were conducted by masters-level thera-pists trained in clinical hypnosis.[18]

In this case, a so-called alternative or complementary healing prac-tice was incorporated within mainstream biomedical research that was conducted at a well-known research university and funded by a US federal government agency. A somewhat different case is suggested by everyday practitioners of hypnotherapy who use it to promote sexual health. At A Time for Change Hypnotherapy in Lakewood, Colorado, the practice is recommended for a wide range of "sex and intimacy issues," including desire and arousal problems, erectile dysfunction, vaginismus, and "unwanted sexual proclivities."[19] The clinic's hypnotherapist is described as "licensed and certified . . . with a diploma from the accredited Hypnosis Motivation Institute."[20] In this case, in contrast with the Baylor study, we see aspiring new professionals entering the sexual health business, but working at some remove from the institutions, traditions, and paradigms of biomedicine.

As I described in chapter 2, a consequential development of recent decades is a more general broadening of who speaks in the name of health—an expansion of cultural authority well beyond the medical profession to encompass a wide array of practitioners and promoters of health and well-being.[21] How should life be lived? What makes it worth living? While doctors once competed for authority over such matters with those, such as clergy, who invoked competing rationales *other than* health, nowadays doctors may at times find their voices diminished or even drowned out within a cacophony of commentary and advice from those who, like them, invoke health, yet do so not from a biomedical standpoint. As Kristin Barker has described in a study of "mindfulness meditation" as a health practice, such developments extend the sway of "health" (or the ideology of healthism) while challenging the specific influence of medical professionals.[22]

With this shift in cultural authority from "medicine" to "health," it has become more difficult to say who is a health expert and why. What are the warrants of authority? What, for example, qualifies an art museum staff member to lead workshops for people with Alzheimer's disease, to "trigger memories using works of art as prompts"?[23] Such questions are particularly acute in the domain of sexual health, which has seen both an intensification of biomedical work and a diversification of expert activities well beyond the medical domain. Indeed, sexual health stands as an especially compelling example of trends that are increasingly visible throughout the medical and health arenas.

The psychologist and sexuality studies scholar Leonore Tiefer has hinted at the new complexities of sexual health expertise by pointing to simultaneous tendencies: at the same time that we witness "the growing visibility of a new cadre of 'sexual medicine' specialists backed by the pharmaceutical industry in the past two decades," we also observe "a growing collection of professionals, other than mainstream health professionals, who offer sexuality advice and treatment (e.g., experts on nutrition, detoxification, yoga, prayer, hypnosis, massage, vitamin injections, and pelvic floor function, not to mention devotees of Primal 'Scream' Therapy or other healing ritual therapies)."[24]

Despite their unconventional beliefs and practices, these new experts "frequently strive for professional status (and remuneration) and use quasi medical model language."[25] Therefore, from Tiefer's perspective, these new experts and aspiring professionals are not posing a meaningful challenge to what she describes as the pervasive medicalization of sexuality. It may be more accurate to say, however, that, as authority moves outward "from medicine to health," these experts are finding non-biomedical routes to the healthicization of sexuality. As biomedical expertise around sexual health grows, but as authority in the health domain simultaneously continues its march well beyond the biomedical, we find both that credentialed experts are staking out terrain around sexual health and that new species of experts are emerging and working to establish their credentials and credibility.

A Plethora of Advice

Some of the most intriguing developments with regard to sexual health expertise concern the rapid expansion of a distinctive niche: providing sex advice to the public. Such advice giving demonstrates especially clearly how experts operationalize sexuality through processes of evaluation—and prescription. Of course, this social role has a long history: I described in chapter 1 how sex advice blossomed in places like the United States in the nineteenth and early twentieth centuries, mostly but not always in the form of popular books published by physicians. In recent decades, sexual health advice has flourished, especially with the advent of new technologies of distribution, and it has diversified in ways that increasingly confound many assumptions about what it means to be an expert. Of course, not all sex advice is framed as being a matter of sexual health, but the same tendencies that lead so many sexual matters to be recoded as health concerns are very much at play in this domain as well.

CELEBRITY DOCTORS AND NONDOCTORS

The format of the radio call-in show, in which listeners pose questions to a host, has presented new opportunities for sexual health advice, especially since the 1980s. Various advice givers, including "Dr. Ruth" Westheimer, "Dr. Drew" Pinsky, and "Dr. Laura" Schlessinger, became celebrities in the United States after taking up this medium. All three adopted the practice of tagging an honorific to their given names, signaling professional credentials alongside approachability. (Pinsky is trained as a medical doctor, Schlessinger holds a PhD in physiology, and Westheimer received a doctorate in education. Interestingly, both Pinsky and Westheimer were raised as Jewish, and Schlessinger, the product of a Jewish-Catholic marriage, later converted to Judaism.) Their programs were highly popular: Schlessinger, for example, claimed a radio audience of twenty million listeners. All three also wrote and published self-help books—a lengthy list, in Westheimer's case, including *Dr. Ruth's Guide for Married Lovers* and *Sex for Dummies*. Yet their perspectives were quite different. Westheimer—feisty and grandmotherly—defended the importance of sexuality while locating its proper placement squarely within the context of marriage, love, and relationships. Schlessinger presented a social conservative counterpoint, decrying the breakdown of traditional gender roles and the extension of rights to LGBT people. Pinsky, who also appeared on MTV's *Loveline* show for many years, offered what was deemed a hipper version of sex commentary for a younger audience.[26]

The range of views among these three pioneers is indicative of how differentiated sex advice has become, with something on offer for just about everyone, regardless of sexual identity, political leanings, or religious beliefs.[27] Nowadays, one can find specialized sexual health advice in every corner of the internet. In the process of developing a market for their advice, however, practitioners have often moved away from any presumption that expertise demands validation and certification via formal credentials or honorifics.

In the United States, one exemplar of the new, deprofessionalized sexual health advice is Dan Savage, a journalist, author, and LGBT activist who, in 1991, launched a sex and relationship advice column called "Savage Love." Originally appearing in an alternative newspaper in Seattle, the column is now syndicated internationally, and, in 2006, Savage expanded to a weekly podcast of call-in advice.[28] In responding to questions posed to him, Savage traverses a wide array of issues related to sexuality, but certainly including sexual health in a number of the senses referenced in this book, including topics such as sexually transmissible infections, sexual dysfunction, the HPV vaccine, the morning-after pill, and sex education. In 2013, Options for Sexual Health, the Canadian organization mentioned earlier in this chapter, named Savage as its "Sexual Health Champion" for the year; its executive director noted that Savage "has done so much for bringing questions of sex and sexual health out of the closet and into everyday conversations."[29]

Savage's positions on casual sex, pornography, same-sex marriage, gay teen suicide, and transgender issues have been controversial both among social conservatives and within LGBTQ communities. Yet his distance from traditional sex advice—and the conventional honorifics accorded to experts—was signaled from the start by his insistence, which lasted until 1999, that each question posed to him be published in his advice column with the salutation "Hey, Faggot."[30]

In more recent years, with the arrival of new technological possibilities for the construction of audiences and the global dissemination of messages, sex advice is increasingly on offer from "social media influencers who share content specifically to break down the taboos surrounding sexual health."[31] Along the way, sexual health expertise has developed in even more deprofessionalized directions. As the headline of a *New York Times* article expressed it in 2016, "The Sex-Ed Queens of YouTube Don't Need a PhD." The article, by Amanda Hess, described sexual health experts such as Laci Green, who began posting videos from her dorm room in 2008, and whose videos had been viewed a combined 131 million times: "She's building a digital empire around what she calls 'sex ed for the Internet,' and she's leading a new generation of amateur sexperts along with her. They earn money from college speaking engagements; ads on YouTube; and by sponsoring products like Durex condoms and the period-tracker app Clue."[32] Green's lack of formal training in sexual health, like that of her young compatriots, was precisely the point: "While Dr. Ruth, Dr. Laura and Dr. Drew telegraphed their academic credentials in their names, modern sex-ed stars make an asset of their amateurism. Eileen Kelly, the 20-year-old Instagram-famous founder of the sex blog and forum Birds&Bees, self-effacingly refers to herself as 'a random girl from Seattle.' The British sex-ed YouTuber Hannah Witton calls herself a 'self-taught expert,' and her lack of credentials is part of her message."[33]

For others who have turned sex advice into a career, the absence of credentials is likewise no impediment, even if it prompts some ambivalence about one's status. "Alexander Cheves isn't entirely comfortable being called a sex advisor because he lacks a formal clinical education or sex therapy certification," observed a columnist in 2019. "But for the thousands of young gay men who know him as The Beastly Ex-Boyfriend he's a touchstone for understanding their kinks and desires from the explosion in popularity of 'pup play' to, well, *use your imagination.*" On his website, Cheves has been "Answering Queer, Kinky Sex & Love Questions since 2014."[34] The case of sex expert Emily Morse is also instructive. Before she began producing the podcast "Sex with Emily," offering a daily two-hour radio show on SiriusXM, and answering questions on Instagram for the benefit of her three hundred thousand followers, Morse had received a bachelor's degree in psychology and had been working as a video producer. When Nekisa Cooper, the vice president of content at the educational platform MasterClass, was asked why she invited Morse to offer online advice, Cooper cited Morse's mastery of her topic but also the fact that "she's so accessible." Said Cooper: "I can totally see myself having a conversation with her about my most intimate things that I never thought I would say, and asking for help and support."[35]

PORN SITES AND PORN STARS

A fascinating further development in the extension of new networks of sexual health expertise is the blurring of boundaries between sexual health advice and pornographic entertainment. At Pornhub, a highly popular source of pornographic materials online, users can also click to the Sexual Wellness Center, a free, online resource that offers informative articles on a range of sexual topics and lists more than two dozen "contributors" to whom questions may be submitted.[36] The company describes its Sexual Wellness Center as "a one-stop shop, available 24/7, to facilitate your needs, be it comprehensive information regarding STIs and safe sex, the latest in sex tech or advice on how to approach a friends with benefits arrangement."[37] Lest any Pornhub visitors misunderstand the purpose, the website carefully explains: "This is for sexual health related questions only. All unrelated inquiries will be ignored."[38]

Needless to say, one function of providing sexual health information in such a venue is to lend legitimacy to a porn site: here again, we see how "health" sanitizes "sexuality." Yet Pornhub's investment in the marshaling of expertise is far from trivial, and it also demonstrates how alternative forums and formats can permit new forms of expertise to flourish. When the service was launched in 2017, Corey Price, Pornhub's vice president, said, "As a leading provider of adult entertainment, we thought it important that we also offer a platform on which carefully sourced information about all aspects of sexuality [could] be made available to our viewers."[39] The experts available for consultation include doctorates in psychology, neuroscientists, OB/GYNs, a certified sex therapist, a photographer, a dating and relationship coach, BDSM practitioners and educators, and a self-described "international sex hacking expert/educator, former top fitness professional, and private celebrity fitness and sex-ed coach."[40]

In the case of Pornhub's Sexual Wellness Center, the link to pornography is primarily the venue itself. In other cases, the boundaries between sexual health and porn are even more elastic. Porn star and sex educator jessica drake (a three-time Adult Video News Best Actress winner, and also a Donald Trump accuser) has produced a series of educational DVDs, with demonstrations by live performers, called "jessica drake's Guide to Wicked Sex." According to drake's website, the videos reflect her "passion for education": "Uniting a lifetime of study with a decade's worth of experiential research, this charming Texan is sharing her expertise with audiences around the globe."[41] Drake has also offered sex education seminars and workshops around the United States, including to a classroom of health professionals and marriage and family therapists at UCLA in 2012.[42]

The Politics of Skepticism and New Articulations of Expertise

WHOM TO TRUST?

Whether it arrives in a professionalized and credentialed form or emphatically not, sexual health expertise is, apparently, omnipresent. New technologies increasingly facilitate its circulation—indeed, new technologies make it possible for sexual health expertise to manifest in novel ways that change its character or ontology. The provision of sexual health advice nowadays by digital assistants such as Apple's Siri and Google Assistant—while not necessarily very accurate, according to an evaluation published in a medical journal in 2017[43]—demonstrates that expertise may be a remarkably heterogeneous confection not entirely bounded by the category "human." Perhaps more reliably, Planned Parenthood's "Roo chatbot," designed to answer the sexual health questions of hard-to-reach teens, also shows how expert knowledge about sexual health is now embedded in and produced by complex assemblages of people and devices.[44]

An inevitable consequence of the diversification and profusion of sexual health advice is anxiety related to assessing the reliability of advice and, in particular, the legitimacy of the expert. Whom should we trust? Of course, this is a fundamental concern about expertise generally, one that acquires particular force at a historical moment when we are ever more suspicious of experts even as we cannot imagine doing without them.[45] In an article posted in 2019 on *Bustle*, the "certified sex educator and writer" Emma McGowan addressed the question in an article entitled "How to Tell If a Sexual Health Resource Is Legit, According to a Sex Educator."[46] While pointing affirmatively to authorities like the CDC and Planned Parenthood, McGowan also acknowledged that "for certain people, like kinksters or LGBTQ folks, these formal institutions may not always have information that is relevant to their specific needs—and sometimes can even feel discriminatory." Hence the need to diversify one's sources of information—but also to "be sure to check and see if your favorite sex educators have any certifications, which are a good indication that they know what they're talking about." Checking on the length of "experience in the field" is also a must, though as McGowan pointed out, "experience" can mean many things, from having hosted workshops, written a comprehensive book, or worked as sex worker.

In the article, McGowan presented her own proofs of expertise, which included being an "SFSI-endorsed sex educator" who had written "all of the copy for the sexual health website 'Sexual + Being' for nearly a decade."[47] Left implicit was McGowan's assumption that her own status as a sexual health expert in itself provided the warrant for her to assess the credibility of other sexual health experts, who, of course, might make claims to expertise on widely divergent bases.

EXPERTISE AND EXPERIENCE

It is hard to assess the impact of the expansion of sexual health expertise. It seems possible that this expansion serves to privilege expertise as a phenomenon more than to valorize the individual experts themselves. That is, the proliferation of kinds of sexual health expertise may circumscribe the authority of any particular expert while reinforcing the idea that sexual health is something about which one might speak authoritatively. Yet it is also possible that the simple evidence that experts come in so many flavors, and the widespread recognition that they often disagree, serves to reduce the credibility of sexual health expertise writ large: it may cast a cloud over the very idea of expertise and privilege alternative modes of speech.

Writing in the late 1990s, the sociologist Joshua Gamson captured some of these cultural tendencies in his analysis of daytime television talk shows, which he found to be theaters of visibility for sex and gender nonconformity, but also stages on which expertise was simultaneously promoted and devalued. On programs like *Donahue, Geraldo,* and *The Jenny Jones Show,* subjects identified as gay cops, cross-dressing hookers, women who love gay men, drag kings, and many others bared their souls and indulged their grievances, while teaching "ordinary" viewers about lives often rendered invisible. These enormously popular and deliberately sensationalistic shows provided a constrained yet meaningful venue for the marginalized—sex and gender outcasts, often also working class and/or people of color—to have their day in the spotlight. But they also leveled the playing field between experts and those whom they purported to know about. Experts on gender and sexuality who appeared on these shows were rarely deferred to, were regularly interrupted, and were generally treated as presenting just another point of view. Schooled expertise struggled to compete with the authority of experience.[48]

NEW COMMUNITIES OF EXPERTISE

The dynamics of expert-lay encounters in forums like daytime talk shows capture certain aspects of a charged relationship, as does the increasing tendency for people to claim the right to name themselves—to apply distinctive sexual and gender identity labels to themselves, or to reject labeling outright, rather than passively wearing the identity "hats" that credentialed experts place on their heads.[49] At the same, an important manifestation of distrust of conventional expertise is the emergence of new varieties of "lay expertise" as the collective, politically engaged work of mobilized communities.[50] This development reflects a commitment to advocacy around sexuality, but it also aligns with an important transformation in the health arena: the increased involvement of patients as information managers, advocates, and activists.[51] While not necessarily challenging a medical perspective, and while often seeking alliances with credential medical experts, health advocacy of this sort typically involves heightened public scrutiny of expert practices. The growing participation in expert domains of people lacking formal expert credentials—educating fellow patients and the public about illnesses and treatments, and even working to transform medical research practices—has challenged conventional notions of expert subfields as discrete and bounded arenas of practice.[52]

In fact, sex is central to this history, and the increased tendency for patients and their advocates to bridge "evidence" with "experience" is exemplified by many community-based organizations focused on sexual health concerns. A defining example comes from the early days of the HIV/AIDS epidemic, when local organizations, rooted initially in LGBTQ communities, sought to educate the public about sexual health risks and remedies. Jeffrey Escoffier has described the sophisticated mobilization of "vernacular knowledge" as a response to urgent need as well as rampant homophobia and stigmatization: "HIV prevention as a public health project among gay men has been shaped by their everyday knowledge of sexuality and community mores and that knowledge's contribution to epidemiological research."[53] As early as 1983, the same year that a possible cause of AIDS was first identified in a laboratory, gay men in the United States had published the first guidelines on safer-sex practices, and the gay press and community-based organizations had begun to circulate crucial advice on how to continue to have sex yet do so as safely as possible.[54]

That these organizations possessed relevant expertise was widely acknowledged. In the midst of the 1984 controversy over whether to close down the gay bathhouses in San Francisco, a state superior court judge hearing arguments on the case mandated the San Francisco AIDS Foundation to define which activities practiced in bathhouses were safe and which were not.[55] Of course, this kind of community-based expertise did not spring out of nowhere; in chapter 3, I described some of the longer history of gay community activism around issues of health and sexuality. However, the brutal necessities of the epidemic (combined with the stark absence, in the United States, of meaningful federal leadership to fight it during the pivotal early years) propelled the development of an extensive network of lay expertise, spread across service organizations and grassroots activist groups. Those who were mobilized as part of this network saw it as their duty to engage in a broad-based project of knowledge empowerment of the community.[56]

Yet the kind of community-based lay expertise that emerges in the context of immediate health risks is just one example. Another noteworthy case is the promotion of lay expertise around sexual health by "sex-positive" feminists. This work has taken shape from the 1970s forward, rooted in second-wave feminism. The recent death at age ninety-one of Betty Dodson, hailed in a *New York Times* obituary as "a feminist sexologist and evangelist of self-pleasure who taught generations of women how to masturbate in workshops, books and videos," called attention to this history.[57] Blending the personal and the political in novel ways, Dodson saw "the do-it-yourself climax as a liberating social force."[58] Through her books such as *Sex for One* (published by Random House and translated into twenty-five languages), but especially via her famous consciousness-raising workshops, held in her home, that involved genital "show and tell" and preached women's right to pleasure, Dodson productively blurred the roles of sex advice purveyor and organizer-activist.[59]

To be sure, Dodson's interests in sexuality extended well beyond what might typically be called sexual health, and her preeminent interest in pleasure threatened to burst the bounds of the sexual health frame. Yet for Dodson, health concerns were often woven into her approach to sexuality: she emphasized what she called "the importance of orgasm to our psychic and physical health," and she described her consciousness-raising groups as being devoted a wide mix of topics, including. "health, yoga, and the martial arts," plus genital hygiene and birth control.[60] Here, again, expertise was rooted as much in the authenticity of personal experience as in claims to specialized knowledge, and it was as much a collective enterprise as an individual endeavor. The sexologist and feminist activist Carol Queen attested to Dodson's broad influence: "Women flocked to her workshops, and some stayed around to develop their own styles of teaching, or activist work, or went back to school so they could be therapists or midwives or whatever style of work that would let them be themselves and make a difference."[61]

Queen herself, a sex-positive feminist and writer with a PhD in human sexuality, became the "staff sexologist" at Good Vibrations, the foundational feminist sex shop in San Francisco.[62] In the early years of the HIV/AIDS epidemic, Queen helped to create and organize a series of intensive and interactive safer-sex workshops called the Sexual Health Attitude Restructuring Process, which employed films, personal sharing, massage, "condom relay races," and blindfolded rituals to promote "sensate focus."[63] Along with Queen, Dodson also influenced a range of sex-positive feminists who became influential sex experts in their own right, including author Susie Bright, one of the founding staff of Good Vibrations; as well as the porn-star-turned-sex-expert and performer Annie Sprinkle, who describes herself as "the first porn star in history to get a Ph.D.," which she earned at the Institute for Advanced Study of Human Sexuality in San Francisco.[64] These various sex-positive feminists in turn provided an example for many alternative sexuality communities that today share information online and advocate on behalf of the safe and pleasurable engagement in a wide range of sexual practices, often challenging biomedical perspectives as well as conventional social norms.[65]

Community-based expertise of this sort spans various boundaries: between expert and lay worlds, between suspicion and embrace of expertise, and between individual advice giving and collective social change. Simultaneously, it challenges many conventional ideas about what it means to promote sexual health. An increasing number of groups are finding it a helpful model for calling attention simultaneously to sexual health needs and erotic rights, using a variety of platforms. In England, for example, the collectively produced *Black Fly Zine*, launched in 2016, has been described as "the foremost sex zine for people of colour."[66] Nominated as Grassroots Organization of the Year at the Sexual Health Awards 2020, the collective behind *Black Fly* also organizes workshops and considers itself as building a "community for sexual wellbeing."[67] As expressed in the group's manifesto, *Black Fly* "centralises the thoughts and feelings of marginalized Black and Brown people in their sexual health"; "seeks to honour and include intergenerational experience"; "believes in messily and vigorously imagined futures"; "is motivated by the collective unpacking of binaries"; and "likes to keep things sticky, rough, raw and open."[68]

While adopting the terminology and label of sexual health, the Black Fly collective presents a radical take on the idea of it that foregrounds both sexual pleasure and anti-racism, conveyed in striking visual terms (fig. 8). According to one participant, Bui Mushekwa, "We work to validate and actively support the experience of ethnic minorities as they

navigate their sexual health within the context of oppressive historical and colonial structures that often hinder the wellbeing of black and
brown people across various identities."[69] One of the founders, Ella Frost,
described *Black Fly* as not so much a "guide" as "a validation to see yourself reflected back."[70] The identities called out for reflection are quite

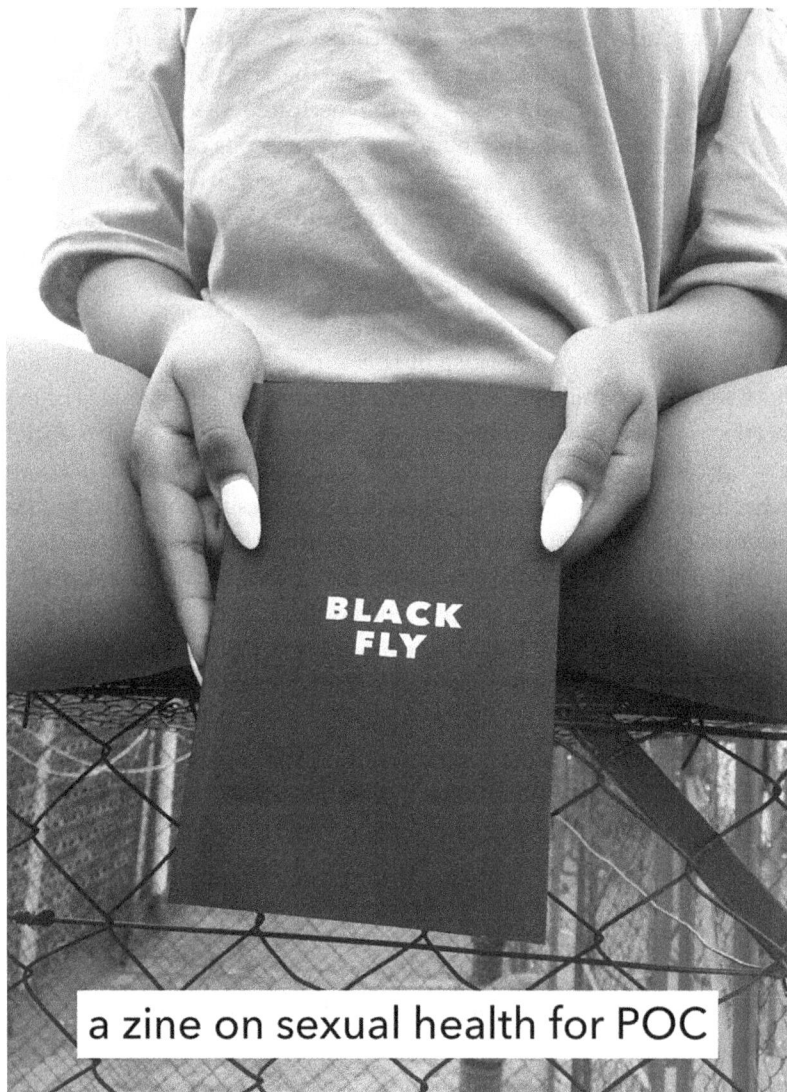

Figure 8: *Black Fly Zine*
Source: *Black Fly Zine* (see https://www.facebook.com/blackflyzine). Reproduced with permission.

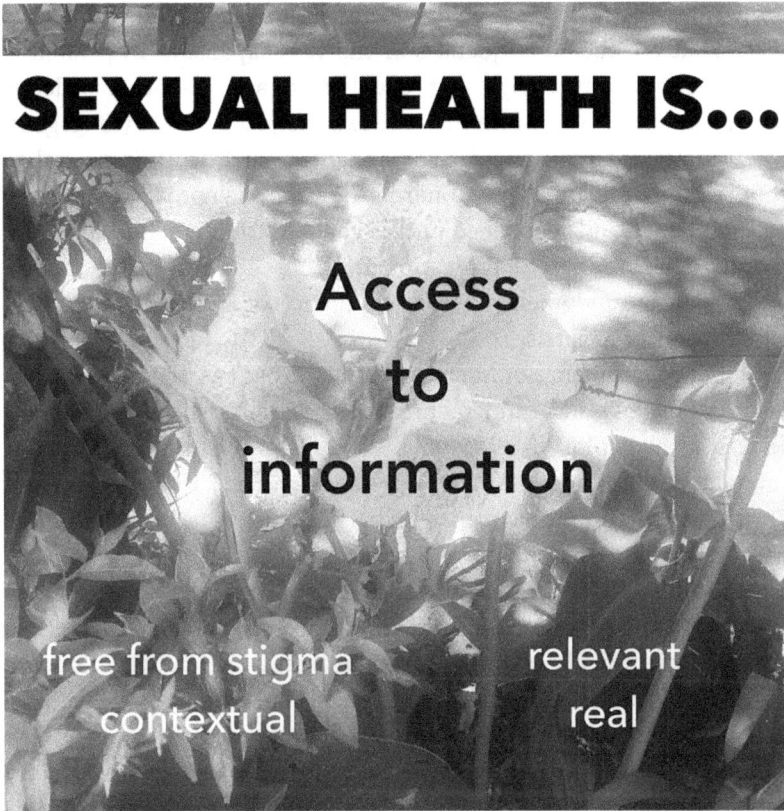

SEXUAL HEALTH IS...

Access
to
information

free from stigma   relevant
contextual   real

Figure 8: (*continued*)

diverse. In a zine called *Swallow It Whole*, produced by Black Fly in collaboration with another organization and devoted to promoting preexposure prophylaxis (PrEP) to prevent HIV infection in Black and Brown women, the authors observed: "We're proud to have made one of few sexual health resources written by and tailored for black women, and to have been able to include contributions from PrEP users, sex worker advocates, trans rights activists, and a range of straight, bi & queer women."[71]

Expertise and the Norm

Traversing the ground from the practitioners of sexual medicine to Dr. Ruth to the Beastly Ex-Boyfriend to Betty Dodson to Black Fly shows how tricky it would be to generalize about sexual health expertise. What are the consequences of the vast expansion in personnel who speak authoritatively about sexual health and produce knowledge or provide services to promote it? If experts prototypically engage in processes of evaluating and advising, and if such work is central to the creation or dismantling of norms, how are such processes affected by the many trends described in this chapter, from credentialing and professionalization, to deprofessionalization, to the rise of resistance against expert judgment, to the emergence of hybrid, community-based forms of expertise?

Under the influence of Michel Foucault, it has been common to understand expertise as fundamental to processes of social control. For Foucault, the explosion of sexual discourses in the modern West was fundamentally connected to the rise of new expert knowledge-making practices in relation to sexuality—in particular, the role of clinical medicine, psychology, psychoanalysis, and sexology in generating new understandings of sexual matters. Crucially, for Foucault, these forms of knowledge and expertise served to "normalize" individuals—that is, to generate scientifically validated norms against which individuals could be compared, measured, placed, and ranked, and thereby judged as normal or abnormal.[72] Here, my analysis suggests both continuity as well as change. In the current era of sexual health, the linkage of sexuality to the imperative of health necessarily continues to locate sexual matters in relation to norms of various kinds: as we have seen in the chapters that make up part 2, forms of sexuality are regularly measured, diagnosed, compared, judged, evaluated and, not uncommonly, found wanting. Yet as I have also shown, the kinds of expertise deemed relevant have also multiplied considerably, even while the boundaries between credentialed and unofficial authorities have blurred. For these reasons, no actor, group, or institution monopolizes the ability to say who or what is "normal" or "abnormal."

The point can be made with reference to a famous distinction offered by the anthropologist of sexuality Gayle Rubin in her canonical article from 1984. Rubin proposed that social space at any given moment could be divided between what she called the "charmed circle" of socially acceptable sexualities (such as vanilla, heterosexual, monogamous, and same generation) and the "outer limits" of abnormal, unnatural, and condemned sexualities (such as S/M, promiscuous, for money, and cross-generational).[73] As a rough heuristic depicted in a diagram, Rubin's formulation has been influential (though also subject to critique for being too culturally specific).[74] Yet—as Rubin herself acknowledged—even in a given society at a specific time, it is probably difficult to determine exactly where the normative boundaries lie, precisely because they are always contested and because, within societies, norms vary to a potentially significant degree.

My point takes this concern further: the effect of the diversification of sexual health and the proliferation of sexual health expertise in recent decades is not to reduce the presence of normalization but to amplify the variability of normative judgments. The multiplicity of meanings that emerge from sexual health projects, and the many kinds of advice offered by sexual health experts of different varieties and inclinations, defy any simple attempt to arrive at a unique categorization of the normative implications. In place of a single hierarchy of sexual valuation, from most privileged to least, we may find a "heterarchy" or "plurarchy" of multiple and competing orderings.[75]

Of course, this does mean that all expert opinions carry the same weight in practice: some experts speak with much more consequence than others. Some have the institutional backing that not only gives their pronouncements more authority but also transforms their views into standardized procedures—which is why a project like a revision of the ICD, carried out under the auspices of the WHO, matters enough for people to fight over the contents. Some have easier access to the communication technologies that will disseminate their messages widely, even as the rise of new technologies offers additional options for distribution. Some have the credentials and diplomas that, even at a time when traditional expertise is often suspect, nonetheless often carry weight. Thus, experts meet on an uneven playing field. But at the same time, ordinary people may often be left with more freedom to choose which experts to heed, though also with the anxiety of knowing that having to choose can itself be a burden. And therefore, when it comes to sexuality and health, the linkages that connect expert judgments about normality with the social and cultural norms that inform conduct show more slippage than a Foucauldian approach might suggest.

Operationalization and Its Many Effects

Over the course of part 2, I have described a range of projects that seek to "tame" sexuality by operationalizing sexual health—an important but difficult task. While it is not uncommon for scientists to encounter difficulties in creating "working objects" for research purposes, the point is that some objects are harder to corral than others.[76] Perhaps sexuality—at least according to the cultural understandings that prevail in modern Western societies—is just too refractory or unruly an object to be easily boxed in. As Fernando Domínguez Rubio has written in a different context: "If docile objects are typically elusive objects of study, unruly objects tend to be highly visible. They are typically described as 'problems,' 'disruptions,' 'glitches,' or 'challenges' that need to be fixed or solved."[77] Hence both the perceived need to impose order and the difficulties in accomplishing it.

This is the vantage point from which to consider the prospects for what, in the preceding chapters, I have called operationalizing sexual health. As we have seen, operationalization works to materialize desires, statuses, and identities relating to sexuality and health by rendering them perceptible and describable.[78] Work of this sort goes beyond the "mere" activity of *defining* sexual health—something that, as became clear in part 1, individuals and organizations may in fact struggle to accomplish. Here, to know sexual health is to take its measure, and this presupposes a series of cognitive and social operations: standardizing, classifying, enumerating, evaluating.[79] Such work is carried out in many domains and at many scales, from interpersonal encounters in the medical clinic to the global health endeavors of the WHO.[80] Operationalizing sexuality may sometimes be necessary in order to transform medicine and health care and provide benefits to patients, clients, and publics, or to produce knowledge using techniques such as surveys that can inform social policy and public health. But operationalizing may also circumscribe and narrow the ways in which those domains grapple with the sexual lives of patients and clients.

Rather than portray the effects of operationalizing in one-sided terms, I have emphasized the ongoing tensions that currently surround and animate it: between the appeals of simplicity and complexity; between the goal of defining normality and the urge to destigmatize sexuality; between the will to know and the will to not know; and between professionalization and lay expertise, or anti-expertise. While the projects of operationalization converge or overlap in many specific ways and may often reinforce one another, one virtue of juxtaposing them is simply to point out they are not all the same—that is, to avoid an

Table 2: Operationalizing Sexuality

Mode of operationalization	How sexuality is construed
Standardized sexual health history	Bundle of risk behaviors
Scales based on patient ratings	Set of functional capacities
Diagnostic classification	Checklists of symptoms corresponding to features of types of individuals
Survey research	Knowable and describable characteristics of a population
Expert advice giving	Behaviors and identities that are perceived as central to lives and relationships

oversimplified reading of what operationalization entails or promotes. To take just one example, across the projects surveyed in part 2, we have seen the very different ways in which social and cultural identities, such as race, ethnicity, gender, and nationality, are conceptualized and addressed. In some cases, they are ignored; in others, they are explicitly determined not to matter; and in still others, differences are made hypervisible as outcome variables, objects of scientific and popular concern, or bases of political mobilization.

Especially clear evidence that not all operationalization is alike comes from how the activities examined in part 2 provide different implicit answers to the same unasked question: *What is sexuality, anyway?* Indeed, in these initiatives, sexuality is construed in remarkably varied ways (table 2). For sexuality to be operationalized as a standardized sexual health history, it must be imagined as a complicated bundle of risk behaviors. For sexuality to be inferred from patient ratings of their behavioral and performative histories and their assessments of satisfaction or dissatisfaction, it must be conceived of fundamentally as a set of functional capacities. For sexuality to be used to sort people into diagnostic boxes, classifiers using checklists treat it as a set of symptoms that refer to either inherent or transient health-related features of types of individuals. For sexuality to be assessed in a survey, it must be conceptualized as the knowable and describable characteristics of a population. And for sexuality to become the object of expert advice, it must be imagined as a constellation of behaviors and identities that are central to people's lives and relationships. It is remarkable that sexuality can be all these different things at once. Yet it makes sense if we follow the approach of the sociologist Stefan Vogler, who likewise found that meanings of sexuality differ significantly by setting depending on the reigning "epistemic logics"—the "institutionalized ways of knowing that guide action in organizational settings and vary based on institutional, cultural, and political factors."[81]

While the ways of thinking of sexuality and sexual health that I have identified are not necessarily mutually exclusive, they do potentially push action and thought in fairly different directions. Once we take these differences into account, then what becomes salient is not the big story of the operationalization of sexual health (or the medicalization or demedicalization of sexuality) but, rather, the *diverse* ways by which experts and professionals of various sorts seek to channel the unruly object that is sexuality and employ it for health-related purposes, and the various consequences that ensue.

Fully understanding the dynamics of operationalization demands a broadened scope. It requires careful assessment of the complex interactions that unfold between "operationalizers" and other actors: policy makers, advocates, the media, and—ultimately and crucially—ordinary people whose sexual health is being weighed, measured, and classified in these various ways.[82] For the taking of a sexual history, it matters not only what doctors ask and how but also how patients answer—how they classify themselves, and which information they deem relevant for disclosure or feel comfortable sharing. In the case of self-administered questionnaires about sexual function, it matters how those selves do the administering—and whether, for example, they feel enjoined by the results to act on the suggestion to ask a doctor whether a particular therapeutic approach is right for them. Diagnoses work to classify people, but those who are called out by the categories may also demand reform of diagnostic systems. Sex surveys depend on truthful respondents and willing funders, but in addition, as we have seen, their results get read by curious people who also may worry about where they fit in relation to the norm, and who may draw moral judgments about their own sexual practices in response to survey results. Experts speak with authority, but those whom they speak about may juxtapose the authority of their own experience. I have provided examples of some of these kinds of responses to operationalization, but clearly this is an area where further study is warranted.

As we widen our focus to capture the many actors who engage with sexual health projects—including governments, the media, social movements, and ordinary people—we also shift away from the concerns of part 2. The rise of sexual health has transformed science, medicine, and health care, but that is not all it has done. To trace the full dimensions of sexual health, our attention must turn to much broader arenas of culture, economics, and politics. This expansion of analytical scope is the purpose of part 3.

Part 3: Under the Sign of Sexual Health

BEYOND THE WORLDS OF SCIENCE AND MEDICINE

As a problem-solving bundle of techniques and ideas, the discourses, practices, and projects of sexual health have proved generative and adaptable. What happens when they travel—when they move more fully into everyday worlds of social, cultural, political, and economic life? In these chapters, I examine what I take to be the three domains into which sexual health has most consequentially extended its presence and been put to use.

First, I propose that through the filter of "wellness," sexual health has emerged as a new arena in which individuals are called on to "optimize" their lives and their bodies, with results that range from self-betterment to commodification to community building. Second, I argue that sexual health has offered tools for the governing of populations and that it sets the parameters of new debates around who counts (fully, partially, or not at all) as a citizen, endowed with rights, prerogatives, and responsibilities. Finally, by tracing how different groups on the political Right and Left use sexual health in order to anchor educational campaigns designed to build better futures, I show how sexual health is employed to reframe political agendas of diverse sorts.

These wide-ranging activities, all enabled in part by the invention of sexual health, demonstrate just how useful sexual health has become as an engine to shape the possibilities and directions of contemporary life. At the same time, the operations of these activities call attention to salient choices about how societies should be organized and lives should be lived.

8 *The Pursuit of Wellness*

A self-described "industry leader in sex education advocacy," the company Tantus Inc. was "thrilled to announce," in 2015, its participation in the second annual Sexual Health Expo, held that year in Phoenix, Arizona. Tantus encouraged attendees to "stop by our table to try our toys, meet members of the Tantus Team, and snag some of your own free Tantus swag." According to the company's advertising, the virtues of its "sexual wellness products"—such as the "VIP Super Soft, the Perfect Strap-On Toy"—extended far beyond their "enticing colors" or the use of a "unique formula of 100% Ultra-Premium Silicone" that is "nontoxic and phthalate free," or the "hours of sculpting, prototyping and testing" that went into their design. More profoundly, Tantus's products came complete with a philosophy that reflected the company's "mission," "values," and "vision": "Tantus was founded on the belief that each person has the right to a healthy sex life and that sexual health encompasses many aspects of physical and mental wellbeing. . . . Tantus believes that a foundation of education will help people live better and happier lives. Tantus believes that our past obligates us to a stewardship for the future of sexual health."[1] These lofty aspirations do more than simply legitimize the sale of sex toys by appealing to a wide array of values and virtues: they locate sexual consumerism in relation to a broader imperative to pursue a lifestyle defined by the goals of health and wellness. By this path, health and wellness are, as the quote suggests, tied inextricably to pleasure, happiness, education, and even the inalienable rights of individuals.

These are not trivial aspirations—and, whatever the motivations for consumption, the size of the financial investment in the so-called "sexual wellness market" also makes the stakes apparent. One estimate by a market research firm valued the global market in sexual wellness products—specifically, sex toys, contraceptives, exotic lingerie and apparels, pregnancy testing products, menstrual cups, and dental dams—at nearly $75 billion in 2019; the report cited the important contribution of emerging economies such as China, India, and Brazil.[2] In the United States, analysts have identified millennials as the driving force in sales, and they have described how "more and more traditional retailers have been updating their sexual wellness sections to include not just family planning and contraceptive products, but also sex toys, devices, lubricants and other items that consumers might otherwise buy online or at competing retailers."[3]

The idea that there might be such a thing as a market in sexual wellness provides one basis for this chapter. But my broader goal is to shed light on the quest to "optimize" one's sexuality—a mission that lies at the juncture of consumption practices and individual self-betterment, and that is authorized, often, by the goals of health and wellness. Such efforts extend beyond the commercial sale of sex toys, lubricants, and contraceptives. Indeed, the most obvious example of such optimization—the case most well discussed and dissected by scholars—is not even included in the above-mentioned market research or estimates of the financial impact of the sexual wellness market: the consumption of Viagra and related "sexuopharmaceuticals" to improve men's sexual function.[4]

In a consequential coincidence of timing, the Food and Drug Administration of the United States (FDA) approved Viagra for sale as a prescription drug in March 1998, just seven months after the agency eased the restrictions that, until then, had forbidden manufacturers from advertising pharmaceuticals directly to the public.[5] Soon Viagra was being pitched to audiences on television, in popular magazines, and on the internet as the preferred treatment for erectile dysfunction—the term that replaced an older, more psychological notion of impotence—prompting millions of men to approach their doctors and request prescriptions. (That such men could then recognize themselves as having a treatable medical problem depended, as well, on the existence and spread of the sexual dysfunction questionnaires that I described in chapter 4, such as the Sexual Health Inventory for Men.) The drug became the top moneymaker for its manufacturer, Pfizer, earning it many billions of dollars.

The positive impact for many men whose ability to have and maintain erections had declined with age should not be underestimated. "You just want to be whole," in the words of one sufferer of erectile dysfunction: "You just want to be like you were before. It's like when somebody has a leg amputated. They get a prosthesis. They can now walk."[6] Proponents of medications like Viagra, such as the urologist Irwin Goldstein, go so far as to compare sexual dysfunction to a kind of death: "These people have horrible lives, they may lose their relationships, and they come in a fairly desperate condition. Some say they'd rather be dead."[7] Yet especially as rival products, such as Cialis and Levitra, came onto the market, observers of pharmaceutical advertising noted a curious ratcheting upward of expectations regarding masculine performance, combined with a chronologically "downward" expansion of the imagined market: a new emphasis on men in their forties and fifties whose erections were simply less than "perfect."[8] "The face of E.D. now is a younger, seemingly much healthier guy," one marketing executive told a reporter for the *New York Times* in 2004. The *Times* article also cited pharma executives' expressed hope of expanding sales of erectile dysfunction drugs to as many as thirty million customers in the United States—that is, about half of all men over forty.[9] By 2017, the *Times* was reporting (in the "Style" section) on the niche marketing of ED drugs to millennials as young as twenty.[10]

Certainly, men's experiences with sexuopharmaceuticals are far from uniform. Use of these medications has varying consequences for their health, sense of masculinity, sexual performance, and relationships with sexual and romantic partners, and no single, overarching story does justice to that diversity of experiences.[11] But the case of Viagra and its cousins captures something about the contemporary quest to optimize sexual health, at least among White, middle- and upper-class men—the idea that, via money (or good health insurance), consumption practices, access to relevant professional expertise, and dedication to self-betterment, one can maximize one's sexual potency and potential, and extend them perhaps indefinitely into the future.[12] To the extent that men with even mild symptoms of ED seek out such drugs, the line blurs between "treatment" and "enhancement."[13]

If the archetypical tales of the present-day optimization of one's sexual health are those of the sexual wellness market on the one hand and the male sexuopharmaceutical industry on the other, then what other stories remain to be told? In this chapter, I seek not just to expand but also to complicate our understanding of the multifaceted pursuit of sexual wellness. I begin by exploring three key concepts—optimization, wellness, and the management of risk—that are intrinsically related to the contemporary commodification of sexual health. Then, after tracing various recent connections between the pursuit of sexual health and contemporary ideas of wellness and well-being, I turn to examples of projects that, perhaps surprisingly, seek to align consumerism and self-optimization with broader political and educational goals. I consider efforts to link sexual wellness consumption with agendas of empowerment and, in particular, gender equality. And I analyze attempts to position sexual optimization at the core of processes of building identity and community while affirming the importance of pleasure. My goal throughout is to emphasize the diverse and double-edged character of these activities of self-actualization and to avoid reductive readings of their complicated effects.

Optimization, Wellness, and the Management of Risk

By *optimization*, I refer to the desire or injunction to treat one's life as a never-ending project of self-improvement, organized particularly around bodily enhancement. Of course, optimizing one's health in general is an important contemporary goal, particularly among those who have the means to pursue it. Treating disease is no longer enough: the modern goal, in the critical view of the bioethicist Carl Elliott, is to become "better than well."[14] Examples are abundant in the domain of sexual wellness: for example, laser vaginal rejuvenation surgery, offered by many cosmetic surgery clinics, promises to enhance vaginal muscle tone and hence improve sexual gratification; while penile enlargement by means of surgery, pumps, pills, creams, or exercises is a concept familiar to most readers of their email "spam" folders. Sex itself is sometimes portrayed as an intrinsically self-optimizing activity. The gender and sexuality studies scholar Kristina Gupta has tracked the scientific and popular press articles that preach the health benefits of engaging in sex—the claims "that sexual activity may increase lifespan, reduce heart attack risk, lower blood pressure, reduce the risk of certain types of cancer, provide pain relief, strengthen immune function, and promote weight loss."[15]

Wellness, the second concept that underlies my analysis in this chapter, "has wormed itself into every aspect of our lives," according to the critical take offered by Carl Cederström and André Spicer in their book *The Wellness Syndrome*.[16] Anna Kirkland has likewise observed the ubiquity of wellness nowadays: "One finds wellness programs, wellness centers, wellness contests, wellness conferences, wellness journals, wellness administrators, wellness awards, wellness tourism, and even a Wellness brand cat and dog food."[17] In the United States, wellness discourses are especially well entrenched in workplace wellness programs, which imagine a "striving, becoming, improving person" as "the ideal employee." These workplace programs seek—sometimes rather coercively and intrusively—to "nudge" employees to adopt healthy behaviors in the hope of reducing health care costs.[18]

But the pursuit of wellness takes many different forms and is often embraced "from below" rather than imposed "from above." Wellness practices have also been called hybrid because of how, according to Justin Lee, they "combine techniques and ideas from across societal sectors ranging from (but not limited to) healing and medicine; psychotherapy and counseling; motivational and personal development practices; fitness and exercise regimes; beauty and personal care services; as well as spiritual and religious movements." Thus, the pursuit of wellness can lead its aspirants to "dabble in a variety of different categories of practices—visiting alternative healers, experimenting with New Age spirituality, reading popular psychological self-help books, trying various fitness exercises, taking nutritional supplements, and engaging personal coaches or psychotherapists to motivate them in life and work."[19]

The growth of wellness industries therefore tracks the more general shift from "medicine" to "health": while the cultural authority of the physician remains strong, the medical profession is now joined by a diverse range of actors who offer diagnoses, treatments, and advice on the business of healthy living.[20] Yet what may often unite the disparate set of activities and motivations that are invoked in the pursuit of wellness, according to sociologist Kelly Moore, is precisely the insistence on optimization of the self. Wellness—which Moore has characterized as the ethos of the "striver class" in a neoliberal historical moment—"is based on the principle of the *optimization* of everything from sexuality, to religious and spiritual life, to sleep, to the speed of our thought processes."[21]

An investment in wellness is a means of anticipating a better future[22]—but it may also reflect, as Nikolas Rose has suggested, the sharp uptick in the "instrumentalizing of anxiety" about health and the body.

As a consequence of the extensive "advertising and marketing in the rapidly developing consumer market for health," Rose has argued, "by the start of the 21st century, hopes, fears, decisions and life-routines shaped in terms of the risks and possibilities in corporeal and biological existence had come to supplant almost all others as organizing principles of a life of prudence, responsibility and choice."[23] This brings me to my third theme: the *management of risk*, and the new emphasis on "responsibilizing" the individual in order to ensure health and well-being.[24] The optimization of health is not only about the pleasures of consumption; it is also about the duties of vigilant self-surveillance in the service of risk reduction (and the consequent reduction of health care expenditures). As new health technologies are introduced, users are exhorted to adopt them in the name of personal, familial, and social responsibility. Yet these responsibilities are often distributed unevenly—for example, in the case of Gardasil, the vaccine to prevent HPV infection, the burden may fall particularly on mothers and daughters.[25]

The management of risk thereby connects to the ideology sometimes called "healthism": the transformation of health into a chief moral imperative of contemporary societies.[26] Especially in recent decades, the goal of achieving health and wellness has provided an apparently inexhaustible source of fuel to normative judgments about how one should engage in the most basic activities of living, from eating to sleeping to exercising to (of course) having sex.[27] In a 1980 article, the sociologist Robert Crawford, lamenting that "a concern with personal health has become a national preoccupation," defined healthism as "the preoccupation with personal health as a primary—often *the* primary—focus for the definition and achievement of well-being; a goal which is to be attained primarily through the modification of life styles, with or without therapeutic help."[28] More recently, in their 2010 volume *Against Health: How Health Became the New Morality*, Jonathan Metzl and Anna Kirkland extended the critique of the moralistic character of health discourses, arguing that "'health' is a term replete with value judgments, hierarchies, and blind assumptions that speak as much about power and privilege as they do about well-being."[29]

While healthism, as noted, permeates discussions of a wide range of social behaviors, the perception of social dangers associated with sexuality leads to an especially strong investment in the idea that that such pleasures must be pursued responsibly: "Don't gamble with your sexual health" is the relevant exhortation, found in any number of promotional campaigns. This idea of managing sexual risk often comes attached to the ideal of self-empowerment and the metaphor of self-investment through the injunction that one should seek to "own" one's sexual health. In a publicity video for OraQuick, an in-home HIV-testing kit sold by OraSure Technologies, Karl Westerberg, also known as Manila Luzon, a drag queen and reality television personality, avers: "One thing I do take seriously is owning my sexual health. And an important part of that is getting myself tested. When my fiancé and I decided to open up our relationship, we made a pact that we would have safe sex and get tested regularly. . . . And it's not just owning my health, it's owning my fiancé's health. And that's why we trust OraQuick, because it's the same test that doctors use."[30] Such messages play on the multiple meanings of "owning," thereby linking a proprietary investment in one's own body with a common idiom for describing the acceptance of responsibility.

Much scholarly work has addressed the contemporary emphasis on risk management in relation to health, including not only the ever-more-powerful diagnostic tools offered by modern medicine to patients and the worried well (including direct-to-consumer genetic testing) but also the self-surveillance enabled by new personal technologies.[31] Natasha Schüll, for example, has analyzed the "quantified self" movement: "In large volumes of self-data, often gathered through digital apps or wearable devices, [adherents] seek to detect patterns and shift habit pathways to increase the chances of personal flourishing."[32] The sociologist Deborah Lupton has drawn the links to the domain of sexuality and sexual health: Lupton describes a wide range of software applications that permit their users to monitor their own sexual and reproductive activities—even to quantify their own sexual performance—and, in some cases, to make their personal attributes available for the scrutiny of others via social media.[33] Risk and responsibility, then, are the "flip side" of consumerist pleasures in the domain of health; together, they stake out the terrain of optimization and the pursuit of wellness.

"Wellness and You"—and Beyond?

Against the din of "sexual health," the phrase "sexual wellness" barely registers. Within the pages of books published in 2019 and digitized in Google Books, for example, "sexual health" appears 162 times as often as "sexual wellness."[34] What does "sexual wellness" connote and when is it invoked? A simple Google search is revealing: the top links, when I performed a search, were to Walgreens, Amazon, and Groupon, while Kmart and eBay also made the top ten. Sexual wellness, in short, is first and foremost a marketing category. The sexual wellness webpage for Walgreens, which is typical in its coverage, lists the following as subcategories: condoms and contraceptives, lubricants and moisturizers, vibrators and adult toys, "mood setters" (such as massage oils and "arousal creams"), sexual wellness supplements (that is, nonprescription products that promise to increase potency), "intimate care" (various cleaning, waxing, and depilatory products), and pregnancy and fertility.[35] Similarly, at the time that I pulled up the page, Amazon listed as its current "best sellers" in the category of sexual wellness products such items as lubricants, condoms, vibrators, dildos, and— clocking in at number 17—"Teeny Peenie Bachelorette Party Sipping Straws."[36] For this diverse assortment of consumer goods, the rubric of wellness performs a bit of cleanup work by linking their purchase to a noble, or at least unobjectionable, goal: after all, who could oppose being well?[37] Online sales also provide a crucial element of privacy as well as convenience, permitting individuals to access sexual products from their computers, tablets, or smartphones with a few clicks, swipes, or keystrokes.

A perusal of popular magazines reinforces the impression of a close link between sexual health and wellness, consumption practices, and lifestyle pursuits. As the sociologist Gary Dowsett has pithily observed, "One of the fascinating things about Men's Health magazine is its collapse of health and sex into one discourse, one framework, one reference, one practice: sex is health; good health is about good sex; good health gets good sex; good sex demonstrates good health."[38] Other lifestyle magazines target sexual matters and sexual products even more overtly, and do so, often, with women readers in mind. The magazine *Sexual Health*, published by SHE Media (and with a readership reported to be 55 percent female), bills itself as "the must-read quarterly guide to sexual wellness for every walk of life." Offering news, product reviews, op-eds, and "interviews with today's sexual wellness experts," the magazine provides "compelling content that balances education and practicality."[39] As suggested by the cover art (fig. 9), *Sexual Health* emphasizes sexual satisfaction as an active pursuit that individuals (often women) can master through proper training. Sandwiched between advertising for sex toys, mostly directed at women, the magazine provides

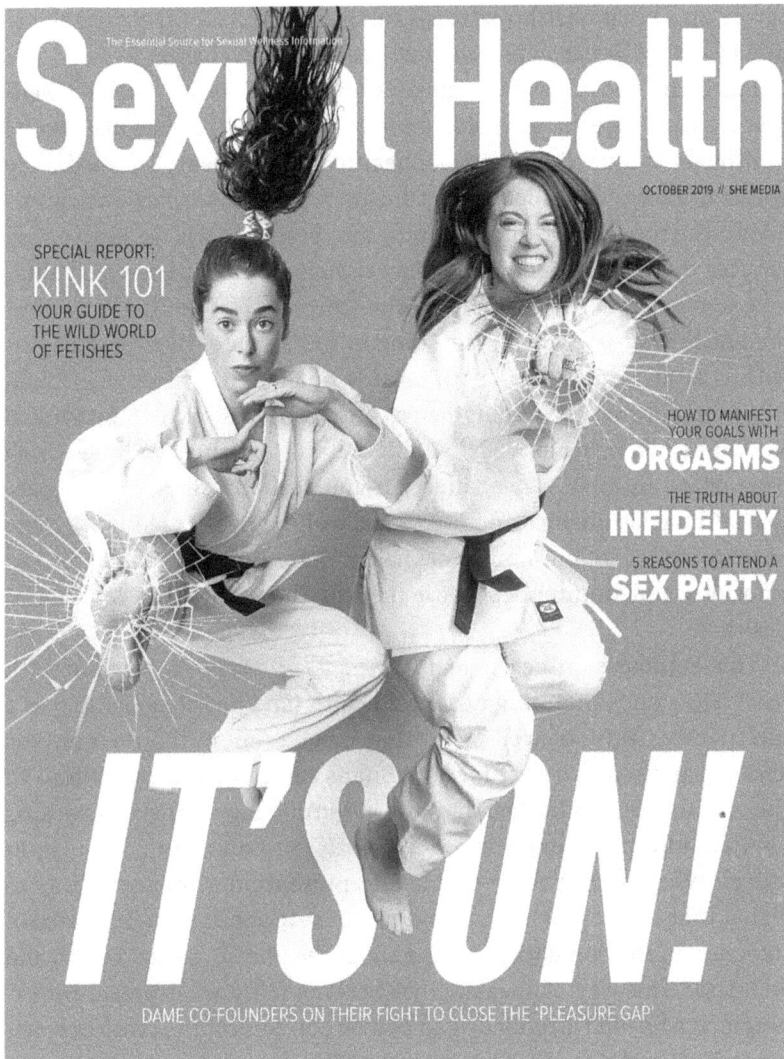

Figure 9: Cover of *Sexual Health* magazine, October 2019
Reproduced with permission of SHE Media.

articles on topics such as "overcoming boredom in the bedroom," "why 'who you are' shouldn't hold you back from sexual exploration," and "new findings on men's versus women's response to sexual stimuli."[40] Such magazines thereby link consumerism to broader aspirations for more satisfying sexual lives. They also represent new opportunities for advice on sexual health matters—further evidence of the diversification of sexual health expertise that I described in chapter 7.

But if the consumerist impulse behind the pursuit of sexual wellness is clearly evident, a consideration of compound phrases like "sexual health and wellness" and "sexual health and well-being" immediately points to a more complicated picture. Both phrases are particularly visible in the names of clinics, centers, and branches within health care services that promise comprehensive or holistic attention to sexuality-related concerns. For example, at the University of Southern California's health center (where, according to the website, "Wellness Begins with U at SC"), the "goal [is] to provide quality clinical services in an environment that is nonjudgmental and respectful of each individual as well as his or her privacy." As its "Sexual Health & Wellness" web page noted in 2017: "Love, affection and sexual intimacy contribute to healthy relationships and individual well-being. But along with the positive aspects of our human sexuality, there are also illnesses, mixed emotions and unintended consequences that can affect our sexual health."[41]

This emphasis on health *and wellness* is, of course, consistent with the WHO's understanding of sexual health (and health generally) as a multifaceted state of well-being that involves more than merely the absence of disease or dysfunction. But as the proclaimed attention to the "U" in "USC" indicates, the shift in terminology signals something else in addition: an explicit concern with the flourishing of the individual. When an STI clinic or a health promotion campaign wants to signal that it cares about *you*, and not merely about reducing rates of infection in the population, it may adopt the phrase "sexual health and wellness." This way of speaking has become fairly widespread. For example, at a forum I attended at an annual congress of the World Association for Sexual Health, a spokesperson for the condom manufacturer Durex—the chief financial sponsor of the conference—explained that "as the number one condom leader, Durex believes not just in sexual health but in sexual well-being. Good sexual health promotes good sexual well-being and also promotes healthy sexual lives."[42] While this may sound like a wordy tautology, in fact the spokesperson's series of equations connecting sexual health, sexual well-being, and healthy sexual lives makes sense if we understand the different goals and meanings that Durex would like its product to signify. On the one hand, Durex appeals to the health-promoting function of condoms in preventing the transmission of infections. On the other hand, Durex aligns its product with an understanding of sexual activity as a positive lifestyle choice for the modern individual—a choice that might risk appearing frivolous, immoral, or even subversive if justified solely as being fun or pleasurable, but which seems valuable and, indeed, healthy once linked to "well-being."

To be sure, the vision of sexual wellness as the lifestyle pursuit of the modern individual invites critique at a time when sex itself seems increasingly packaged as an individualized consumer object—in the form of pornography, of course, or perhaps in the predicted near future of ubiquitous "sex robots."[43] More generally, critics of the ideology of wellness have called attention to the downside of the worship of individualism—and the corresponding decline in the investment in health as a public good. Anna Kirkland makes the point clearly in her appraisal of corporate wellness programs: "Wellness promotes a conservative, individualistic health ideology, thereby undercutting communal, structural, redistributive, and sympathetic approaches to health. The more health is framed as within personal control, the more it will seem that everyone deserves his or her place in the health hierarchy. Wellness is thus poised to help push American health politics farther to the right."[44]

As a characterization of the programs she studied, Kirkland's assessment may be justified. Yet as we have already seen, the nexus of sexual health, wellness, and well-being encompasses a considerable variety of approaches and activities, from commercial websites to health clinics, and it is hard to generalize about their ideologies or effects. That sexual wellness consumerism can embrace the political in varied ways was demonstrated in 2017 by the "sexual health and wellness" brand Unbound, whose makers launched a campaign to send vibrators to members of Congress to protest a health care bill that threatened to defund Planned Parenthood.[45] Indeed, even when sexual health and wellness practices tend toward individualization and privatization, they may, paradoxically, also align with social and political action.

These tensions are nicely encapsulated in the example of a vending machine that was installed on the University of California, Davis, campus in April 2017. Dubbed the "Wellness to Go" machine, it offers, where soft drink options might more typically be arrayed, a mix of products for sale, including "the morning-after pill as well as condoms, pregnancy tests, tampons and over-the-counter medication such as Advil."

Promoted by a college senior who campaigned for student senate with the pledge to "make Plan B [emergency contraception] more afford-able and accessible," the vending machine commodifies wellness but also destigmatizes sexuality. "I really value the anonymity of having a vending machine," one student commented: "A lot of students like the judgment-free space and don't have to feel the pressure of interacting with people."[46]

To be sure, it is easy to scoff at the idea that "wellness" might be made available "to go," like takeout restaurant food. Yet college officials at UC Davis who initially opposed the Wellness to Go machine and sug-gested that its products could simply be sold at the campus bookstore missed the point that a technology of privatized consumption also af-forded privacy (and, as it happened, a lower price) in obtaining items like Plan B—a medication that has been the object of significant push-back from religious conservatives and others who oppose sexual and reproductive rights.[47] Indeed, the machines, which have also since been installed at Stanford, Pomona College, Brandeis, and Yale, have been sharply criticized by some conservatives, who refer to them as "abor-tion vending machines" based on an inaccurate portrayal of Plan B as an abortifacient.[48] Thus, Wellness to Go is a political critique and an outreach campaign, tightly packaged inside the consumerist contours of a vending machine.

Women's Turn at Pleasure?

Societal attention to the needs and desires of older men—in particu-lar, older men with economic means or good health insurance cover-age, who tend to skew wealthier and whiter—has been much remarked on with respect to the marketing of Viagra and related drugs. Yet it is striking how often sexual wellness optimization activities nowadays target women—though again, often women of a certain social class or, at least, ones with disposable income.

CONSUMPTION, EMPOWERMENT, AND GENDER EQUITY

A good example is the rhetoric surrounding the many products and activ-ities made available at the Sexual Health Expo (or SHE), self-described as "America's premier sexual wellness event," which has traveled to various cities across the United States. (Recently, the event has been redubbed the Sex Expo, but it remains connected to SHE Media, identified just earlier as the publishers of *Sexual Health* magazine.) According to its promoters: "SHE will showcase the best products to spice up your sex life. From lubricants to innovative pleasure products, this unique, curated approach to product exhibits invites attendees to leave their inhibitions at the door and explore today's top intimacy products." While publicity materials claim that the expo attracts a "diverse crowd" that includes "couples and singles of all genders and sexual orientations," photos on the website predominantly feature women—much as the event's acronym would suggest—and most of the guest speakers are women as well.[49]

Although the expo can be attended free of charge, repeated references to the "upscale venue" and the "chic backdrop" in promotional materials hint that the lifestyle being advertised here is one that aligns women's sexual freedom with status aspirations and conspicuous consumption. Yet the focus is also squarely on education and sex-positivity. The event pairs the display of products with lectures and workshops on a wide array of topics related to sex and relationships, including advice on how to engage in and safely enjoy specific sexual practices, from anal sex to rope play. Thus, the expo reflects the melding of multiple goals and interests, from consumerism and status attainment, to empowerment, to education and "responsibilization," and it relies on forms of community-based expertise, described in the previous chapter, that have developed out of progressive social movements.

Venues like the Sexual Health Expo exemplify trends found more generally in the increasing marketing of sexual wellness products to women. As Lynn Comella has described in her book *Vibrator Nation*: "Many adult entertainment companies, from sex-toy manufacturers to retailers, are recalibrating their business practices with an eye toward wooing female shoppers. Traditional brick-and-mortar retailers, for example, are removing their video arcades, painting their stores to make them lighter and brighter, hiring female staff, and placing a greater emphasis on stocking quality products and offering attentive customer service."[50] Yet Comella's main interest as an analyst is not in the repurposing of the mainstream sex products industry to attract women but in the feminist sex shops that such repurposing threatens to displace. Comella tells a story, dating back to the 1970s, of how stores like Eve's Garden in New York City and Good Vibrations in San

Francisco "brought an unapologetically feminist standpoint to the sexual marketplace." Without ignoring the complications of mixing commercialism with feminist politics, Comella lauds this feminist model for having "created a viable counterpublic sphere for sex-positive entrepreneurship and retail activism, one where the idea that the personal is political is deployed in the service of a progressive—and potentially transformative—sexual politics." Comella quotes the feminist sex advocate Susie Bright's characterization of Good Vibrations as a "sex education kiosk" where the customers who stopped in could learn about all kinds of sexual topics while also buying their vibrators.[51]

Feminist sex shops do survive into the present—Good Vibrations now calls itself a "sex-positive sexual health and wellness toy retailer"[52]— but as the sociologist April Huff has described, these shops "envision part of their business goals to be the act of packaging feminist rhetoric of self-empowerment to the technologies being sold." Employing a rhetoric of "liberation through pleasure" and endorsing practices of "ethical consumption," the owners of these shops seek to "balance politics and profits" and help their customers draw "connections between personal liberation and the larger field of sexual and feminist politics."[53]

These complicated stances are suggestive of a broader arena of women-friendly marketing, almost always accessed online, that operates under the sign of sexual health and wellness. As Shelly Ronen has observed in a study of the "moral standing" of sex toys, heterosexual women's desire has nowadays been positioned as "central to the moral legitimacy of sex toy consumers," and heterosexual women have been "constructed as superior sexual consumers—as more sexually worthy than men." As Ronen points out, these formulations valorize women's sexual desires while simultaneously reproducing a double standard: male desire is understood to be "raunchier," while women's "is acceptable and high-class."[54]

In this environment, a range of so-called sex-tech companies practice "sex-positive entrepreneurship," and their staff also see technologies as agents of personal and social transformation. Nuelle, a self-described "women's personal health and wellness company focused on delivering groundbreaking solutions for women's sexual well-being and intimacy," has emphasized the goal of redressing gender inequities in access to commodities and hence access to sexual pleasure. "While technology over the years has focused predominantly on the needs of men, now women and couples are also seeking more innovative options to address their physical and emotional needs," Nuelle claimed in a press release announcing the company's latest product, "Fiera Personal Care Device + Remote" (priced at $249, and available at Amazon and other venues). Indeed, Nuelle signaled an activist sensibility by reporting that the company had "recently partnered with leading organizations in the health and education space to launch LegalizeV, a movement that advocates for open and honest dialogue regarding women's sexual health."[55] (LegalizeV opposes censorship of the word "vagina" in public discourse.[56])

One might reasonably ask whether Nuelle's stances on gender politics signify commercialism in the service of social change, or just positioning in the service of sales. The question of how well the new optimization of sexual health truly accords with gender equity and women's empowerment has similarly emerged in the domain of pharmaceutical licensing and marketing. However, in this case, involving the pharmaceutical drug flibanserin, popularly understood as a kind of "female Viagra," different groups of women's health advocates have staked out opposing positions.

"FEMALE VIAGRA" AND THE GENDER POLITICS OF PHARMACEUTICAL DRUG DEVELOPMENT

Approved by the FDA in 2015 and sold under the brand name Addyi, the drug flibanserin has been billed as a victory in a long quest to provide a biomedical solution to the problem of female sexual dysfunction. The condition being treated has gone by various names, including "hypoactive sexual desire disorder in women" in the DSM-4 and "female sexual interest/arousal disorder" in the DSM-5. Regardless of name, the phenomenon has attracted critical scrutiny of how biomedical experts, in Alyson Spurgas's terms, construe femininity "as elusive, mysterious, and in need of direction," and women as properly receptive to men's sexual desires.[57]

While previous, unsuccessful attempts to treat the condition had sought, following the model of Viagra, to increase blood flow to the genitals, flibanserin instead targets the brain.[58] Yet the drug has a checkered history. Originally developed as an antidepressant and then repurposed by the company Boehringer Ingelheim, flibanserin was rejected by the FDA in 2010 and again in 2013 as a result of concern about side effects, such as low blood pressure and fainting, and insufficient evidence of efficacy in promoting sexual desire.[59] The drug was picked up by Sprout Pharmaceuticals, self-described as a women-directed company, which refiled a new drug application with the FDA. Sprout, whose website featured a photo of six determined-looking female employees, arms crossed and facing the camera,[60] presented evidence from clinical trials showing that flibanserin brought about an average increase of one "sexually satisfying event" per month in premenopausal women taking the pill daily, compared to similar women who took a placebo.

The subsequent debate and the FDA hearings that led to FDA's licensing reflected a battle between competing representatives of women's interests. On the side in favor of approval of flibanserin was a coalition of organizations brought together under a banner called "Even the Score"—an entity created by a former director of the FDA's Office of Women's Health, who had been retained as a consultant by Sprout.[61] (Even the Score declined to answer questions from a *New York Times* reporter about how much of the coalition's budget came from Sprout or other pharmaceutical companies working on female sexual health products.[62]) With members that included the American College of Nurse-Midwives, the Black Women's Health Imperative, the International Society for the Study of Women's Sexual Health, the National Hispanic Medical Association, and the American Sexual Health Association (ASHA), Even the Score made a simple argument: men enjoy many pharmaceutical options to treat sexual dysfunction (which have been approved despite significant potential side effects); women have none; therefore, in the name of what they called sexual health equity, any medication that even slightly benefits women should be approved. The organization's publicity materials urged supporters to contact Congress, sign a petition, share their stories, and "join the movement."[63] Even the Score also produced a widely circulated mock television ad that claimed women had been "left high and dry" by gender inequity in sexual dysfunction medications.[64] At the urging of Even the Score, eleven members of Congress led by California representative Jackie Speier wrote to the FDA on March 26, 2015—the seventeenth anniversary of the approval of Viagra—to complain that flibanserin "has not been afforded the same priority [as Viagra received] despite having much less severe side effects." The members of Congress wrote: "We firmly believe that equitable access to health care should be a fundamental right, regardless of whether you are a man or a woman. But when it comes to sexual health—and, in particular, sexual dysfunction—that's just not the case."[65]

On the other side, against approval of the drug, were arrayed well-established women's health organizations such as the National Women's Health Network and the Boston Women's Health Book Collective (which produces the touchstone text *Our Bodies, Ourselves*), along with a group called the New View Campaign, which, since its founding in 2000, has opposed the medicalization of female sexuality and the reliance on pharmaceutical solutions to sexual problems.[66] These opponents pointed to the limited efficacy of flibanserin as well as the fact that the drug was linked to fainting, especially when combined with alcohol; they argued that a bad drug was of no benefit to women. Some, such as Thea Cacchioni, a sociologist and professor of women's studies, also questioned the diagnostic category of hypoactive desire and wondered how much it reflected a capitulation to social expectations about women's abilities to satisfy their partners.[67] An online petition authored by Leonore Tiefer, a psychologist and organizer of the New View Campaign, argued that "politics and marketing are endangering women's sexual health" and called on the public to "reject the dishonest use of feminist language such as 'choice' and 'gender equality.'"[68]

After its expert advisory committee voted 18–6 in favor of licensing flibanserin, the FDA approved the drug on August 18, 2015, for premenopausal women suffering from hypoactive sexual desire disorder.[69] The agency required a boxed warning on the medication label for Addyi, advising women to abstain from alcohol while consuming the product because of the risk of fainting.[70] Two days later, Sprout announced the sale of the company to Valeant Pharmaceuticals for a price of $1 billion.[71]

The FDA defended its decision as evidence based, though agency officials also acknowledged differences of opinion among the review team about whether licensing was warranted (not an uncommon event in itself).[72] By February 2016, the already-minimal claimed benefits of the drug had been adjusted further downward, as pooled data from clinical trials suggested that the average boost from flibanserin was more on the order of one-half a sexually satisfying event per month.[73] Defenders of flibanserin, such as columnist Sonia Sodha, writing in the *Guardian*, denounced what she called the "anti-flibanserin feminist brigade" for seeking to rob women of their freedom to choose a treatment that might work for them.[74] Less stridently, Lynne Barclay, the president and chief executive officer of ASHA, also emphasized the virtues of letting women make their own informed decisions: "Let it be between a woman and her provider. Let them decide, is this a good thing for her or not? It's not up to me to decide that."[75] But female sufferers of hypoactive sexual desire disorder, and their doctors, appeared largely to agree with the skeptics: while Viagra had racked up more than half a million prescriptions in its first month alone, Addyi generated only four thousand in half a year.[76]

Much more might be said about a controversy that raises questions that are simultaneously scientific, political, cultural, and economic. There is, to be sure, nothing especially unusual about the presence of sharp debate about how to interpret clinical trial data, how to use such data for regulatory purposes, or how much to defer to patient choice when doing so.[77] Yet in this case it seems reasonable to be skeptical about the wisdom of supporting, in the name of gender equity and freedom of choice, a drug with at best modest efficacy—especially when financial incentives seem to have played an outsized role in the story at several turns. There is certainly a danger of too quickly "admonishing the strawman of 'Big Pharma,'" as Alyson Spurgas has suggested in reference to this case.[78] Yet at a minimum, the story of flibanserin sounds a warning signal about how the pursuit of sexual optimization may create incentives for action that are more to the benefit of the pharmaceutical industry than to individuals (of any gender) who are in search of sexual health and satisfaction.

"Healthysexuals" on PrEP: New Stories of Identity and Community

In 2017, Gilead Sciences, a biopharmaceutical company based in Foster City, California, invented—and trademarked—a new sexual identity: the "healthysexual."[79] Visitors to the "healthysexual" website on the Tumblr platform were exhorted: "Own your own sexual health. Start with Being Healthysexual." Cute graphics, sexy photos, and an abundance of hashtags spread across several pages on the website encouraged a range of behaviors and attitudes associated with the adoption of a healthysexual lifestyle:

> "Healthysexuals show it off. And get their health on."
> "Healthysexuals protect themselves. Know your prevention options."

"Do it again and again and again . . . Getting retested every 3–6 months can feel so good."

"Look good doing it. Knowing your prevention options can help you feel confident."

"You can be healthysexual. Whatever you're into."

While being a healthysexual apparently encompassed the performance of many possible activities to prevent the spread of HIV and other STIs, including using condoms and getting tested, anyone who clicked a few links on the site would likely find their way to information about one prevention method in particular: preexposure prophylaxis, commonly known as PrEP, which involves the repurposing of antiviral medications for use not as treatment for HIV infection but rather as prevention. The idea, validated by clinical trials, is that uninfected individuals who take antiretroviral medication can avoid having an infection take root even if they are exposed to HIV. In 2012, the FDA approved Gilead's drug Truvada, a combination of two antiretroviral drugs, as a daily pill to be used for just this purpose. By 2019, Gilead had also marketed a second drug combination, Descovy, as preexposure prophylaxis for HIV. In the United States, consumers of PrEP include long-term partners of people who are HIV-positive, but especially at the outset, it was mostly associated with sexually active gay men.

Of course, it was doubtful that the moniker of healthysexual would gain much traction as a way for people formally to label themselves or understand their sexual identity. While sexual identity categories are less stable and more differentiated than is often supposed,[80] their elaboration is complex cultural work involving, typically, reciprocal interactions over time between experts who engage in labeling and individuals and groups who take up those labels and work with and rework them—doing so because the labels resonate with self-understandings and prove useful in negotiating social and sexual interactions.[81] Yet even if few, if any, people call themselves "healthysexuals," the point ultimately is that Gilead may succeed in capitalizing on a set of cultural, sexual, and biotechnological developments that, for gay men, have created an equation between optimizing sex and optimizing health.

For much of the history of the HIV/AIDS epidemic, sex and health have been pitted in tension with each other. In the earliest years, gay men were advised simply to stop having sex, and public health authorities focused on closing venues, such as bathhouses, that were perceived as promoting sexual opportunities and the spread of infection. Through grassroots AIDS education campaigns pioneered originally by gay community–based organizations, the equation between sex and death was powerfully challenged, as activists asserted the virtues of sexual pleasure and sexual freedom while educating the community about techniques of prevention.[82] Yet despite attempts over the years to more closely align health promotion with the pursuit of sexual pleasure—for example, through valiant efforts to "eroticize" condom use—the tension between these goals has persisted. But in recent years, PrEP has changed the equation. The official word, promoted by public health organizations and the FDA, is that PrEP is not supposed to substitute for condoms but rather accompany their use. In practice, the appeal of PrEP on the street lies to some degree in the possibility of tossing out an unwelcome latex barrier and engaging in what is often referred to as a more "natural" form of sex (although here, of course, as with, in a different way, Viagra, the natural is enabled by the pharmacological).

Initially, these possibilities ignited a range of debates within gay communities—debates that, once again, complicate our understanding of the repercussions of attempts to optimize sexual health. On the one side, with the advent of PrEP, some criticized the rise of what they called "Truvada whores": men who supposedly were looking to a pharmaceutical license to indulge in sexual promiscuity. (Others worried about the risks of pharmaceutical side effects and the implications of enhanced medical scrutiny of gay men's bodies.) But on the other side, defenders of a liberated sexuality accused these critics of engaging in what they called "slut shaming" as a way of shutting down conversation about sexuality and risk. Some gay men quickly proceeded to adopt the label of "Truvada whore" as a badge of honor, or perhaps even, with the online spread of a T-shirt emblazoned with the phrase, as a political fashion statement.[83] The San Francisco Public Health Department, working with community-based HIV prevention organizations, declared PrEP to be "Our Sexual Revolution" in a splashy advertising campaign featuring an ethnically diverse assortment of energetic and celebratory individuals (fig. 10).

The public health scholars Ronald Valdiserri and David Holtgrave have maintained that it is precisely by taking a "sexual health" approach to PrEP that progress can most likely be made, both against

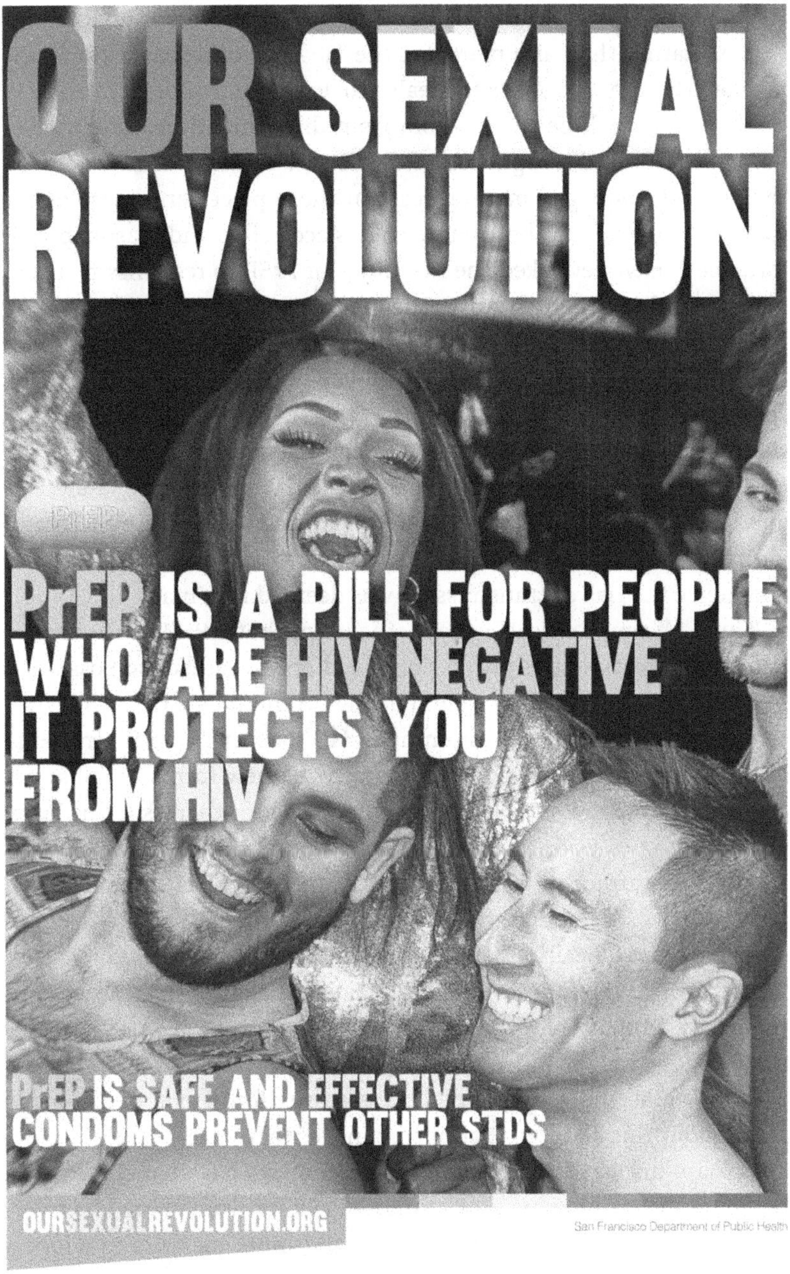

Figure 10: "Our Sexual Revolution" (San Francisco Department of Public Health)
Source: San Francisco Department of Public Health promotional campaign, 2017.

HIV and "as part of an overall strategy that empowers individuals to thrive." Rather than aim merely at the "absence of disease," they have invoked the concept of sexual health to warrant an approach that valorizes overall well-being, freedom from discrimination, assurance of human rights, and recognition of diverse sexualities.[84] And in fact, on the ground, some gay men (at least in those places and parts of the world where PrEP has been more or less accessible and reasonably affordable[85]) have reworked the meanings of PrEP to resignify forms of identity and community. An article in the *Huffington Post* in 2014 cited the emergence of new HIV-related identity statuses to complement the familiar "positive" and "negative," including "negative, on PrEP" and "poz, undetectable."[86] While "negative, on PrEP" signified a willingness, thanks to chemoprevention, to countenance a range of potential sexual acts regardless of the potential partner's HIV status, "poz, undetectable" signaled that partners need not fear infection because successful antiretroviral treatment had rendered one's viral load undetectable, and hence the risk of transmission was deemed minimal.

Thus, pharmaceutical options, including both PrEP and what is known as "treatment as prevention," held open at least the possibility of healing a long-standing wound in gay communities: the divide over serostatus and the sexual shunning of HIV-positive men.[87] Some analysts have therefore cautiously endorsed the new forms of "pharmaceutical citizenship" enabled by PrEP.[88] However, others, such as Jason Orne and James Gall, have suggested that the benefits of PrEP come with "strings attached": these analysts connect "PrEP citizenship" with new forms of surveillance that dictate behavioral norms for a "responsible, moral, and healthy HIV-negative individual that indefinitely continues PrEP as a public good."[89] It is plausible that both of these contradictory tendencies will continue to be in play as PrEP use becomes more widespread.

Meanwhile, the example of PrEP also reinforces the point, made throughout this chapter, that opportunities to "optimize" one's sexual health are unevenly distributed. Some analysts have concluded that public health campaigns that promote PrEP for women are less tolerant of sexual risk for that population and more inclined to adopt a discourse of responsibility.[90] At the same time, sexual health educators working with women of color have found that many of them presume that PrEP is intended essentially for men who have sex with men, given the public messaging around it.[91] Organizations such as the Black Women's Health Imperative, which introduced a "Let's Talk about PrEP" campaign, and Planned Parenthood of Greater New York, which targeted its "PrEP for Women Too" campaign at Black and Latina women, have sought to change the dynamics of access through grassroots outreach.[92] However, these groups face an uphill battle in reversing the disparities that both put ethnic minority groups at higher risk of infection and reduce their access to information and quality medical care.

Indeed, in the United States, only a fraction of those who might benefit from PrEP currently receive it, although a new federal program introduced in 2019 has sought to provide the medication for free to those who lack prescription drug insurance coverage, provided they have a doctor's prescription for PrEP.[93] As Clay Davis has suggested, the perception of the ideal PrEP user as being simultaneously at high risk of infection but also "poised to adhere perfectly to an intervention" creates space for justifying underrepresentation on the argument that those leading more "marginal" lives are less likely to use the medication responsibly.[94]

The Dilemmas of Optimization

These possibilities of new pharmaceuticalized lives, like other stories in this chapter, suggest the many sides of the optimization of sexual health and wellness—and complicate any simple analysis or critique. Without question, these activities suggest how sexuality nowadays has become subject to a "healthist" impulse as we are all enjoined to be sexually "well." Yet the motivation is not only to lead healthier lives but also to lead lives that are more fulfilling, more pleasurable, and perhaps more consistent with political values of various sorts. These examples demonstrate, once again, that sexual health constitutes more than just a medicalizing (or "healthicizing") of sexuality, precisely because the pursuit of sexual health aligns, potentially, with so many different values and goals.

The push to optimize one's sexual health is everywhere. Yet as we have seen, such optimization, performed at the juncture of consumerism, self-improvement, and risk management, holds together contradictory impulses in a state of tension. Optimization has the potential to promote inequities or redress them, to privatize the pursuit of health or safeguard health as a public good, to commodify sexuality, or to infuse it with new and politicized meanings—and competing tendencies are sometimes embedded in the very same projects and products. I continue the discussion of the multiple political valences of sexual health in the next chapter.

9 *Social Risks, Rights, and Duties*

GOVERNING VIA SEXUAL HEALTH

On October 31, 2018, shortly before the midterm elections in the United States, news outlets reported a Trump administration move to ban "sexual health." More precisely, the US State Department was considering a ban on official uses of the term. As reporters for the newsmagazine *Politico* explained: "U.S. diplomats may soon be prohibited from using the phrases 'sexual and reproductive health' and 'comprehensive sexuality education' under a proposal being floated by Secretary of State Mike Pompeo." According to one source, US officials would instead be obliged to use terms such as "reproduction and the related health services." Described as "being pushed by a handful of conservative political appointees at the State Department and other agencies," the proposed ban, it was predicted, "could lead to more contentious negotiations at the United Nations."[1] Indeed, the previous week, US diplomats ultimately had backed down when their demands to cut the phrase "sexual and reproductive health" from a declaration issued at a global health conference met with resistance.[2]

Through these and other related actions (actual or threatened), Trump administration officials sought to police language use as a tool to promote conservative policy goals with regard to gender and sexuality—especially to oppose access to abortion and contraception, but also to undercut efforts to curtail sexual harassment and protect LGBTQ (and particularly transgender) people from discriminatory treatment. As reported in *Foreign Policy* alongside the news of the potential ban on "sexual health," US diplomats had recently sought to "strike references to the word 'gender'" from resolutions before the UN General Assembly.[3] This followed quickly on the heels of news reports of an effort by the

US Department of Health and Human Services (HHS) to establish a new legal definition of "gender." The goal was to restrict the options to "male" and "female" and treat gender as an invariant characteristic of an individual—exactly as recorded on the birth certificate and determined by supposed "immutable biological traits."[4] Previously, in his first days in office, Trump had reinstated the so-called Mexico City Policy (known to critics as the "global gag rule"), which bars US aid to international organizations that provide or promote access to abortion, and also denies funding to organizations that simply advocate for access to safe abortion or for the liberalizing of abortion laws. Other recent Republican presidents had also enforced the policy, but under the Trump administration it applied not just to family planning grants but to all global health funding.[5]

In point of fact, the US government could not will sexual health out of existence, or make gender politics disappear, or treat transgender, gender nonbinary, or intersex people as fictional, no matter which words it chose to employ or proscribe.[6] Yet the State Department's effort to prohibit the phrase "sexual and reproductive health" is noteworthy in light of the two-decade-long evolution of what I will call "sexual health governance." At the dawn of the new millennium—and also under a Republican president—US Surgeon General David Satcher had issued the landmark Call to Action to Promote Sexual Health and Responsible Sexual Behavior.[7] At least since then, sexual health has been an acknowledged object of governmental scrutiny and policy making in the United States, and it has been deemed a key linkage point between individual conduct and social membership. That is, government agencies have sought to encourage various ways of being sexually healthy and responsible and have undertaken projects to actively promote and try to ensure sexually healthy outcomes. By the Obama years, the notion that the government had a stake in the promotion of sexual health had become thoroughly regularized as official policy. The HHS designated "sexual health and responsible sexual behavior" as one of ten leading health indicators, and sexual health was featured as a chief goal in important federal planning documents, including HHS's National Prevention Strategy.[8] These policy emphases and others related to sexual health remained in force during the Trump administration, State Department actions and pronouncements notwithstanding.

This history raises important questions about how agencies of the state address matters of both sexuality and health—and how bringing sexuality and health together authorizes new projects of governance. Specifically, this chapter asks: How, and in what ways, have US agencies made sexual health both an object of governance and a tool for governing? Which visions of sexuality and health have they incorporated into those projects? What forms of self-governance on the part of individuals have been encouraged by these governing efforts? Which imagined ways of being a "good citizen" or a "bad citizen" are associated with, or run contrary to, sexual health governance? How have such governance efforts differently addressed groups of citizens who can be distinguished according to race, class, gender, sexuality, and nationality? And finally, how have these plans, actions, and imaginaries varied depending on changes in political circumstances (and presidential administrations) in the United States? I will explain how sexual health governance has juxtaposed distinctive ideas of rights and responsibilities and created new, if unevenly available, possibilities for social inclusion.

I begin with reflections on helpful ways to conceptualize state action and citizenship in this case. I then take the US federal government as my case study, tracing the evolution of sexual health governance from the late 1990s through early 2021, through the administrations of Bill Clinton, George W. Bush, Barack Obama, and Donald Trump, and up to the start of the Biden administration.[9] Toward the end of the chapter, I briefly consider how we might turn to other countries to add nuance to the analysis.

Conceptualizing State Action and Citizenship in an Era of Sexual Health

As Kimberly Morgan and Ann Orloff capture with their metaphor of the "many hands of the state," what we often, as a matter of convenience, call "the state" is far from being the cohesive and unitary actor that the term implies—and still less one that remains stable over time.[10] Morgan and Orloff propose "an understanding of states as encompassing multiple institutions, varying forms of interpenetration with civil society, multiple scales of governance, and multiple and potentially contradictory logics."[11] Such a perspective proves crucial in understanding how, for example, the Department of Health and Human Services may promote sexual health even as the State Department seeks to ban the very term. Taking my cue from these scholars as well as others who have called for the "disaggregation of the monolithic entity of the state,"[12] I approach "the state" through attention to the particular actions of particular agencies and offices, but without reducing "stateness" to that: "States are more than bundles of governing institutions, because of their claim to embody the will of a collectivity."[13]

This perspective on the state also raises questions about our ability to ascertain its boundaries in any sharply defined sense, given that the practices carried on within state agencies may sometimes merge seamlessly with ones conducted "outside" the state. Recognizing the fuzziness of the dividing line between "state" and "society" is a move consistent with various bodies of scholarship: research that reveals how the evolution of the state in the modern West has been linked to scientific and technological development;[14] work that examine the links between governance and self-governance;[15] and studies that recognize that social movements are sometimes found "inside" as well as "outside" state agencies.[16] All these considerations are helpful in considering how state actors have taken up questions of sexual health.

While it has been well understood that matters of health are of direct concern to state governance, by contrast, one issue that has been underexamined by scholars until fairly recently is the place of sexuality in the workings of modern states. Yet there is reason to treat matters of sexuality as anything but marginal to how states administer populations. The historian Margot Canaday has made the point forcefully in her analysis of the reverberating relationship, over the course of the twentieth century, between the rise of the administrative capacities of the US federal government and the consolidation of nonheteronormative sexual identities such as "gay" and "lesbian."[17] The sociologist Stefan Vogler likewise has analyzed how state-sanctioned legal processes, such as asylum hearings and sex offender commitment procedures, become sites where sexuality is known, detected, and administered.[18] More broadly, though in a different national context, the sociologist Jyoti Puri has called for attention to the myriad ways by which "sexuality easily affects every aspect of the assemblage abbreviated as 'the state,'" and she has emphasized that "engaging the state critically means attending to its constitutive elements, that is, the discourses and micro practices of governance, reports, documents, interactions, procedures, and more."[19] These insights align closely with my approach in this chapter to tracking how state agencies have sought to define and institutionalize specific orientations toward the promotion of the sexual health of the population.

To develop the arguments in this chapter, I also adopt an expansive conception of citizenship—one that goes beyond a focus on legal status (however consequential) to describe a more general concern with political belonging as reflected in rights, responsibilities, and identities.[20] Citizenship in this sense is not an either-or: in place of a static notion of citizenship as something one either fully possesses or fully lacks, it makes sense to understand the boundaries of citizenship as the outcome of multiple ongoing struggles that reflect "constantly shifting relationships of power."[21] As many scholars have described, the history of citizenship as a category of universal membership is simultaneously a history of exclusion, and citizenship has been defined in practice by means of the creation or dismantling of a wide range of social divisions and hierarchies.[22]

In recent years, many scholars have paid increasing attention to the embodied or health-related aspects of citizenship ("biocitizenship"), while others have considered the dimensions of citizenship that relate to sexuality and sexual identity ("sexual citizenship"). In this chapter I adopt Aaron Norton's term "biosexual citizenship" to join together these two sets of concerns.[23] Briefly, sexual citizenship refers to the claim to rights,[24] and also the assumption of responsibilities, associated with the multiple dimensions of exclusion or incorporation that stem from sexual practices, identities, norms, and attributions.[25] While sexual citizenship may be something one actively claims, it may also arrive as more of an imposition—a consequence of "discourses, programs, and other tactics aimed at making individuals politically active and capable of self-government," in Barbara Cruikshank's terms.[26] Somewhat analogously, biocitizenship (and its cousins, including biological citizenship, biopolitical citizenship, genetic citizenship, therapeutic citizenship, and so on) refers to the varied ways in which one's bodily or biological characteristics becomes a basis for political claims or for the assertion of rights or assumption of responsibilities.[27] Here again, in contrast to these bottom-up accomplishments, biocitizenship can also describe a more top-down process in which (as the medical historian Jonathan Metzl expresses it) "new selves and citizens are created by . . . health rhetoric, and . . . non-selves and non-citizens are constructed and then left out."[28]

Taking up Norton's neologism of biosexual citizenship helps me to expand the concept of biocitizenship by emphasizing the place of the sexual, but also to expand sexual citizenship through greater attention to health, biology, and the body. I define biosexual citizenship as differentiated modes of incorporation of individuals or groups fully or partially into a polity through the articulation of notions of rights and responsibilities, in cases where biological and health-related processes are brought into some relation with sexual meanings or identities. This conceptual intersection of biocitizenship and sexual citizenship calls attention to how embodied pleasures and risks associated with sexuality figure in the worlds of biomedicine and public health, as well as how public health officials, in engagement with others, participate in defining sexual rights and responsibilities.

A Call to Action: The Discourse of Responsibility

Appointed in 1998 by President Bill Clinton to serve as surgeon general and assistant secretary for health, Dr. David Satcher turned his attention to a variety of social problems. His office proceeded to issue reports on mental health, youth violence, smoking, and suicide prevention. By 1999, Satcher had also trained his gaze on sexuality. In December of that year, Satcher convened a "dialogue conference" of more than one hundred people, who were described by one participant as being "from a wide range of disciplines, opinions and value systems," to discuss the feasibility of a national strategy on sexual health. A second conference the following July brought together 130 individuals representing ninety organizations to draft a set of concrete recommendations.

Eli Coleman, former World Association of Sexology President and director of the Human Sexuality program at the University of Minnesota, served as "scientific editor and special advisor."[29] Yet Coleman recalled his discomfort with Satcher's initial framing of the initiative as a discussion of "responsible sexual behavior"—not sexual health. He also recalled the general nervousness about the whole endeavor on the part of Satcher's staff, some of whom pointed to Clinton's dismissal of a previous surgeon general, Joycelyn Elders, in 1994, after she had waded into controversial waters surrounding sex education.[30] According to Coleman, however, Satcher returned from an appearance at the International AIDS Conference held in Durban, South Africa, in July 2000 committed to the idea that, despite political risks, the strategy

document should adopt the phrase "sexual health."[31] The episode suggest the centrality of the AIDS epidemic to the push for a national
agenda. Yet "sexual health" was not merely a euphemism for HIV/AIDS;
rather, it was conceived from the start in more expansive terms.

According to John Bancroft, the director of the Kinsey Institute, who
was an insider to the process, the report was originally scheduled to be
released in late 2000 or early 2001 in the waning days of the Clinton
administration. However, upon the election of Republican president
George W. Bush—whose administration seemed far less disposed toward open talk of sexuality—the project was put temporarily on hold.
"To our pleasant surprise," wrote Bancroft afterward, "David Satcher
held firm to his commitment," even if the rollout was "a little delayed."
On June 28, 2001, Satcher declared sexual health a national health priority in his Call to Action to Promote Responsible Sexual Health and
Responsible Sexual Behavior. In the face of criticism of the document
from religious conservatives, Bancroft recalled, "the White House remained awkwardly silent."[32]

Yet the Call to Action was far from radical in its approach to sexual
matters. While alluding briefly to "the many positive aspects of sexuality," Satcher quickly turned his attention to "undesirable consequences." Pointing to "alarmingly high levels of sexually transmitted
disease (STD) and HIV/AIDS infection, unintended pregnancy, abortion, sexual dysfunction, and sexual violence," Satcher called for "a
mature national dialogue on issues of sexuality, sexual health, and responsible sexual behavior."[33]

As Alain Giami has observed in an analysis of this episode, Satcher's
discourse diverged in important ways from the working definition associated with the WHO: In place of the WHO's capacious definition
of sexual health that lauded the autonomous pursuit of sexual well-
being, Satcher emphasized the key theme of "responsibility" that had
attracted him from the outset.[34] In fact, the words "(ir)responsible"
and "responsibility" appeared forty-six times in the sixteen-page main
text of the document. By contrast, these terms do not appear at all in
the thirty-three-page WHO report from 1975, except in quite different
contexts. (However, many references to "responsibility" do appear in
subsequent WHO reports, such as the 2002 "Defining Sexual Health,"
which opens with the claim that "sexual and reproductive health and
well-being are essential if people are to have responsible, safe, and satisfying sexual lives."[35])

Writing much later, in 2017, and reflecting on the Call to Action, Satcher and coauthors noted that the term "responsible" was "not intended to be normative or prescriptive, and they maintained that "being responsible could mean differently things in different contexts."[36] Indeed, throughout the document, Satcher sought to weave together the imperative of responsibility with a respect for diversity and commitment to inclusivity. His message to HIV-positive Americans in his cover letter was typical of this approach: "We realize that you are not the enemy. . . . At the same time, it is also important that you realize you have an opportunity to partner with us in stemming the spread of this illness; to be responsible in your own behavior and to help others become aware of the need for responsible behavior in their sexual lives."[37] According to Satcher, "sexual responsibility should be understood in its broadest sense," encompassing the individual's responsibility to cultivate awareness, respect, and tolerance, but also the community's responsibility to promote access to sexuality education and sexual and reproductive health care and counseling."[38] Yet as the title of the document suggested, Satcher most immediately was exhorting the nation to engage in "responsible sexual behavior," understood fundamentally with reference to the prevention of STIs and unplanned pregnancies.

Moreover, "responsibility" was a resonant watchword of the era, and not just for conservatives: in 1996, Clinton had signed into law the Personal Responsibility and Work Opportunity Act, described as putting an end to "welfare as we have come to know it." Thus, Satcher's discourse was broadly consistent with a neoliberal emphasis on self-management and the declining faith in the capacity of government to distribute resources effectively.[39] Invoking responsibility may have seemed a safe route to garnering broad support for the initiative across the political spectrum. At the same time, in the context of the backlash against welfare, the discourse of personal responsibility may have held the door open for racial and class-based connotations with regard to sexual health that Satcher himself did not intend. After all, the critique of welfare was all too often articulated as a denunciation of supposed sexual irresponsibility on the part of poor women of color, who were seen as bearing "too many" babies;[40] and the welfare reform bill, along with imposing new work requirements for recipients, also instituted initiatives specifically to promote marriage. According to Teresa Kominos, these steps problematically "introduced a goal-based system of incentives and penalties that assume a welfare mother has control over her lifestyle, or, more frankly, that she chooses to be poor [and] that if given the proper incentive, she can also choose not to be poor," in part by choosing marriage.[41] Thus, the many connotations of "responsibility" signal divergent approaches to governing the sexuality and reproductivity of the population.

Institutionalizing Sexual Health Governance

Looking backward in 2013, Satcher would lament the limited progress in achieving sexual health in the United States and would point to his earlier agenda as "a dream deferred."[42] Displaying similar disappointment, academic commentators writing in the *Journal of the American Medical Association* in 2010 complained that "the United States lacks an integrated approach to sexual health" and observed critically that not a single reference to sexual health appeared in the one thousand pages of the Affordable Care Act.[43] Such observations highlight not only the ever-precarious and "illegitimate" status of sexual matters, but also the uneven character of attention to sexual health within the branches and agencies of the federal government: it is not surprising that legislators defending an already-controversial health care overhaul would steer clear of sexual topics.

Yet the years following Satcher's Call to Action did see important steps to making a sexual health agenda central to public health governance, particularly during the Obama administration. Public health officials gave weight to Satcher's goals by incorporating "responsible sexual behavior" as one of ten leading health indicators in "Healthy People 2010," which laid out the nation's preventive health agenda for the first decade of the new century.[44] According to the document, these indicators "reflect the major public health concerns in the United States and were chosen based on their ability to motivate action, the availability of data to measure their progress, and their relevance as broad public health issues." A decade later, in "Healthy People 2020," a revised list of twelve leading health indicators included "reproductive and sexual health."[45] In addition, the nation's first National HIV/AIDS Strategy, issued by the Obama White House in 2010, described itself as "[providing] an opportunity for working together to advance a public health approach to sexual health that includes HIV prevention as one component."[46]

In 2011, one of Satcher's successors, Surgeon General Regina Benjamin, launched the nation's first "National Prevention Strategy," which identified seven health priorities for the nation, of which one was repro-ductive and sexual health.[47] The strategy document called for increased preconception and prenatal care, greater support for reproductive and sexual health services, the provision of effective sexual health education, and enhanced early detection of HIV, viral hepatitis, and other STIs.[48] In a section called "Partners Can," it identified a host of potential allies for these efforts, including include state, tribal, local, and territorial governments; businesses and employers; health care systems, insurers, and clinicians; schools, colleges, and universities; community, non-profit, and faith-based organizations; and individuals and families.[49]

Of the various HHS component agencies in the Obama years, the Centers for Disease Control and Prevention (CDC) proved especially committed to the theme of sexual health. A key figure in this effort was Dr. Kevin Fenton, the director of the CDC's National Center for HIV/AIDS, Viral Hepatitis, STD, and TB Prevention. A public health specialist and medical epidemiologist, Fenton was born in Glasgow and educated in Jamaica, and he then completed his postgraduate studies in London. With a particular interest in "race, ethnicity, and the epidemiology of sexually transmitted infections" (the title of his doc-toral dissertation), Fenton has appeared on the "Root 100," an annual list of "the most influential African Americans." As a dynamic and rela-tively young center director at CDC, Fenton was, as he recalled, one of only three directors who were kept on in the transition from the Bush administration to that of Obama.[50]

With the Bush administration, Fenton later observed, "we had to move really carefully . . . to build trust. . . . When I came in, there was a complete lack of trust between the administration and the CDC on issues related to HIV and sexual health, and sexual health wasn't even mentioned." However, the transition in administrations soon presented new opportunities—even if sexual health remained "a big deal" and, as he recalled, "we didn't want to push our luck." Convinced that success-ful change would of necessity be incremental, Fenton set out to "land sexual health as a concept," grounding the effort in several key prin-ciples: "Number 1, move slow and move deliberately. . . . Number 2, en-sure that what we do is based on good evidence. Number 3, ensure that what we do is co-produced, and that we set an agenda of radical in-clusion and collaboration because we need to build a constituency. . . . We needed to get the churches on board, which included . . . evangelical churches because we wanted the Black churches. We needed to get researchers who were reticent about this in addition to those who were really advocates."[51]

Some of the fruits of this effort became apparent in April 2010, when, over the course of two days, staff employees at the CDC sat down with sixty-seven invited experts and stakeholders to hash out an agenda for the nation's sexual health. Fenton called for a "radically inclusive" public health approach to promoting sexual health, one that would "bring new partners to the table."[52] The group of attendees was, in fact, diverse and included leaders from the National Coalition of STD Directors, the National Coalition for LGBT Health, and the National Alliance of State and Territorial AIDS Directors, along with representatives of the Ford Foundation's Sexuality, Reproductive Health and Rights Program, the Navy and Marine Corps' Sexual Health and Responsibility Program, and the Metropolitan Interdenominational Church.

The CDC's two-day consultation reflected an explicit effort by the agency to build consensus on a science-driven sexual health agenda that would propel, but extend beyond, its efforts to prevent STIs. Connected to this goal was the CDC's process of elaborating its own definition of sexual health. "It was important for us to have a definition that worked for the U.S., and that was owned by the U.S., and that was palatable in the U.S.," Fenton later recalled.[53] When it finalized its definition of sexual health in 2012, the CDC's Sexual Health Workgroup affirmed that "sexual health is an inextricable element of human health and is based on a positive, equitable and respectful approach to sexuality, relationships and reproduction that is free of coercion, fear, discrimination, stigma, shame and violence." Notably, and in keeping with the broader emphases of the discipline of public health and Fenton's own sympathies, the new definition distinguished individual-level determinants of sexual health, such as attitudes and behaviors, from determinants at the societal level—what it called "socioeconomic and cultural contexts."[54] The workgroup's definition also balanced the "risks and responsibilities" of sexual behavior with its "benefits," and likewise balanced "adverse outcomes" with "the possibility of fulfilling sexual relationships."[55]

But there were limits to this progressiveness: the word "pleasure" did not appear as one of those potential benefits of sexuality, and, indeed, references to pleasure are essentially absent in contemporary sexual health governance discourse. Fenton described "many, many [internal] debates on pleasure" during his time at the CDC, but recalled concluding that "it is about winning the battle and not losing the war":

> I remember saying to the team, "Okay, we'll drop pleasure now in the definition. It doesn't mean that it can't be in our program and in the work that we do, and it doesn't mean that in three to five years' time when you come back to update your definition, that you can't [include pleasure]. But let's not fight over this and then not be able to progress."[56]

FROM SOCIAL HYGIENE TO SEXUAL HEALTH GOVERNANCE

In chapter 1, I described one of the genealogical precursors of sexual health: the social hygiene movement that lasted from the end of the nineteenth century through the First World War. The varied efforts under the umbrella of social hygiene brought together public health officials, military leaders, physicians, social workers, and moral reformers working with various nongovernmental organization. Uniting medical science with a vision of a healthier society, promoters of social hygiene trained their attention on sexually transmitted diseases, perceived as a threat to the white American mainstream brought by various outsiders, and as a risk to the country's moral fiber and military readiness. Through disease prevention campaigns, new ideas about sex education, and legal and regulatory efforts directed especially at prostitution, reformers sought to create sexually responsible citizens and a healthier society. A comparison between that era and the period of sexual health governance in the United States in the early twenty-first century is instructive, provided that one eschews both simple tales of social progress and easy judgments of fundamental continuity.

In both periods, political actors from government as well as civil society organizations have promoted broad agendas that link sexuality to health; in both cases, those agendas have addressed social problems by tying matters of state governance to the governance of the self. To be sure, the social hygiene movement had a deeper—and more punitive—impact, and the cause of sexual health has not resulted in formal legislation to the degree that social hygiene prompted.[57] By comparison, sexual health governance to date is patchy, incomplete, and often more evident at the level of exhortations than accomplishments (and, in certain respects, as I have indicated and will discuss, has been under attack in recent years).

There are interesting resonances that connect the two eras: notably, the consistent language of "responsibility" reflects an abiding interest in the forging of "good" biosexual citizens—and in determining who counts as a "good" or "bad" sexual citizen. Yet it is important not to give too much weight to individual words, outside of their broader semantic contexts: "responsibility" can mean many different things. In the modern era of sexual health, a lack of responsibility often connotes "excess" and the inability to self-regulate, as suggested, for example, by social concerns over promiscuity and sexual "compulsivity" or "addiction."

A complicated question of continuities and discontinuities concerns the specificity of racial difference in assessments of risk and responsibility. More than a century ago, the social hygiene movement explicitly linked racial otherness to sexual risk via discourses of eugenics, and sex education efforts during that time functioned, as Julian Carter has described, as "a social technology for the normalization of ideal modern whiteness."[58] More recent discourses and practices of sexual health governance in the first decade or so of the twenty-first century—promoted in some cases by public health officials of African descent, such as Satcher and Fenton—have rejected such links. Fenton, for example, sought to disrupt racial stereotyping while delivering resources to communities of color; his emphasis on the social determinants of health led him to identify the "stark and social and economic disparities" found in the United States as the cause of "sexual ill health," and he criticized the "laziness" of attributing it to race and ethnicity without examining issues of "access and privilege and power."[59]

Yet in the broader culture, ideas about who is sexually "responsible" or "irresponsible" may often invoke racialized fears, whether explicitly or implicitly[60]—as described above, in relation to the discourse around "welfare mothers." Public attention to the presumed HIV-transmission threat stemming from Black men "on the down low" is another recent example of a long history of pernicious stereotyping of African Americans in hypersexualized terms—as moral subjects who lack a capacity for proper impulse control and whose sexuality therefore must be "managed" by others.[61]

Somewhat similarly, Jenny Brian and coauthors have described how recent efforts to promote the use of long-acting reversible contraception

(LARC) reenact longtime practices of constructing a "responsible sexual citizenship" that is "racialized, classed, and gendered"—complete with presumptions about the irresponsibility of young, poor, racial and ethnic minority women.[62] Arguably, projects of sexual health governance in practice can never fully extricate themselves from these invidious histories. Describing the programs that promote LARC to young Latina women, Chris Barcelos has noted not only the long history of white social anxieties about "responsible" reproduction among women of color but also the glaring absence of a concern with sexuality as a domain of pleasure and desire.[63]

Yet this is not the whole story when considering the broader outlines of sexual health governance, and again, comparison with the social hygiene era helps to make the point. Importantly, sexual health governance in recent decades, as distinct from the earlier social hygiene era, has also counterposed responsibilities with *rights*, thereby balancing—at least potentially, and at least for some—the two opposing tugs of citizenship. This approach presumes not only the rise and success of social movements that have demanded rights around sexual expression and sexual identity but also the broader valorization of the sort of individual that rights discourses themselves presuppose—a modern individual who is deemed capable of self-knowledge and who can be exhorted to make responsible choices.[64]

In addition, the nature of the interest in promoting biosexual citizenship has also changed since the social hygiene era, with the moral dimensions of the discourse transformed—at least during the Obama administration—by a partial and tentative embrace of the virtues and benefits of sexuality, the endorsement of the idea of a right to sexual expression (within fairly well demarcated bounds), a more straightforward repudiation of a sexual double standard between men and women, and a much greater openness than in the past to diversity with regard to sexual identity. (Of course, greater openness at the level of rhetoric is no guarantee of changed practice.) These differences in moral and political valences between the two eras cannot be understood absent a consideration of how certain sensibilities of late twentieth- and early twenty-first-century social movements—particularly civil rights, feminist, and LGBTQ movements—came to percolate not only through the broader society but also through government administrative agencies, especially in the Obama years.[65]

One sign of the influence of social movements is the recent emphasis on inclusivity and consensus in building bridges between government, civil society, and individual citizens. To be sure, in promoting projects such as sex education, moral reformers in the social hygiene era sought to enlist not only public schools but also "families, churches, [and] civic institutions," as the historians John D'Emilio and Estelle Freedman have described.[66] But the aspirations of recent sexual health governance are even broader. Consistent with his assembling of a wide array of participants from academia, religious institutions, foundations, and public interest groups at the technical consultation in 2010, the CDC's Fenton called for incorporating "new, diverse, and dynamic partners" to the table in building a "holistic coalition."[67] These emphases reflect a political environment in which government health officials perceive the expectation that they reach out to advocacy groups and other so-called partners and stakeholders that may claim a right to participate in the process of addressing social problems.

Still, sexual health governance in this sense appears to be at least as much top-down as bottom-up. Even while the recent era of sexual health governance is more formally inclusive than that of the earlier era of social hygiene and more respectful of the rights-bearing individual, nonetheless the kinds of citizenship offered in the name of sexual health frequently appear to involve the invitation to adopt authorized ways of behaving responsibly so as to be granted access to the status of the good citizen.

Similarities and differences also surface when considering the pragmatic interests of military officials during the two historical eras. Much like the preoccupations of the military during the First World War, the Sexual Health and Responsibility Program (SHARP) of the Navy and Marine Corps (founded in 1998) directs its educational efforts at "the consequences of sexual risk-taking," not just for the individual sailor or marine but also for the efficiency of the organization. Writing in a special issue of *Public Health Reports* in 2013 that featured sexual health, the program manager, Michael R. (Bob) MacDonald, provided statistics to emphasize the burden placed on the military by health care costs and lost-duty days as a result of STIs and unplanned pregnancies. Yet the program's motto, "Chart a Safe Course" (symbolized by a lighthouse logo) was intended to affirm "that individuals have both the right and responsibility to make choices about their health, and that sexual health decision-making is a lifelong and dynamic process because a person's life circumstances and relationships may change over time."[68] Thus, the more blatant moral rhetoric of the social hygiene era was mostly absent, replaced by a discourse of "responsibilization" that locates the individual moral actor as the person who has both the right and responsibility to make health-promoting choices.

In a further indication of social change, MacDonald hailed the repeal of the military's "don't ask, don't tell" policy as "a new opportunity to more openly address issues of HIV risk among gay and bisexual men in uniform."[69] Here again, we see how certain tropes associated with recent social movement activism around gender equality, LGBTQ rights and HIV/AIDS destigmatization have made their way into health governance and even military organizations, resulting in new emphases on inclusiveness, choice, and agency. Yet the exercise of choices and rights inevitably runs up against limits in the context of a military organization. Indeed, the careful balancing of rights with responsibilities in the discourse of SHARP suggests a perception that there may be only so many potential "safe courses" that might be charted while still ensuring that—so to speak—the sailor makes it safely back to port.

HEALTH DISPARITIES AND LGBTQ INCLUSION

An additional point of contrast between the two eras concerns the kinds of political opportunities that emerge at a time when the reduction of health disparities is an important official goal of government health agencies as well as a guiding frame for health advocacy groups. Especially since the late 1980s, through the efforts of a tacit coalition that encompassed activists, health professionals, and government health officials (importantly including Surgeon General Satcher), HHS agencies have embraced the mandate of reducing and eliminating health disparities, especially by race, ethnicity, and gender.[70] Often accompanying the goal of targeting health disparities is a corresponding emphasis on providing "culturally competent care," in accordance with HHS's "National Standards for Culturally and Linguistically Appropriate Services (CLAS) in Health and Health Care."[71] These policy frameworks subsequently have provided important new possibilities for advancing biosexual citizenship claims under the banner of LGBTQ health—or increasingly, "sexual and gender minority" (SGM) health—

which has come to be understood as another domain where health disparities regularly surface.

In response to lobbying by LGBTQ organizations, federal health agencies began turning their attention to health concerns affecting sexual and gender minorities in the late 1990s (in the waning years of the Clinton administration), as LGBTQ people crossed the symbolic boundary from "outsider" to "citizen."[72] This new emphasis ebbed during the George W. Bush administration but picked up steam again with the publication in 2011 of a lengthy Institute of Medicine report on LGBT health that had been commissioned by the NIH, as well as by the establishment of an Internal LGBT Coordinating Committee within HHS.[73] In 2015, the NIH released its inaugural Strategic Plan for Sexual and Gender Minority Health Research and created a new Sexual and Gender Minority Research Office, located within the Office of the NIH Director and tasked with coordinating SGM research activities across the agency.[74] Then, in October 2016, the NIH formally designated sexual and gender minorities (or "SGM populations") as "a health disparity population for research purposes."[75] That same year, an NIH web page was devoted to "NIH Pride Celebration 2016," a set of activities organized by three NIH units: the Office of Equity, Diversity, and Inclusion, the Sexual and Gender Minority Research Office, and the National Institute on Minority Health and Health Disparities.[76] All these efforts came about through the interplay between health officials and LGBTQ advocacy organizations, particularly those focusing specifically on rights to medical care and rights to sexual freedom.[77]

To be sure, matters of LGBTQ health may often concern issues unrelated to sexual behavior and sexual health per se—focusing instead, for example, on health effects of social stigmatization or, in the case of transgender people, effects of hormones. Yet while earlier moves, in the 1990s and 2000s, toward promoting LGBTQ health often sought to bypass controversy by downplaying sexuality altogether,[78] more recent attention has treated sexual health as an intrinsic component of the overall health of sexual and gender minorities.[79] (For example, the Institute of Medicine report specifically reviewed not just the impact of the HIV/AIDS epidemic but also, as a separate category, the sexual health concerns of LGBTQ individuals.[80]) Thus while the emphases of LGBTQ health advocacy extend beyond questions of sexuality, in practice the new attention to sexual and gender minorities reflects, in part, their incorporation within an inclusionary framework of biomedical and sexual governance and citizenship that targets health disparities while aligning with sexual health.[81]

The Trumpian Turn

Donald Trump's election as president in 2016 quickly sparked alarm among many of those committed to the broad agenda of sexual health governance in the United States—not to mention many others concerned about sexual and reproductive freedoms. Alongside the enforcement of the "global gag rule," there were additional worrisome indicators of a changed atmosphere. Trump appointed Tom Price, a physician and Republican member of Congress from Georgia, as his first secretary of HHS, prompting critics to note his staunch opposition to reproductive choice and LGBTQ rights, among other issues.[82] In Trump's first year, HHS cut grants to eighty-one organizations whose programs aim at pregnancy prevention, and the administration proceeded to favor abstinence until marriage as the preferred framework for sexual health education.[83] The administration's perceived indifference to the course of the HIV/AIDS epidemic led six members of the Presidential Advisory Council on HIV/AIDS to resign in June 2017; Trump then fired the remaining members of the council in December, reportedly without explanation and in letters delivered by FedEx.[84]

Efforts continued to remove "sexual health" language from United Nations resolutions. "We do not support references to ambiguous terms and expressions, such as sexual and reproductive health and rights in UN documents, because they can undermine the critical role of the family and promote practices, like abortion," HHS Secretary Alex Azar told the UN General Assembly in September 2019.[85] A number of other actions and policies supported by the administration or the Republican-controlled Congress aimed to reduce reproductive choice, for example by restricting access to health plans that cover abortions.[86] The health of LGBTQ people also seemed at risk, with a new rule permitting health care providers to discriminate against them based on religious motives.[87] One press report from shortly after the inauguration in January 2017 described how the CDC had postponed indefinitely an LGBT youth health summit that had been in the works for months.[88] Later, advocates protested when it was learned that questions concerning sexual orientation were to be removed from a federal health survey of the elderly population.[89] "If they don't count us, we don't count," LGBTQ health advocates warned; ultimately, HHS officials responded to pressure and added the questions back to the survey.[90]

Soon afterward, President Trump announced by tweet a ban on transgender soldiers in the military, supposedly driven by concern over the costs of their health care—although, as many commentators noted, the amount spent by the military on gender-affirming medical care for transgender troops was less than one-tenth of the $84 million it devoted to erectile dysfunction medications.[91] While the presence of transgender soldiers was deemed to threaten "unit cohesion," the vision of sexual health connoted by Viagra seemed to signify "readiness" in a way that aligned happily with a conservative vision of military—and masculinist—ideals.

Yet another threat of erasure, widely discussed in 2017, concerned a list of words that reportedly had been "banned" at the CDC, including "transgender" and "fetus," among others. The move was widely condemned, and transgender health advocates cited the CDC's own research that pointed to the greater health risks encountered by transgender people.[92] It later became known that agency officials had not so much forbidden the words as warned employees that it would not be strategic to use them in funding requests.[93] However, this clarification did not allay concerns.

When released toward the end of the Trump administration, Healthy People 2030, the government's decennial health plan, appeared to demote issues of sexual (or sexual and reproductive) health, which had been featured in the two preceding plans. The phrase didn't appear, and the only related issue to make the list of "leading health indicators" was the objective of increasing the proportion of people who know their HIV status. However, Healthy People 2030 did list sixteen objectives relating to the goal of "improving the health, safety, and well-being of lesbian, gay, bisexual, and transgender people" and twenty-two objectives relating to sexually transmitted infections.[94]

An analysis of the strategic plans issued by HHS every several years also suggests a more restrictive approach to sexual health on the part of the Trump administration.[95] To be sure, none of the recent strategic plans that I reviewed (from 2004 forward) contain the phrase "sexual health." Yet the plans issued in 2004, 2007, 2010, and 2014 all contain multiple references to sexually transmitted infections, unprotected sexual activity, and sexual risk behaviors, and the 2010 and 2014 plans also refer to issues of sexual orientation and the health concerns of LGBTQ individuals. By contrast, the 2018 plan uses the word "sexual" only twice, both times in reference to sexual violence. The words "gay," "lesbian," "bisexual," and "transgender" do not appear.[96]

OUTSIDERS AND CITIZENS

In other ways, too, the rhetoric and practice of the Trump administration strengthened the possibilities for the drawing of sharp lines between "good" and "bad" sexual citizens.[97] Anti-immigrant policies and the stoking of overt xenophobia and white nationalism raised the prospect of potentially significant changes in sexual health governance and biosexual citizenship. In an essay I first drafted during the Obama presidency, I observed: "while xenophobic and anti-immigrant sentiments continue to be widespread in the broader society, in the era of social hygiene and eugenics they were part of the official discourse, while (again, at least up through the Obama years) they have been de-linked from sexual health governance, at least in any overt fashion."[98] Yet even my tempered optimism demanded some rethinking after the President himself invoked sexualized rhetoric by branding immigrants as "rapists."[99] Trump's florid language made clear that the deformations of sexual health governance during his term were not simply those of the censorship or silencing of sexual health concerns. Rather, as Michel Foucault noted long ago in his *History of Sexuality*, silencing is just one tactic among the many modes by which sexuality is set in motion and endowed with powerful performative effects.[100]

DILEMMAS OF SCIENCE AND EVIDENCE

Trump and his supporters also cultivated suspicion of scientific expertise—in general, but including around sexual health. This populist revolt against expert "elites" also prompts consideration of the longer historical trajectory.[101] What has "science" meant in the governing of sexuality and health, and what notions of science have been invoked?

During the social hygiene era, reformers placed their faith in technocratic rule and in the person of the expert. With the institutionalization of sexual health governance, appeals to science clearly remained a crucial legitimating rhetoric, yet faith in the person of the expert was displaced, or supplemented, by insistence on the evidentiary basis and methodological warrants for proper action to promote sexual health.[102] Government documents and articles referred, for example, to "scientifically tested and proven interventions"; "scaling up evidence-based practices"; "the CDC-recommended, evidence-based, six-step model for working with patients to reduce sexual risk behavior"; and "formal government recognition of the need for an evidence-based public health approach to the promotion of sexual health . . . in the U.S."[103] This emphasis on locating the government's sexual health advice within the framework of evidence-based medicine and policy was accompanied by an interest in developing nationally representative surveys and surveillance systems that would permit public health officials to track progress toward sexual health goals.[104] "Robust data provide the cornerstone for an effective public health response," wrote the CDC's Fenton in 2010 in the *Journal of Sexual Medicine*, describing the need for population-based surveys of sexual health and behavior.[105] Thus, modern sexual health governance presupposed the development of the formal scientific tools to "operationalize" sexual health that I described in part 2.

In these ways and through these various means, the "good biosexual citizen" was imagined as someone who acts in accordance with the best available evidence and divulges truthful information about his or her sexuality. While the original WHO discussion of sexual health made no mention of evidence, the emphasis on evidence-based "interventions" assumed that matters of sexuality should be addressed from the standpoint of outcomes, and more specifically that sexual health practices require validation of a particular sort, derived by testing an intervention in a prospective manner using a control group.[106] As Fenton also observed, the appeal to evidence "fit with the culture of the CDC" and immunized his efforts against any perception of "being sort of touchy-feely."[107]

Indeed, public health officials' insistence on evidence has been an important tactic in countering attempts to impose policies that are driven, first and foremost, by narrowly political or ideological concerns—always a particular risk when the topic is sexuality, and certainly so during the Trump administration. Notably, another of the terms deemed controversial at the CDC, along with "transgender" and "fetus," was "evidence based"—and the suggestion that evidence was now deemed irrelevant or contrary to good policy struck most observers as astonishing—or in the words of the chief executive of the American Academy for the Advancement of Science, "ridiculous."[108] At a so-called post-truth moment when scientific evidence was being deemed less persuasive than ideological commitments, yet another cornerstone of the discourse around sexual health governance seemed at risk of being dislodged.[109]

When the very idea of evidence seems under attack, there is a natural tendency to respond by ratcheting up the defense of evidence-based policymaking. Yet overreliance on narrow conceptions of evidence can also be problematic for sexual health governance. The policy emphasis on validating sexual health interventions and disseminating those that are "evidence based" has been controversial insofar as it typically imposes the model of the randomized clinical trial—drawn from pharmaceutical drug testing and epidemiological research—onto the domain of sexual practice, where it may fit less well.[110] Prioritizing evidence may also privilege narrow but testable understandings of sexuality and sexual health over more complex renderings that are less easy to operationalize and test.[111] Finally, the turn to evidence as the final arbiter of "responsible" sexual practice may have the effect of demarcating the bounds of legitimate participation in decision making about sexuality by restricting it to those who have the expertise, credentials, and experience deemed necessary to produce and evaluate evidence. The Trumpian moment therefore raised the stakes in considering the complicated question of how one might mount a robust defense of scientific reasoning around sexual health without presupposing which forms of science, or which blends of expertise and democratic participation, are most appropriate for the purpose.

CONTRADICTIONS OF SEXUAL HEALTH GOVERNANCE

Certainly, the approach to sexual health during the Trump administration suggested a sharp turn, if not a reversal, in the course of sexual health governance. Yet some caveats are in order. It bears notice that the rightward movement in relation to sexual topics in fact harked back to earlier episodes in the George W. Bush administration. Flash points from those years included an unwillingness on the part of the CDC to endorse the efficacy of condoms in preventing the spread of HIV; a decision by the FDA to overrule its expert advisory panel and ban a morning-after contraceptive pill; the institution of an HHS policy limiting attendance by government scientists at international AIDS conferences; and advice by NIH program officers to researchers that they might escape scrutiny by Republicans in Congress by avoiding certain terms in grant applications, including "sex worker," "men who have sex with men," "anal sex," and "needle exchange."[112] Yet those developments nonetheless coincided with the early phases of the establishment of sexual health governance as described in this chapter. Thus, on the one hand, developments under Trump may constitute less of a break with the recent past than they first appear, when compared with a previous Republican administration; and on the other hand, every administration is at least somewhat internally inconsistent in its policy approaches, much as my theoretical discussion of the disunity of "the state" would predict.

Indeed, even while, under Trump, the State Department sought to ban the phrase "sexual and reproductive health" and some federal agencies deleted online references to LGBT concerns, the NIH Sexual and Gender Minority Research Office continued to operate and to advertise its goals, activities, and funding calls on its website and listserv. In 2019, the office released an expanded definition of sexual and gender minority populations, which now included lesbian, gay, bisexual, asexual, transgender, two-spirit, queer, and intersex persons, among others.[113] And in the last months of the Trump administration, the office released its strategic plan for the coming five years, featuring an affirmative message from NIH's director Francis Collins.[114] The NIH even continued, throughout the Trump years, to mark the annual celebration of LGBT pride with a dedicated web page.[115]

At the level of the Department of Health and Human Services, actions in support of sexual health governance also continued right up to the final weeks of the Trump administration. In December, HHS released the first-ever Sexually Transmitted Infections National Strategic Plan, specifying goals and strategies for the coming five years. (My comparison of the final plan with the draft released for public comment a few months earlier suggests that advocates were successful in inserting language on topics related to sexual and gender minorities.[116]) As noted, Healthy People 2030, while downplaying sexual health generally, nonetheless retained sixteen health objectives linked to the topic of promoting LGBT health.[117] More generally, key policy documents like the National Prevention Strategy remained in place, ensuring at least an official commitment to the promotion of sexual and reproductive health, as US Public Health Service officials themselves asserted.[118] The judicial branch of government also pushed back, for example by rejecting the administration's attempt to exclude LGBT people from key protections under the Affordable Care Act.[119] In short, while state administration of sexual and health matters clearly passed through a dangerous phase, it is a complex matter to make sense of continuities and breaks in sexual health governance.

Beyond the United States:
Varied Contexts of Sexual Health Governance

I described in earlier chapters how a concern with sexual health spans national borders, so it is not surprising that other countries have also sought to advance sexual health agendas and promote sexual health strategic plans. These include countries as diverse as New Zealand, Cambodia, and Mauritius.[120] One oft-cited effort—the United Kingdom's National Strategy for Sexual Health and HIV (released in July 2001) was contemporaneous with the Surgeon General's Call to Action.[121] But at least one other such initiative—the Canadian government's adoption of "the terms 'sexual health' and 'healthy sexuality' . . . to support the positive integration of sexuality and the prevention of sexual problems"—preceded the US Surgeon General's Call by several years.[122]

I cannot do justice here to the details of these various governance projects.[123] But in general, the diverse emphases of sexual health governance around the world reflect not only the polysemous nature of sexual health that I described in chapter 2—that is, the adoption of the term to characterize and signify a very wide variety of activities and goals—but also the particular preoccupations in different national contexts and the cultural, political, and institutional features of those societies. No doubt some assumptions and inclinations of sexual health governance have diffused across national borders. Yet both the wide variation in how health care is organized and paid for (not to mention large differences in how government is structured in general) and the differences in attitudes about sexual matters necessarily affect how sexual health governance and biosexual citizenship play out.

For example, as Alain Giami has described, the UK National Strategy was intended specifically to rationalize sexual health service delivery within the centralized National Health Service. Very much in contrast to the United States, it adopted a "harm reduction" perspective that included open discussion of access to condoms, contraception, and abortion.[124] In a different case, the Inuit Five-Year Strategic Plan on Sexual Health (released in 2010) was produced by a national representative organization of Inuit women across Canada, and the focus was largely on the prevention of HIV/AIDS and Hepatitis C.[125] By contrast, in Argentina's Programa nacional de salud sexual y procreación responsable (National Program for Sexual Health and Responsible Procreation, known as *Salud sexual* for short), the emphasis is on family planning, and the history of legislation promoting this effort reflects the complexities of gender and class politics in that country.[126] In Iran, the National Document on Sexual Health Training, produced in 2019, cited the WHO's working definition of sexual health yet also stated the aim of "using an Islamic approach" to "promote awareness and education on sexual health and sexual abuse."[127]

Although it is beyond the scope of this book, it would be a fascinating project to consider and systematically compare the varying ideas of "good" and "bad" sexual citizens that have been promoted by sexual health governance activities in countries around the world. No doubt both similarities and differences are worth exploring. In New Zealand, for example, critical analysis of national sexual health programs has pointed to concerns, also relevant to the United States and presumably many other countries, about how dominant discourses of risk may perpetuate histories of stigmatization of ethnic minorities.[128] In England, a newer "Framework for Sexual Health Improvement" adopted in 2013 emphasized sexual health across the life course, and was one of the first governance documents to call attention to sexual health issues for people of older age.[129]

It would likewise be valuable to relate the different visions of governance and citizenship to broader, nation-specific patterns and histories of knowing, studying, and regulating sexuality, health, and the body. Such a comparison might further shed light on the particularities of sexual health governance by examining (among other things) the roles of different branches of government, the kinds of alliances struck between state actors and civil society organizations, and the degree of reliance on discourses and practices of evidence-based medicine and policy.[130]

Rights and Duties of Citizenship:
What Sexual Health Governance "Does"

Sexual health governance clearly varies by country. It also varies by state and region within the United States, and, at the federal level, it is orchestrated differently by different agencies of government. That is, by focusing on HHS, I have provided an incomplete picture of the terrain of sexual health governance, given the "disunity" of modern state apparatuses. We might ask, for example, What does sexual health governance look like for the 1.4 million people who are held in prison in the United States? The continued refusal in many jurisdictions to countenance basic projects of safer-sex promotion, such as condom distribution, within US prisons suggests how certain key state agencies reinforce an approach to sexual health governance defined essentially in terms of neglect and callous disregard, if not outright punitive and racist intent.[131]

Even when restricting our attention to public health agencies, it appears that the institutional and political practices relating to sexual health have multiple consequences and repercussions. Some of these have to do with sexuality and health specifically: establishing new visions for what constitutes health, and prescribing what constitutes acceptable sexual practices—or challenging such assertions. However, other effects are broad ranging and demonstrate some of the new uses to which sexual health may be put. They include providing templates for the—often partial—incorporation of individuals and groups into the broader society; drawing boundaries between those who are deemed to "belong" and those deemed not, according to race, ethnicity, sexual identity, immigration status, and so forth; and "managing" groups deemed problematic. In other words, sexual health governance is meant to solve sexual problems, and health problems, but *not just* those problems. Most abstractly, the issues at hand include: How should people behave? How can social order be maintained? How can individual desires for freedom coexist with social order? What are the rights and duties of citizenship? This broad array of concerns makes evident that much more is at stake in sexual health governance than the question of whether sexuality has become "medicalized." Sexual health governance can be pursued in the service of a wide variety of ends, and the imperative of being healthy is ultimately just one of them.

In aiming to bring about a distinctive national future, projects of sexual health governance provide examples of what Sheila Jasanoff and Sang-Hyun Kim have termed "sociotechnical imaginaries": "collectively imagined forms of social life and social order reflected in the design and fulfillment of nation-specific scientific and/or technological projects."[132] My analysis has revealed how, in the United States, such projects have been addressed through both contestation and consensus, and through consideration of both responsibilities and rights. Given the recent official emphases on inclusiveness and the participation of designated stakeholders, and following the diffusion into worlds of governance of rights-based language promoted by social movements, it appears that advocacy groups demanding sexual rights—including a right to sexuality as a form of pleasure—have become important and recognized voices in the public sphere (though not, of course, without pushback). Moreover, the polyvalent discourse of sexual health often provides such groups with "cover" to raise taboo topics in a socially legitimate language.

However, advocacy groups rarely set the terms of discourse or policy in a domain increasingly governed by a fairly limited set of authoritative frameworks: biomedical risk, social responsibility, and evidence-based practice. As I have noted, these frameworks do not inhere necessarily in modern conceptions of sexual health and indeed were much less present in the original WHO-sponsored definition. But they have often been central to what I have termed sexual health governance, at least in the US context (though probably beyond). Furthermore, it seems clear that the worrisome developments in sexual health governance that followed the election of Donald Trump as president constituted a powerful pushback against the gains of progressive social movements. Even in the Biden administration, these developments may herald a more constrained environment for promoting sexual health and may inscribe invidious distinctions between those deemed truly to "belong" to the polity and those imagined as threats, problems, or outsiders.

This study of sexual health governance makes evident just how central matters of sexuality and health have become to everyday understandings of the scope and purpose of politics. The next chapter develops this argument even further by exploring how, across the political divide, the goal of sexual health proves politically efficacious by suggesting competing visions of a better future toward which we might work.

10 *Bridges to the Future*

REPOLITICIZING SEXUAL HEALTH

Three years after leaving his government post, the former surgeon general David Satcher embarked on what might be the most quixotic campaign in the history of sexual health. Having issued the landmark "Call to Action" on sexual health, Satcher had retained his interest in the issue and had founded a sexual health program at the Morehouse School of Medicine in Atlanta. Then, in 2004, seeking to overcome what he called an "environment of polarization," Satcher contacted the leaders of twenty-eight nonprofit organizations from across the political spectrum that focus on sexuality policy, and he invited them to meet to come to agreement on just what would constitute sexual health, how it should be pursued, and how it should be researched. Twenty-five of the groups, including the Black Women's Health Imperative, the Medical Institute for Sexual Health, the National Council of Churches, and the Planned Parenthood Federation of America, accepted the invitation and sent representatives to a series of meetings over the course of eighteen months.[1]

Coming to consensus proved difficult. Seven of the advocacy groups—including Focus on the Family and the Traditional Values Coalition on the Right, and the Lambda Legal Defense and Education Fund and the Gay, Lesbian, and Straight Education Network on the Left—withdrew before the process was complete because of what were later described as their "divergent perspectives." However, in 2006, Satcher released a fifty-page interim report that outlined the areas of agreement among the eighteen organizations that stuck with the process, along with what were politely called the "areas of current non-agreement." Said the report: "We have dared to touch a '3rd rail' in what some describe as the US cultural wars and discovered that it is possible to reach some areas of significant agreement, while not compromising deeply-held values, beliefs or commitments about which we may continue to disagree."[2] In his own public comments at the time, Satcher struck a more modest note: "I'll leave it to other people to say whether it was a success. [But] if you can get people to come together and listen to each other, that's an achievement."[3]

The participants reached consensus on a statement of best practices for research on sexual health that would ensure reliability, internal validity, external validity, replicability, and statistical significance—that is, an agreement that was more procedural than substantive, though many participants hailed it an important accomplishment.[4] In addition, the report described a common "vision for sexual health": "We envision a society in which individuals, families and communities are encouraged to understand human sexuality and to cultivate sexual health and responsible sexual behavior. In a society committed to the sexual health of all people, individuals would understand and respect their own sexuality and that of others. Norms for responsible sexual activity must promote individual and community health in ways that are respectful of the varying and deeply-held perspectives on these sensitive matters within our communities."[5]

This was a relatively bland compromise; it is not hard to imagine the words ("rights," "marriage") that ended up on the cutting-room floor. The "areas of non-agreement" among the participants who stayed with the process particularly included beliefs about sexual orientation, strategies to address HIV/AIDS and other STIs, and frameworks for sexual health education—that is, many of the places where the rubber hits the road in sexuality and health policy.[6]

As an exercise in what the report called "respectful listening," the so-called National Consensus Process proved modestly successful, perhaps beyond what many of its participating group leaders anticipated.[7] "I didn't expect anything to come from it," recalled Sharon Camp, the president of the Guttmacher Institute. "I thought I'd go to the first few meetings, but I got hooked."[8] But as an attempt to forge consensus on a sexual health agenda for the United States, this endeavor, not surprisingly, fell victim to the wide divergence in political visions that "sexual health" has been invoked to describe.

The Strategic Utility of Sexual Health:
The Politics of Articulation

It is not news that sexuality often lies at the crux of conflict between the Left and the Right in the United States. Same-sex marriage, sex trafficking, abortion, the availability of contraception, and the question of who uses which bathrooms are just a few of the many sexuality-related topics that have been staples of political debate in recent years—sometimes as substantive concerns, but often as symbolic politics and the means to foment moral panics.[9] Sex education (often called "sexual health education") for young people is a telling example of the fiercely competing character of analyses and proposals: on one side, calls to reorient educational programs in ways that recognize rights, pleasure, and desire, under the banner of "comprehensive" sexuality education; on the other hand, a focus on "sexual risk avoidance" and the promotion of "abstinence-only until marriage," with pleas for attention to responsibility, sexual "integrity," and the risks of unhealthy outcomes.[10] Although my focus in this chapter will be the United States, many scholars have noted the global dimensions of these sorts of political struggles over sexual beliefs, practices, identities, and policies.[11]

Rather than recap the long history and broad dimensions of the politicization of sexuality (or, for that matter, health) in the United States, I take a different and more specific approach: I examine how the recasting of such issues as being matters of *sexual health* permits varied political actors to use sexual health as a bridge to broader critiques and visions of a better future.[12] This approach continues the emphasis of part 3 of this book on the crucial question: once sexuality and health have become connected, what *other* agendas—located some distance from traditional health and medical domains—can now be pursued?[13]

In other words, I explore the strategic utility of sexual health projects—but not just insofar as they affect sexuality or health. I provide a number of examples of what I will call "bridging work," although I focus on two in particular: among the Christian Right, bridging from a critique of sexuality deemed unhealthy to efforts to reinforce traditional family forms and patriarchal gender relations; and on the Left, bridging from the problem of sexual assault and nonconsensual sex to a broader critique of gender inequalities. Although the perspectives on sexual matters could not be more different, my point is that political actors on both the Right and the Left have been laying claim to what they call sexual health. And in both cases the forging of a connection between sexual health and a broader political vision has proved strategically useful in a struggle to gain allies, influence public opinion, and bring about social change. Both are examples of what political theorists Ernesto Laclau and Chantal Mouffe called "the practice of articulation," which involves constructing new, albeit temporary, alignments of discourses and practices across the social and political terrain.[14] Not coincidentally, both efforts involve a concern with "education," broadly construed—not just sex education in the formal sense (though certainly that), but also more general efforts to educate the public about sexual health matters in an effort to shape visions of a better society.[15]

DEPOLITICIZATION VERSUS REPOLITICIZATION

There is a sense in which my focus on "bridging" marks a break from the kinds of examples used elsewhere in this book. I have offered many descriptions of how people invoke the discourses and practices of sexual health in the hope of sanitizing potentially controversial topics relating to sexuality—containing sex safely in the embrace of health and granting it legitimacy by doing so. Such sanitizing, I have also suggested, may sometimes go hand in hand with *depoliticizing*, where the goal is to fly under the radar and escape unwanted attention. Yet sometimes, people find that the label and discourse of sexual health offer an effective lever to move their concerns front and center in the political landscape. They may invoke sexual health not to depoliticize an issue but rather to *repoliticize* it—to characterize its political significance in a new and different way, precisely by bringing to bear the apparent weight of expert authority, or at least, the cachet of health as a social good. By this route, as opposing groups organize, mobilize, and promote or resist social change, sexual health may become a battleground—a site of struggle over competing visions of our collective futures.[16]

Of course, the choice of whether to use sexual health to depoliticize or to repoliticize is itself a strategic one, and the best way forward may not always be obvious. This was the dilemma that confronted Planned Parenthood in 2019 when its new director, Leana Wen, sought, according to some commentators, "to significantly reorient the group's focus away from the abortion wars and more toward its role as a women's health provider." By emphasizing that the agency's work represented proper health care, pure and simple, Wen (herself a physician) sought to insulate the organization at an especially difficult political moment. "This is health care" was the straightforward name of one advocacy campaigns launched under Wen's tenure. Yet at a time when abortion rights seemed especially vulnerable and the Trump administration and Republicans in Congress had, in effect, placed a target on the back of Planned Parenthood, many within the organization sought a more forceful political advocate at the helm—leading, in part, to Wen's rapid departure from her post.[17] That is, Wen's critics within the organization sought not to take refuge under the protective shadow cast by "health" but rather to bridge from sexual health to a broader political agenda.

FRAME BRIDGING

How does sexual health enter the domain of the political? How are new "bridges" built? To explain how this happens, I adopt some of the vocabulary of scholars of social movements who use the concept of framing to call attention to the ways in which groups with political agendas actively engage in signification processes—how they seek to shape representations of reality and say what the world is like.[18] The polysemy of sexual health facilitates this process, making it an especially adaptable term and object for pursuing political goals of various sorts, or for becoming rhetorically linked to other concerns.[19]

One of the common means by which political actors invoke connections across issues and bring frames into alignment with the perceived interests of potential adopters is through what analysts of social movements call "frame bridging": linking together two different frames that were previously unconnected but that can be presented as ideologically congruent.[20] Such bridging work is most glaringly apparent when the two concerns being linked have not historically been seen as related in an appreciable way—say, for example, the promotion of sexual health and the legalization of marijuana use, two agendas which some advocates have sought to unite under the banner of the "cannabis sexual health movement."[21] Or consider an editorial that appeared in 2009 in the *Lancet*, the prominent medical journal based in the United Kingdom. Entitled "Sexual and Reproductive Health and Climate Change," the editorial fleshed out what, at first glance, might seem an unlikely union of topics. In essence, the editorial maintained that attention to population control would become ever more important around the globe in order to mitigate the likely consequences of climate change. Therefore, for those interested in promoting greater access to contraception, climate change increased the urgency while presenting new opportunities to get out the message: "perhaps it is time for the sexual and reproductive health community to use the climate change agenda to gain the traction women's health deserves."[22]

In other cases, frame bridging demonstrates the aspiration to forge connections and alliances across constituencies. In 2015, for example, the National Coalition for Sexual Health promoted the hashtag #BlackSexualHealthMatters. In an article on its website (reprinted from the website BlackDoctor.org), the organization used the hashtag to describe "a call-to-action to increase the use of essential preventive sexual health care services in the Black community"—most specifically, the use of PrEP, or preexposure prophylaxis for HIV. While making a cogent case for the need for enhanced HIV prevention efforts in Black communities based on epidemiological trends, the article, in effect, "leaned on" the contemporary visibility and political salience of the Black Lives Matter movement to confer both topicality and urgency on its message.[23]

Pairings such as these suggest how advocates might strategically link the most diverse sorts of concerns. These examples begin to suggest the important political possibilities for individuals and groups from across the political spectrum to bridge from sexual health to other political programs. In the next two sections, I focus on a few especially salient illustrations, first from the political Right and then from the Left.

Frame Bridging on the Christian Right: Sexual Health, Wholeness, and Social Responsibility

While it is well known that evangelical Christians associated with political conservatism have had much to say about sexuality, it may come more as a surprise to learn that they are also invested in what many of them call sexual health. On the one hand, sex is a frequent topic of discussion in advice books and columns, in blogs, and in online resources aimed at evangelical Christians, and these cultural sources offer guidance about how to integrate a "healthy" sexuality into a moral life. On the other hand, sexuality is an immediate concern of numerous advocacy groups that seek to apply Christian principles—alongside what they herald as scientific evidence—in the development of a conservative political agenda. Between these two worlds—that of advice and counseling, and that of collective political action—I argue that the elastic discourse of sexual health provides an important bridge.[24]

In chapter 1, I emphasized the long history of sex advice in the United States, as well as the diverse beliefs about healthy sexuality that those proffering such advice held and sought to promulgate. Then, in chapter 7, I analyzed the more recent rise of new manifestations of sexual health expertise, often engaged in the advice business. The distinctive makeup of present-day evangelical Christian sex advice is a fascinating case in point that has begun to receive significant scholarly attention. Correcting a common misunderstanding, the historian Dagmar Herzog has pointed out that "the Religious Right is . . . hugely sex-affirmative with respective to marital sex." Indeed, "since at least the mid-1970s, evangelical Christians have been pushing the good word that evangelicals have more fun—that godly sex is the most fabulous sex."[25]

As the sociologist Kelsy Burke and the religious studies scholar Amy DeRogatis have both observed in recent years, the internet, and popular culture generally, is awash in evangelical commentary about sexual matters. Rather than imagine a uniform prudishness among Christian conservatives, this scholarship suggests, "many American evangelicals have come to believe that good marital sex is not just ordained by God, but is healthy and leads to strong self-esteem, financial prosperity, and heightened spiritual awareness."[26] DeRogatis describes sermons on appropriate sexual behavior delivered from pulpits across the United States, as well as a burgeoning industry of Christian self-help books offering sex advice.[27] (Although DeRogatis emphasizes the fundamental "whiteness" of the evangelical target audience, as depicted in illustrations of White couples but also in notions of sexual purity as being "lily white," she also devotes a chapter to "books and blogs about sexuality and salvation geared to evangelical people of color."[28]) Burke goes further in her analysis of communication to consider "a wide range of digital media, including online sex toy stores, online message boards, blogs, podcasts, and virtual Bible studies that discuss a plethora of topics related to marital sex."[29]

According to Burke, "BetweenTheSheets.com, LustyChristianLadies. com, LovingGroom.com, AffectionateMarriage.com, StoreOfSolomon.

com, and MaribelsMarriage.com are all examples of Christian sexuality websites—sites that are easily recognizable as Christian with content focused specifically and explicitly on positive expressions of sex/sexuality within marriage."[30] Through their engagement with these websites and their products, Burke argues, Christians "present themselves as sexually modern rather than prudish, distancing themselves from stereotypes about conservative religion and sex."[31] Indeed, Burke finds evidence of positive assessments by at least some evangelicals of a wide range of sexual practices extending as far as erotic cross-dressing and "pegging" (a woman's use of a strap-on dildo to anally penetrate a man). These practices are deemed acceptable, at least by some, with the crucial proviso that they are performed by a husband and wife in the service of promoting marital intimacy. In these online discussions, participants "draw upon God's approval of sexual intimacy and pleasure within marriage relationships to make decisions about the appropriateness of non-normative sex" and, sometimes, find ways to "imbue kinky acts with alternative meanings."[32]

My own research into that subset of evangelical Christian discourse that specifically references "sexual health" revealed a somewhat tamer world, with a greater measure of policing accomplished via normative invocations of "health." However, I did find some spirited defenses of marital sexual pleasures. For example, the website Christian Sexual Health, which offers "practical help in areas of Christian sexuality in the hope that husbands and wives would fully enjoy each other in the God ordained union of marriage,"[33] insists that sex is part of God's plan. "If you have been brought up to think that sex is dirty and were not presented with the model of sex being a wonderful blessing within marriage," the website advises frankly, "you may need to get some help."[34] The website's authors acknowledge domains of doctrinal uncertainty—masturbation, for example, "is a gray area" about which the Bible "is strangely silent"[35]—and go so far as to suggest that "a virgin bride will find sexual intimacy far more enjoyable if she has been physically preparing in the months leading up to the wedding" (that is, using her fingers in a daily regimen of gradually stretching the hymen).[36]

More generally, however, conservative Christian sexual health advice is a hybrid mix of several diverse elements: conservative religious doctrine, complete with references to biblical passages; a broadly psychological discourse about healthy relationships and the place of sex within them; and appeals to scientific evidence about forms of health

and disease linked to sexuality. This mixture bears out Herzog's contention that "no matter what the topic, arguments for greater sexual
conservatism today invariably come wrapped in the language not just
of physical health but especially also of psychological well-being."[37] In
particular, I found that, in conservative Christian discussions, sexual
health is often equated with other terms that suggest psychological, but also spiritual, well-being, such as "sexual integrity" and "sexual wholeness." Moreover, and not at all inconsistently with Herzog's
point, conservative Christians are keen to find and invoke scientific
experts whose views support their own stances—and thereby to position themselves as critical participants in a modern world of reasoned
discourse.[38]

On his website, Gary Thomas (self-described as "a bestselling author
and international speaker whose ministry brings people closer to Christ
and closer to others") offers advice that exemplifies Herzog's point
about the psychotherapeutic framing of evangelical prescriptions. In
his discussion of the "marks of a healthy sexual relationship," Thomas
maintains that "Christian sex is always relational sex. . . . Healthy sex
serves a relationship; unhealthy sex becomes the relationship which is
asking too much of sex."[39] This commitment to health—understood simultaneously as sexual, relational, and spiritual—permits Thomas to
take a firmer stance against deviations from "vanilla" marital heterosexuality. He argues, for example, that "allowing your husband to wear
your undergarments or indulging some other fetish so that he's not
shamed by it is sort of like holding a needle while he injects himself
with heroin."[40] Setting aside the unabashed commitment to "a biblical
view of sex," the discourse of wholeness and authenticity results in assessments of sexual "unhealthiness" that, at least in certain instances,
might as easily have originated from secular sources, including some
well to the left on the political spectrum: "In unhealthy sexuality, the
sexual experience leaves you feeling empty, alienated, almost like you're
role-playing or an object."[41]

Other online sources similarly frame their prescriptions from the
standpoint of sexual health. The website of the Christian Association
of Sexual Educators (a project of Sexual Wholeness Inc., based in Su-
wanee, Georgia) promotes training sessions designed to "equip and
empower ministry leaders," who will then "be confidently commissioned to permeate all facets of their church with sexual health and

preventive wholeness."[42] In its vision statement, entitled "Cultivating Sexually Healthy Churches," the organization offers "a practical theology of sexuality based on Biblical truth that emphasizes God-reflective intimacy, chastity and covenant monogamy," along with "sexual wholeness," "practical and accurate sexual information," and a commitment to "nurturing the sexually wounded, encouraging hope, healing and restoration."[43]

Yet sources of evangelical Christian sexual health advice share not only a psychotherapeutic sensibility and an instinct to invoke the goal of "health" but also a cultural critique and lament: the perception, common to evangelical discourse more generally, of being beleaguered defenders of traditional morality in a world where social supports have broken down, threats to moral order run rampant, and narcissistic individualism trumps a commitment to the greater good.[44] Specifically, with regard to sexual matters (which are seen as especially symptomatic), commentators point to the decline of traditional family forms, the lingering effects of the sexual revolution, increasing social acceptance of sexual and gender minorities, "a hook-up culture that promotes porn,"[45] and "our hyper-sexualized culture" that reaches nearly everyone via the internet and cable television.[46] This cultural critique is significant because of its relation to my main point—that, for evangelicals, the discourse of sexual health offers a bridge between sex advice and political action. In other words, the same threats that imperil healthy sexuality at the level of the individual and necessitate advice and counseling also demand a collective response and an intervention in social policy.

Close attention to a key "para-church" organization on the Christian Right—Focus on the Family—helps to clarify this point. Founded in 1977 by the psychologist James Dobson, the Colorado Springs–based organization with more than six hundred employees promotes a fundamentalist agenda on issues of abortion, gambling, LGBT adoption, same-sex marriage, transgender rights, and substance abuse, among others. Its daily half-hour radio show is broadcast on two thousand radio outlets in the United States and many others around the world (and is available as a podcast), and its associated political arm, Family Policy Alliance, lobbies on a range of political issues.[47] The organization, which spent more than $92 million in 2018,[48] continues to be influential and well connected: in 2017 Vice President Mike Pence was an honored guest at its fortieth anniversary celebration, where he took the opportunity to declare that President Donald Trump was "an unwavering ally" of the group.[49]

Focus on the Family conceives of itself, in part, as a resource for individuals in need of advice and crisis intervention, and it offers information, referrals for "licensed Christian counselors in your area," and a free consultation "with one of our licensed or pastoral counseling specialists."[50] Its website also makes available an abundance of life advice geared at individuals, some of it under the framework of sexual health. Indeed, for Rob Jackson, who identifies himself on the organization's website (in a series of articles from 2004) as a father of two young children and as a therapist specializing in sexual health, "the topic of sexuality is second only to teaching our child about God."[51] Jackson takes the goal of health seriously: "we want to emphasize that sexual health is part of an overall approach to wellness." Jackson explains: "We teach our children the importance of hygiene and how to take baths that clean the body. We must also teach them how to take emotional and spiritual showers for the mind and spirit."[52]

According to Jackson, "the foundation for sexual health and integrity is loving God and finding satisfaction in His spiritual beauty," and marital sex is "a foretaste of the spiritual connection between Christ and His Church." The implications for Christians, as spouses and as parents, are clear, in his view: God "has empowered us as males and females to express sexuality in gender-specific ways, and he has placed those expressions in the sacred context of marriage."[53] While offered with a scriptural warrant, Jackson's claims, in his view, are also consistent with good science: "Research has shown greater sexual satisfaction within monogamous marriages."[54] Pointing to the hypersexualized "world they are living in"—where children are constantly exposed to sexual images and discourse, Jackson warns his readers: "We had better equip our children."[55]

Elsewhere on its website, Focus on the Family offers its ideas about other sexual and gender-related matters, again by taking a personal approach and proposing practical advice, under headings such as "How Did We Get to This Gender-Confused Place," "Public Restrooms—Your Privacy and Safety," and "When Homosexuality Hits Home for the Holidays."[56] But Focus on the Family's efforts to promote what they consider sexual health do not end with the proffering of advice or individualized counseling. Just as centrally to its mission, Focus on the

Family is a political advocacy organization that seeks to change US society by shaping public opinion and influencing the mass media as well as government officials, legislators, and courts. Thus, the organization takes a strong stand against reproductive choice and in favor of abstinence-only sex education in schools; they seek the defunding of Planned Parenthood; and they oppose civil rights protections for LGBT individuals.[57]

The idea of sexual health is an important framing device for this advocacy work as well. For example, in 2010, Chad Hills, the "sexual health analyst" at Focus on the Family, proposed that "preserving the sexual health of their children" is a policy priority on which Democrats and Republicans could both agree, and cited a survey that purported to show that nearly as many of the former as the latter supported abstinence-only education.[58] The reference to the survey is significant: whereas the sex advice side of Focus's sexual health efforts invokes psychological discourses to bolster religious claims, the advocacy side is more inclined to align the dictates of religion with the mantle of science and mainstream public health. (However, many researchers have complained that the organization has distorted their findings.[59]) Thus, for example, an article on the organization's website about sex education maintained that the abstinence-only approach is better characterized as "sexual risk avoidance," which "is actually a term taken from public health."[60]

The fact that Focus on the Family indeed has a "sexual health analyst"—that they would dedicate a staff role to this purpose—is noteworthy in itself: it demonstrates not only the polysemy and adaptability of the term "sexual health," but also the significance of this framing of sexual matters to at least some aspects of the organization's policy work. I first encountered the staff position in 2007 when April Huff, my research collaborator in a study of public responses to the HPV vaccine, interviewed Linda Klepacki, Focus's sexual health analyst at the time.[61] Armed with both a nursing degree and a master's in public health, Klepacki described her engagement with sexual health policy as grounded in a careful and exhaustive reading of relevant scientific studies: "I am scientific in my approach myself. I do *prolific* research." When asked about her belief that Focus had been mischaracterized in the mass media (specifically, that the organization had been portrayed as being unreflexively opposed to HPV vaccination on the logic that the availability of the vaccine would promote teen promiscuity), Klepacki replied: "There seems to be a longing to characterize people of faith as not . . . having a scientific basis for their arguments or their thoughts or their beliefs. We are an organization that bases any thought or belief on science. That's interwoven with our faith. So any [position] having to do with pharmaceuticals, vaccines, any kind of . . . medical basis for an intervention is *100% based on science*."[62]

In 2013, intrigued by Focus on the Family's commitment to the discourse of sexual health, I traveled to the organization's sprawling, forty-seven-acre complex—which is large enough to have its own zip code in Colorado Springs, Colorado. After receiving a VIP tour of the facilities (including the office suites, radio studio, and space dedicated to hosting the birthday parties of children in the community), I sat down with sexual health analyst Chad Hills, as well as Jeff Johnston and Glenn Stanton, two other staff members who work on issues related to sexuality, gender, and the family.[63] When I asked these men what the term "sexual health" meant to them, their answers were delivered in a mixture of the strands of discourse that I have described: religious, psychological, and scientific. Johnson (who has written of his personal "struggle with sexual addiction and homosexual attraction"[64]) observed that "woman was drawn out of man," and therefore sexuality is "that desire to reconnect what . . . once got separated." "Health" therefore describes a state where this "hunger to connect" is grounded in a marital relationship that preserves traditional conceptions of "our maleness and femaleness": "That's what we would call 'health': when things are kept in their proper sphere." For Stanton, "sexual health would be . . . full human integration," and its opposite is disintegration. Hills, the sexual health analyst (who has training in microbiology and chemistry), did not disagree with his colleagues' formulations but added to the mix his knowledge about neurotransmitters in the brains of "animals who bond for life as a pair, versus other animals who mate with whoever."

I followed up by asking Hills, Stanton, and Johnston for their views on the WHO's working definition of sexual health (which I read to them). They took exception to several aspects, bristling particularly at the emphasis on "rights." Not only were these presumed rights uncoupled from a conception of responsibility, they argued, but discussion of them painted a picture of (in Johnston's words) a "brave new world" in which "it's almost like, 'I have the right to sex so you gotta give it to me.'" But perhaps the most revealing moment came when I asked why they adopted the "sexual health" framing of their activities in the first place. Why not use an alternative phrase that might more immediately signal their concerns? "Why aren't you the 'sexual morality analyst,'" I asked Hills.

"I think that's because science doesn't listen to morals," Hills replied. "[The] CDC doesn't want to hear about sexual morality." Johnson and Stanton chimed in to clarify that the language the organization uses in its policy work "has to resonate" with legislators and the mass media, as well as with "unbelievers." In other words—consistent with my arguments, in chapter 2, about how and why the discourse of sexual health has become so widely disseminated—the very fact that their interlocutors describe sexual issues by reference to sexual health makes it strategic for representatives of an evangelical Christian political advocacy organization to adopt the same phrase. Yet as the conversation continued, Hills, Stanton, and Johnson also sought to reclaim "health" from a religious standpoint. That they would do so is not surprising: the religious studies scholar Lynne Gerber has also described, in her ethnographic study of evangelicals, how they employ the concept of health "to engage secular culture while reshaping the category's meaning to encompass moral demands of faith." Evangelicals "[infuse] this seemingly secular category with meanings that complement, rather than oppose, the moralization of a category like sin."[65]

"There are different ways to look at 'healthy,'" observed Stanton, pointing to the term's elasticity, and suggesting that Focus on the Family's religious and moral take on "healthy relationships" was just as legitimate a rendering of the term as any other. In short, policy experts at Focus on the Family find a "sexual health" framing of their outreach activities to be attractive and useful because of the phrase's malleability, its familiarity, and its broadly positive associations with scientific evidence and healthiness—an alignment that gives them traction when speaking to external audiences. At the same time, when speaking to individual Christians and offering advice about their life problems, the organization's spokespersons also find "sexual health" a suitable framing, one that allows them to express their ideas about wholeness and integrity. Conveniently, "sexual health" provides a bridge between these two different missions of the organization.

That matters of individual behavior and broad social policy should be so closely tied to one another is also not altogether surprising, considering the significance attached to sexual choices in the eyes of evangelicals. As DeRogatis has described, "how you have sex, when you have sex, the amount of sex you have, when you have children—even the smallest act within an evangelical marriage can have these larger-than-life meanings."[66] Yet there is surely some irony in the conservative adoption of its own version of what those on the Left, since the 1960s, would describe as the principle that "the personal is political." Religious conservatives are often critical of what they perceive as "political correctness" on the Left—an insistence that personal behavior be aligned with larger political aims. Moreover, the idea that the personal is political might appear to them to bespeak the kind of expressive individualism that, in their view, has caused so much harm to contemporary society—not least with regard to sexual mores. Yet for evangelical Christians who seek to improve lives and change society, the personal and the political are indeed stitched together in the alternative way that I have described, and the language of sexual health helps, at times, to provide the suturing.

Frame Bridging by Progressives in the #MeToo Era: Sexual Health, Consent, and Gender Relations

In 2019, the prominent sex education organization Sexuality Information and Education Council of the United States (SIECUS) announced a "rebranding" after fifty-five years in operation. Going forward, the organization would be known as SIECUS: Sex Ed for Social Change. In the words of the president and chief executive officer Christine Soyong Harley: "we are pushing the sex education conversation beyond the benefits it can have on an individual's sexual health. . . . We are encouraging our field, our supporters, and ourselves to continue to explore the large-scale culture shift that sex education has the power to create in this country."[67] This aspiration is a textbook case of what I have called bridging work. The idea here goes beyond the claim that promoting sexual literacy will result in sexually healthy lives—an idea already suggested by the now-frequent billing of sex education as "sexual health education." More profoundly, sexual health is positioned here as a mediating term between the individual and the social—a lever to translate individual sexual literacy into broader social, cultural, and political transformation. Needless to say, this vision of social change differs dramatically from the bridging work on the Christian Right—even while both seem dedicated to uniting the personal and the political.

The zeitgeist that SIECUS's rebranding tapped was one defined, in no small measure, by the powerful social movement against sexual harassment and sexual assault that had come to be known as #MeToo. As SIECUS's state policy directory, Jennifer Driver, speculated in 2019: "Imagine what the #MeToo movement would look like if people everywhere started to rethink sex education. We would have an entire generation of folks that could clearly articulate and define consent. We would have more people who understand what sexual violence is. We would have young people coming of age with an ingrained respect for their own and other people's right to bodily autonomy. And we would have a society that can frame and respond to sexual violence in a way that does not further traumatize, shame, or blame survivors, but instead, places the blame squarely on the perpetrators."[68]

These weighty aspirations for what sexual health education might accomplish also corresponded with many educators' perspectives on what was sorely lacking in the standard curricula. One public health expert commented in 2019 on the frustrations experienced by young people whose sex education amounted to little more than information on how to not get pregnant and how to not contract diseases: "In my own experiences teaching sexual health classes to high-schoolers, teens expressed concern over the numerous cases of sexual assault, harassment, and rape being discussed on tv and online. . . . They were not just interested in avoiding pregnancy or STIs, but how to communicate better and have healthier relationships—whether they included sex or not."[69] Sexual health education, in short, needed to be reconceived in light of #MeToo. A clear sign of the salience of these concerns came in 2020, when a Washington state referendum calling for mandatory sex education in public schools was hotly debated, yet passed with the support of nearly 58 percent of voters in the state: the referendum specifically required that students be educated about "affirmative consent" and that they be "taught to spot the signs of sexual violence and safely intervene if possible."[70]

In other words, the agenda articulated by those reflecting on sex education bridged from a focus on individual sexual health to a broader concern with the very nature of interpersonal relationships and social institutions in US society in the early twenty-first century. In so doing, this agenda presupposed that "sexual assault, harassment, and rape"—issues that might, at first blush, seem properly to belong in the sphere of law and criminal justice—may, in fact, be conceived of as matters of wellness and health. This was not a brand new idea: the sociologist Jaimie Morse has analyzed how, in recent decades, sexual violence has come to be understood as a social problem located at the interstices of medicine and the law, concretely symbolized by the sexual assault medical forensic exam (or "rape kit").[71] Reflecting such developments, the WHO's working definition of sexual health references "the possibility of having pleasurable and safe sexual experiences, free of coercion, discrimination and violence." Yet while such ideas have been in place for some time, it takes political work and "rearticulation" to mobilize them in the service of a specific agenda for social change.

These new discussions of sex education and sexual violence raised a range of concerns relating to the dynamics of sexual situations—including both wanted and unwanted encounters, as well as the many lying in the gray zone between. But they pointed as well to the broader distribution of power in society. As debates over sexual violence have played out since the emergence of the #MeToo movement in 2016, commentators in the United States have noted the many intertwined issues that necessarily come into play: the sense of entitlement to sexual favors expressed by the rich and privileged, especially those who control access to career advancement; the legacy of the long history of racialized sexual violence that dates back to slavery, when the ownership of Black women's bodies included the presumption of their sexual availability; and the vicissitudes of gender and sexual relations in a society where men often coerce women into unwanted sex, but so also, sometimes, do women with men, and men with men, and women with women (not to mention those who reject binary gender categories). The point is not just that sexual violence is experienced differentially, in ways shaped by the intersection of various forms of oppression. In addition, challenging sexual violence is made difficult by the numerous entrenched hierarchies—organized by social class, race, gender, and sexual identity—that are implicated in its perpetuation.[72] Again, what is especially intriguing here is the idea that this remarkably broad array of sociopolitical concerns is intrinsically connected to health, and that education around sexual health provides a critical space to intervene.

The #MeToo movement has called out instances of sexual harassment and violence found all throughout US society, but an especially salient site of sexual health bridging work has been the terrain of the college campus. (This is no surprise at a time when all the major cultural and political clashes in the broader society seem to play out in microcosm on campus.) Much scrutiny has focused on the promotion of "affirmative consent" policies for sexual interactions among students—with a fair bit of overemphasis in the media, as Elizabeth Armstrong and coauthors have pointed out, on some of the most exacting but least representative of such policies.[73] Much debate has also swirled around the perceived fairness or unfairness of the campus investigative and judicial procedures that come into play following the lodging of complaints of sexual violence.[74] Finally, many scholars and pundits have considered potential causal ties between sexual assault and changing sexual mores among young adults, particularly the effects of the so-called "hookup culture."[75] Perhaps less attention, however, has been given to attempts at colleges to create pedagogical spaces where education on "healthy" relationships is combined with a broadly progressive or feminist political agenda.

For example, at my own university, Northwestern, a group called Sexual Health and Assault Peer Educators "provides education, organizes events, and generates campus dialogue about sexual health and sexual assault." (Again, the seamless movement here from sexual health to prevention of sexual assault is itself noteworthy and marks the rise of a particular understanding of how to think about sexual violence.) Student peer educators, after completing a training class, organize presentations and hold workshops at fraternities and with other campus groups, plan outreach events, and offer advice to fellow students—all in the service of the group's mission "to increase students' comfort about sexuality, encourage them to learn and adopt healthy sexual behaviors and help them recognize and address unhealthy and dangerous behaviors and attitudes regarding sexuality."[76] On campuses elsewhere, students and staff have organized theater productions on the relations between alcohol use and sexual assault, and have offered classes in self-defense.[77]

Such moves reflect a shift toward finding ways of changing campus cultures to prevent sexual assault in the first place, rather than emphasize punitive responses after the fact.[78] Of course, the simple invocation of "sexual health" or "healthy sexual behaviors" as part of sexual assault prevention efforts does not guarantee any bridging to a more substantive political agenda. It is common enough for initiatives on campus (and elsewhere) simply to reference sexual health as a goal that encompasses the absence of sexual coercion, among other things.

Yet as the scholars Jennifer Hirsch and Shamus Khan have suggested in a detailed ethnographic study of sex, power, and assault on campus, sexual health can also be the opening wedge in the fostering of "sexual citizenship," denoting "the acknowledgment of one's own right to sexual self-determination and . . . the equivalent right in others."[79] Their research project, called the Sexual Health Initiative to Foster Transformation, located the propensity for sexual assault within a broader "ecosystem": rather than accepting overly broad and simplistic diagnoses such as "toxic masculinity," they directed attention at the patterns of sexual interactions and alcohol use on campus, the organization of physical space, and the complexities of power dynamics according to gender, race, socioeconomic status, and age.[80] Their analysis points to the importance of sexual health education, not only in college, but necessarily beginning much earlier, as a precondition for building a world with greater gender equality (and equality more generally).[81] It thereby links "education" in the specific sense used by sex educators with a broader vision of political education and social change.

Such projects, as Hirsch and Khan have proposed, treat sexual citizenship not as "something some are born with and others are born without," but rather as a goal that must be fostered by shoring up the enabling conditions "that promote the capacity for sexual self-determination in all people."[82] They therefore direct attention at the social conditions "upstream" that foster self-determination as well as those that set the stage for sexual violence—rather than focusing "downstream" on individual behaviors and their immediate consequences.[83] Hirsch and Kahn thereby align themselves with progressive strands of public health that not only favor "prevention" over "treatment" but also seek to change the society, rather than reform the individual, in order to promote health. Thus, while Hirsch and Khan, like so many others, are addressing social problems through the prism of sexual health, their orientation reminds us, once again, that "health" can mean many different things and can animate many different agendas.

Porn as a "Public Health Crisis"?
The Complexities of Political Alignment

Clearly, the kinds of bridging work attempted by proponents of sexual health vary dramatically across the political spectrum. Yet despite the intractability of conflict between the political Left and Right over sexual health issues, it is important not to oversimplify our understanding of the terrain of politics. Sometimes the configurations around a particular debate defy our conventional categories of political ideology. An interesting example concerns recent attempts in the United States to declare pornography a "public health problem." Here, we see how the rhetorical power of the goal of health provides a new license to intervene and take action to combat a sexuality-related social problem—yet in a way that creates strange political bedfellows.

In April 2016, Utah's governor Gary Herbert signed a nonbinding resolution that made just such a declaration concerning the health effects attributable to porn. According to Todd Weiler, the Republican state senator who sponsored the resolution, pornography is an "epidemic that is harming the citizens of Utah and the nation." Supporters proposed that porn may be "biologically addictive" and attributed a number of distinct harms to this epidemic spread, including low self-esteem and body image issues among adolescents, the hypersexualization of teens, and effects on brain development including "deviant sexual arousal." Others offered analogies between the porn industry and the tobacco industry.[84] A few months later, in July 2016, these anti-pornography arguments moved to the national stage: shortly before the Republican National Convention began in Cleveland, Republicans added an amendment to a draft of its platform that described Internet pornography as a "public health crisis."[85] By 2019, resolutions decrying pornography as a health crisis or epidemic had passed at least one branch of the legislatures of seventeen different states.[86]

In this example, we see how politicians can advance a political agenda with regard to sexuality by recasting a social problem as a health issue and redescribing the goal as one of fighting a growing epidemic. These actions have come in the wake of growing attention to the centrality of pornography to modern life online—even if the frequently quoted estimates about the high percentage of internet searches devoted to porn may in fact be overstated.[87] And they coincide with, and feed off of, a more widespread critique of the effects of exposure to pornography, which is often seen to promote an unhealthy "addiction."[88] As the title of an article published in *Newsweek* in 2018 expressed the concern, readers need to learn "How Porn Addiction Is Harming Our Sexual Health."[89] While such views have become widespread, the recent declarations by state legislatures amp up the discourse by invoking not just the addiction metaphor but also those of "epidemic" and "crisis."[90]

Importantly, while Republicans have been more inclined to push the characterization of porn as a public health crisis and while the states associated with this initiative are among those generally considered more conservative, in fact this agenda has drawn on arguments advanced by advocates across the political spectrum. Those advocates also have invoked a range of ideological arguments and scientific and medical claims.[91] For example, the Utah senator Weiler was influenced, on the one hand, by a Utah-based organization called Fight the New Drug, all of whose founders are Mormons,[92] and on the other hand by Gail Dines, a self-described radical feminist activist and professor of sociology and women's studies at Wheelock College in Boston, Massachusetts. Dines argued in an op-ed in the *Washington Post* that the question of whether porn is immoral can be sidestepped if we instead acknowledge that porn is a public health crisis: "As the research shows, porn is not merely a moral nuisance and subject for culture-war debates. It's a threat to our public health."[93] Dines pointed to a range of academic studies that find the consumption of pornography to be "associated with" various negative attitudes, behaviors, and outcomes.[94] Dines also founded an organization called Culture Reframed that characterizes pornography as "the public health crisis of the digital age."[95]

The alliance, whether explicit or tacit, that brings conservative (often religious) opponents of pornography together with some within the ranks of radical feminism should make us suspicious of any presumption that political debate over sexual futures necessarily lines up along conventional Left-Right lines. Indeed, the complex alignments around pornography are not new: they recall the "porn wars" of the 1980s, which provoked bitter divides among the ranks of feminists and scholars of gender and sexuality at the time.[96] However, a key difference in the current discourse is the much greater tendency nowadays to name "public health" as the social concern that must be defended and as the guiding rationale for considering pornography's effects. Somewhat similarly, recent efforts to combat sex trafficking have led to unlikely alliances between religious conservatives and what the sociologist Elizabeth Bernstein has called "carceral feminism," which seeks criminal justice solutions to problems of sexual and gender inequality. In that example as well, advocates may invoke public health rationales, such as violence prevention and HIV/AIDS prevention and treatment, in order to build constituencies of support across conventional political divides.[97]

In light of these wide-ranging attempts to invoke health as a motive for targeting sexuality-related social problems, it is interesting to recall my description in chapter 8 of the effort by the online site Pornhub to launch its own "Sexual Wellness Center." Pornhub's alternative rendering disrupts the connection between porn and social harms by linking the consumption of pornography to wellness and education. That idea is worlds apart from the view that porn constitutes a public health crisis—yet strikingly, what both formulations share is the presumption that "health" is the master discourse that legitimizes and propels political and practical agendas with regard to sexuality.

Politics and the Futures of Sexual Health

Once again, in this chapter, "sexual health" is hard to catch hold of because of the astonishing variety of work accomplished in its name. Along the way, much as I have also demonstrated in previous chapters, both "sexuality" and "health" take on a diverse set of meanings. Yet here we see various maneuvers undertaken not just to reposition sexuality and health but also, by that means, to reshape the space of politics and the content of the political imagination.

For evangelical Christians who speak of sexual health, sexuality is a God-ordained guarantor of marital intimacy, wholeness, and generational reproduction, while health is a state of physical, mental, and spiritual cleanliness. For #MeToo feminists and those targeting unwanted sex, sexuality references a set of capacities for pleasure and self-expression that are threatened by force, inequality, injustice, and the absence of consent, while health describes a state of well-being to which individuals and societies are entitled and which structural change in society can help promote. And not surprisingly, the participants in Satcher's National Consensus Process, who brought these and other understandings to the table, failed to clarify the ontology of either sexuality or health beyond acknowledging their definitional complexity.

The divergence in meanings suggests the stakes in political struggles. To advance the cause, political actors of all stripes expressly invoke the label of sexual health to reframe a manifestly political agenda and shape a conception of political education. This repoliticization, as I have shown, depends on "frame bridging" in order to construct connections to issues of concern to particular constituencies. The different examples I have analyzed are yawningly far apart from one other—in some cases, diametrically opposed. But they hold at least one thing in common: they demonstrate at least an implicit recognition that connecting one's agenda to the promotion of sexual health is strategically useful. Whether sexual health is yoked to the defense of rights, or gender and sexual egalitarianism, or moral responsibility, or personal wholeness, or the integrity of relationships, or the critique of misogyny in pornography, in each case sexual health discourse provides a potent way to speak to one's constituents. Even more importantly, it offers possibilities for speaking to the not yet converted—perhaps, to those who stand in the "middle" between the sexuality-related agendas of Left and Right—as well as to the mainstream and alternative media that might help spread the word.

Sexual health, then, is a gateway to the future—however that future is conceived. The very idea of sexual health has become central, perhaps indispensable, to the formulation of political visions. What are the benefits, and what also might be the costs, of construing politics—as well as knowledge, and selfhood, and our embodied desires—in these terms? I explore this question more fully in the conclusion.

Conclusion: Whither Sexual Health?

Sex and Health under Lockdown

The weird, anomalous, and painful year of 2020—a year of physical distancing and the suspension, deferral, and reimagining of so many aspects of "normal life"—is a strange time to draft the conclusion to a book on sexual health. In my graduate seminar on health, illness, and biomedicine—converted on the fly, in April, to online Zooming, the students scattered from Buenos Aires to London—we read Andrew Lakoff's book *Unprepared: Global Health in a Time of Emergency*. Published a couple of years before the advent of COVID-19, Lakoff's book examines "the tacit regimes of knowledge and intervention that experts bring to bear to address situations of urgency and uncertainty."[1] Having worked my own way to the end of a book that is likewise about the rise of new modes of knowledge and intervention, I find it hard not to reflect on the entanglement of global health security with matters of sexual health. "Sex" does not appear in Lakoff's index, but HIV/AIDS plays a pivotal role in the history he recounts: the emergence of the AIDS epidemic punctured the convenient myth—present at least in the global North—that rampant infectious disease was a concern of the past that modern medicine had gloriously transcended.[2]

Perhaps more than any other single cause, the course of the AIDS epidemic explains why health institutions began to take sexuality seriously, and how sexuality and health became so closely intertwined. However, the relations between sexual health and pandemics extend beyond the historical—and continuing—impact of HIV/AIDS: life under lockdown has sparked its own ruminations about sex, safety, health, and disease. This was true from the earliest days of the pandemic in the

United States. "Phone sex is safe sex," read the title of an op-ed in the *New York Times* published in March 2020. "Saying no to sex right now doesn't make you the Nancy Reagan of the COVID-19 era," wrote the author, Philip Dawkins, recalling the first lady's famous advice to America's teens to "just say no" to premarital sex. As a positive model, Dawkins pointed to the gay hookup app Sniffies, which had urged its users not to hook up to slow the spread of coronavirus.[3] Soon after, the *Wall Street Journal* described the anxieties of "sex in the time of coronavirus," with experts proposing "mindful sex techniques [to] help calm the nervous system and allow people to better focus on connecting with a partner."[4] Other experts of various sorts eventually weighed in as well. Jera Brown, a self-described "queer kinky polyamorous Christian," offered advice on *Rebellious*, an online magazine, about how to create one's own risk profile and decide what degree of exposure to the virus was acceptable and comfortable.[5] Meanwhile, specialists in sexual health drew diverse connections to the new epidemic—such as the suggestion, in the *Journal of Endocrinological Investigation*, that COVID-19 can impair sexual and reproductive health by causing erectile dysfunction, and conversely, that erectile function might serve as a "quick and inexpensive" surrogate marker of overall cardiovascular and pulmonary health among COVID-19 survivors.[6]

Not surprisingly, gay health organizations also were quick to rethink matters of pleasure and safety in the new medical context: they issued provisional guidelines much as they did in the earliest years of the AIDS epidemic, well before the full details of viral transmission had been established by scientists.[7] In a blog post called "Sex & Covid-19: Get the Facts," Howard Brown Health Center, which has served Chicago's LGBT community since 1974, explained little-discussed aspects of knowledge about the novel coronavirus ("It has not yet been found in semen or vaginal fluid") and gave practical advice about reducing the number of sex partners, washing sex toys, and disinfecting shared keyboards.[8] One commentator, the columnist Stephen Petrow (author of books on etiquette), reflected on the awkwardness of replacing traditional handshakes and air kisses with elbow bumps and "jazz hands," and compared the challenge to the striking behavior changes promoted by community-based AIDS organizations in the 1980s, such as the normalization of condom use in sex between men.[9]

All these conversations acknowledged the profound and multiple links between sex and health, which seemed only amplified in the context

of a pandemic that upended so many aspects of everyday life and ne-
cessitated endless assessments not just of absolute risk but also of
complex trade-offs. In December 2020, an op-ed writer complained in
the *New York Times* about the "nasty Puritanism" in the United States,
as reflected in the "deluded implication that all of us who failed to
partner up by March 2020 should live without meaningful connection until there is a vaccine." The author contrasted the "unrealistic
and inadequate" advice from experts in the United States with views
from abroad that specifically juxtaposed the competing risks to health
and well-being: "In Holland, officials advised coming to an arrangement with a sex buddy. Denmark's health chief said: 'Sex is good, sex is
healthy. As with any human contact, there is a risk of infection. But of
course one must be able to have sex.'"[10]

These discussions demonstrate—yet again—how much we now
think of sex and health in the same breath. They show—yet again—
the wide-ranging uses to which ideas of sexual health can be put as
circumstances demand, and as new opportunities permit. They make
evident just how central the marriage of sex and health has become
to modern life in its most diverse aspects—to what we know, believe,
trust, and do, and to our basic understandings of what constitutes
risk, safety, and our obligations to others. Moreover, the emergence of
concerns at the nexus of sex and health in the midst of the new life-
and-death dilemmas of the COVID-19 pandemic—and all the ways in
which those concerns invoke the history of the HIV/AIDS epidemic—
remind us of the strong perception of crisis that pervades so many
sexual health projects and initiatives.

Sexual health matters. At the start of the third decade of the twenty-
first century, the sexual health of humanity (understood in the very
many ways described in the preceding chapters) stands in a precarious
position. The problems have profoundly global dimensions, much like
health disparities generally: the sharp global inequalities that produce
disparate health outcomes also provide unequal access to resources to
confront and overcome health challenges. Yet even in a wealthy country
like the United States, the trials are acute and multifaceted. Far from
being a leader in sexual health, the United States lags behind many
other countries on key indicators: unplanned pregnancies, for example, account for almost half of all pregnancies, while in many US states
between a quarter and a half the population lives in what have been
termed "contraception deserts."[11] As rates of STIs have soared in recent

years—manifested in trends that include a rising number of cases of syphilis in babies, born to women whose infections went undetected—federal funding to support STI prevention has been slashed.[12]

Meanwhile, a surging concern with sexual coercion and harassment has broken a long history of relative silence on the issue, yet a presidential candidate who had been recorded bragging about his freedom to commit sexual assault with impunity was subsequently elected to the highest office. Over four long years, that president and his legislative and judicial collaborators proceeded to promote the systematic denial of sexual and reproductive rights, supported what has been termed a "war on sex,"[13] and sought to reinforce traditional conceptions of gender and reverse progress toward transgender rights. They also set out to undermine a fragile system of health care provision. Although the Trump administration put forward a plan to end the HIV/AIDS epidemic in the United States by 2030, it simultaneously supported budget cuts for HIV research, treatment, and prevention both at home and abroad. It stigmatized some of the groups most at risk, while ignoring the growing threat of HIV infection in the rural white regions presumed to favor Trump at the polls.[14] The ouster of that administration in the 2020 elections presaged new directions on many of these fronts, but with uncertain prospects in addressing the underlying issues.[15]

The omnipresence and polysemy of "sexual health" is a symptom of these many challenges. It is also a valuable but incomplete strategic response to them. At a time when the meanings of both sexuality and health are substantially up for grabs, and when both lie at the crux of debates about the sort of society people want to live in, it is not surprising that so many speakers should continue to invoke the aspiration of something called sexual health. The analysis in this book offers critical tools for understanding the contemporary conjoinings of sexuality and health; for assessing their complex effects; and for imagining alternatives. These final pages ask what the various configurations of sexual health can accomplish: What hopes and risks are entailed in such projects? What can these projects tell us or do for us, and what, perhaps, can they *not*?

What Have We Caught?

Sexual health is elusive and hard to pin down, but there is much we can now say about it. To begin with, the quest for sexual health matters in three fundamental ways. It has immediate practical implications and touches directly on many people's lives. It alters how we conceive of sexuality more generally, while transforming what it means to be healthy. And because the benefits and harms of sexual health are unevenly distributed, the question of how its pursuit can best address the needs of everyone is part of a larger conversation about pathways to social equality and justice.

"Sexual health," as we understand it today, did not spring out of nowhere. As I have shown, the roots of our contemporary understandings of sexual health can be traced back over a couple of centuries to encompass the proffering of health-related sex advice, the development of the field of sexology, and the efforts to promote social hygiene. From these early moments, the crisscrossing links between sex and health gradually drew strength from authoritative pronouncements, scientific research programs, projects of governance and self-governance, and the rise of a consumer market around sexual knowledge and commodities. In the mid- to late twentieth century, specific conditions of possibility related to the social organization of sexuality and the modern significance of health brought these concerns to the surface, and aided motivated actors who promulgated an initial working definition of sexual health under the auspices of the WHO in 1974. An unexpected pairing of terms was articulated, and this odd coupling proved ever more generative.

What could not then have been predicted was the subsequent "buzzwordification" of sexual health. Against the backdrop of significant social and biomedical developments such as the devastating spread of the HIV/AIDS pandemic, and alongside the rise of a broad-ranging cultural and economic investment in health as a terrain that extends well beyond the biomedical, "health" has been invoked consistently, across a wide array of networks that overlap only partially, to legitimize and sanitize sexuality. Functioning as a discursive engine to power initiatives of the most differentiated sort, sexual health is the all-purpose solution to a growing range of social problems. Yet these renderings of sexual health construe both "sexuality" and "health" in diverging ways.

The ambiguity of sexual health and the proliferation of kinds of expertise in relation to it challenge any simple, overarching story of a tidal wave of "medicalization" overtaking sexuality: the changes that are unfolding are too multiple and contradictory to be captured by the term, and the relations of influence between sexuality and health are also best conceived as bidirectional. The diversification of sexual health also raises questions about whether anything fundamentally connects its many strands beyond the simple concatenation of the two terms. However, in recent decades, a number of organizations have sought to stitch together different threads of meanings of sexual health, assembling new entities such as "sexual and reproductive health and rights." They also have promoted a more comprehensive definition of sexual health that seeks to unify many of the prevailing understandings and agendas and locate them under a capacious sexual health umbrella.

Meanwhile, as the centripetal and centrifugal tendencies of sexual health do battle, the various unfolding projects of sexual health promotion prove consequential. Not only do they target critical deficiencies and real-world dilemmas related to sexuality and health, but they also underscore the interpretative flexibility in just what we take "sexuality" and "health" to mean—that is, they take sides, implicitly or explicitly, in the struggle to say what sexuality and health *ought* to look like. Moreover, the goal of sexual health has proved useful in the service of many ends, some of them quite broad and significant. As the chapters of this book have shown, the impact of investment in the promotion of sexual health is especially evident in four domains: the "operationalizing" of sexual health for various purposes of scientific knowledge making, diagnostic work, and medical treatment; the adoption of the aspiration of sexual health as a motivator for self-improvement; the imbrication of sexual health into practices of governance and the promotion of a healthy citizenry; and the leveraging of sexual health education projects by political actors who seek to connect them to more expansive conceptions of political education and broader visions of a better world. Across these various projects, we find a host of social and cultural developments, some of them competing with one another and some of them aligning. These include new modes of marketing sex, new communication forums for providing sex and health advice, new visions of the patient-provider relationship, new strategies for managing risks, new struggles between experts and nonexperts, new ways of drawing social divides, and new visions of human rights.

CONSEQUENCES

It is easy—and important—to assert the many benefits of the invention and evolution of sexual health. Projects to promote sexual health have challenged the deep fears and stigmas that continue to surround sexual topics and have provided important alternatives to punitive approaches. These projects have also given ordinary people the tools, information, and treatments that can improve their lives, avoid illness and suffering, and extend their agency and control. By bringing sexual issues more squarely into the purview of ordinary medical practice, these projects also propose a new conception of medical care and the patient-provider relationship. More abstractly, the spread of discourses and practices of sexual health have broadened conceptions of human rights and social justice.

Yet each of the activities spawned by the goal of sexual health is complex enough to give birth to its own dilemmas, tensions, and contradictions—and thereby to suggest the double-edged character of sexual health. The work of operationalization promises concrete improvements in health and the destigmatization of sexual differences, but it may oversimplify and standardize, while investing in controversial notions of the normal and the universal. The pursuit of an optimized sexual wellness may imbue sexual matters with political meanings, or it may commodify sexuality and reinforce the idea that health is something available for purchase by those who can afford it. Governance valorizes the exercise of sexual rights but seems tied to particular understandings of risk and responsibility that may stigmatize some populations and groups and may constrain the exercise of sexual citizenship. The bridging of sexual health to visions of the future may take such diverse forms across the political spectrum that the work ends up merely reproducing social conflict. All of these activities demonstrate the productivity and utility of sexual health, but none of these provides a simple argument in favor of the virtues of the concatenation.

Moreover, all of these activities cut differently for different groups, with potential benefits for some and costs for others. Across the many projects of sexual health described in this book, questions of race and ethnicity, social class position, immigration status, gender identity, sexual identity, differences in degree of sexual desire (including that deemed "too much" or "too little"), disability, and location within global hierarchies of nations have surfaced repeatedly, though in complicated ways. The encounter between transgender people and sexual health institutions is a useful one to consider: I have shown how trans people are often ignored and not infrequently pathologized, yet sometimes, as in the case of the new edition of the ICD, positioned as pivotal in processes of social change and biomedical reform. The axes of race and class reveal at least as much complexity. In some situations, such as the sexual health survey results that found higher rates of condom use among Black and Latinx people, those inhabiting "marked" social identities are called out as model sexual citizens, and in other cases, such as in the development of community-based sexual health expertise, those who are socially marginalized may develop strength through sexual health promotion. But in many other cases, sexual health projects have treated the socially marginalized as sexual health's problematic "other," in need of monitoring and regulation—or have simply ignored their presence.[16]

Social inequalities raise important questions about who is treated as objects of coercion, and who is seen, instead, as agents of their own destinies. Inequalities also point to corresponding concerns about access: Who is able to obtain Viagra, or emergency contraception, or PrEP, or a safe abortion? In short, an analysis of sexual health that takes into consideration the various forms of social stratification that cause sexual persons to differ (as well as how such statuses intersect) sharply complicates any simple assessment of effects.

Clearly, it remains a challenge to define and assess sexual health. The resonance of the concept as a way of visioning healthy bodies, citizens, populations, and nations reflects its capacity to be so many things to so many people—a vehicle for addressing social problems, a gateway toward consideration of an ever-widening range of contemporary concerns, and a screen for projections of diverse needs, hopes, and desires. Yet it continues to be an object in formation—still not fully institutionalized, still struggling under the weight of the stigma that surrounds sexual matters, and still capable of evolving in different possible directions. Only over time will we learn how the very meanings of health have changed as biomedical research and health care practices become "sexualized." And only over time will we learn how the meanings of sexuality have been reshaped as sexual norms, practices, and identities are "healthicized."

The analysis developed in these pages, in other words, does not afford any oracular insights into the future. It is difficult, if not impossible, to know whether the various social problems construed as matters of sexual health will prove resolvable, ameliorable, or intractable. It is likewise difficult to predict how the term itself will come to be employed. We are "catching" sexual health in the midst of its initial stabilization following a turbulent period of emergence. What new areas, practices, and bodies will "sexual health" illuminate? In the long run, the malleable concept of sexual health conceivably may become more simplified and less polysemous, perhaps (though not necessarily) converging in a more conventionally biomedical or public health direction. Or, perhaps, advocates of a comprehensive and synthetic vision of sexual health will succeed in stitching together the different threads of meaning (as organizations like the World Association for Sexual Health clearly hope and intend). Alternatively, the tensions between competing meanings and projects of sexual health may cause the term to collapse under the weight of its own multiplying significations. But for now, the more divergent the programs that are pursued in parallel under the rubric of sexual health, the more that sexual health itself comes to be seen as a social priority and an unassailable virtue. And the greater the uptake, the more it creates pressure for others to adopt it as a term du jour that will be instantly recognizable to grant proposal reviewers, journals editors, and funders of clinics, training programs, and advocacy campaigns.[17]

MOVING ANALYSIS FORWARD

In providing a window into and assessment of the worlds of sexual health, the investigation presented in these pages has obvious limits. I have described the globalizing pretensions of sexual health as well as some of its differential effects, but I have not been able to examine systematically or comprehensively how the discourses and practices of sexual health call out to people differently, according to geographic region, demographic subpopulation, or biomedical risk group around the world. Nor have I been able to examine deeply, in an on-the-ground ethnographic fashion, the many ways in which different people, in different institutional and organizational settings, respond to sexual health activities—neither the full dimensions of popular uptake nor the diverse and ingenious pathways of resistance. This study therefore opens up more doors of investigation than it succeeds in closing, which I would propose is a good thing.

While other sexual health stories remain to be told, from an intellectual standpoint the example of sexual health is analytically useful in suggesting angles for approaching a problem I sketched in the introduction: how we might proceed to study complex objects whose characteristics, connections, and implications cause them to transgress the boundaries of neat analytical categories. Rather than assert a unitary theoretical "take" on sexual health, I have relied on kaleidoscopic refraction—and the diverse theoretical resources of sociology, sexuality studies, and studies of science, technology, and medicine—to figure the object in multiple ways. Each chapter is the product of a different spin of the conceptual kaleidoscope, providing insights into genealogies, social problem frames, buzzwords, conceptual umbrellas, operationalizing practices, unruly objects, self-making, governance, citizenship, and political education.

These various renderings of the same reality are pieces of the same puzzle, and they connect in ways that have permitted me to tell a continuous story. The chapters certainly imply one another, and many of the same organizations, objects, and individuals move across them and stitch them together. For example, some of the tools for assessing sexuality that are described in chapter 4 have been adopted to serve the individual pursuit of wellness (chapter 8) as well as the ends of governance (chapter 9). Yet, perhaps, at the end of the day, these interlinked pieces cannot be assembled into a fully coherent whole.

I believe an analytical strategy such as the one I have pursued here could fruitfully be applied elsewhere. The potential generalizability of the approach is perhaps most immediately evident to me when considering other projects that implicate "health." After all, other "kinds" of health typically imagined as unitary may also consist of relatively distinct strands that scholars should disentangle, and may also be sufficiently boundary spanning to lend themselves to kaleidoscopic analysis.[18] "Global health" is a case in point: the anthropologist Didier Fassin has characterized global health as a frustrating concept precisely because its "content and [contours] are extremely variable."[19] "Environmental health," which as the sociologist Sara Shostak has demonstrated, encompasses such disparate concerns as environmental justice and gene-environment interactions,[20] may also consist of different strands or domains. Other compound terms, such as "women's health" and "mental health," may similarly merit investigation that both decomposes the term and sheds light on the concept from diverse theoretical angles.

The point, of course, is not merely to reveal conceptual diversity where some have imagined unity. Beyond that somewhat academic

finding are likely to lie critical questions that point to practical implications: Who gets to lay claim to the agendas for promoting these
various domains of health and illness, such as global, environmental,
women's, and mental health? Whose needs take primacy in the push
to safeguard such forms of health? These questions point us forward
to a consideration of broad arenas of health and illness—but they also
return us to key considerations of this book.

The Double-Edged Sword

What, then, is the goal of the movement for sexual health? The analysis presented in this book should prompt skepticism about the use of
the definite article *the*: clearly, there are many goals and many movements, some of them intertwining and some diverging. Yet it's worth
considering some straightforward attempts at a clear answer to this
question. At the close of his plenary presentation at the National
Sexual Health Conference in 2019, Dr. Kevin Fenton, longtime sexual
health advocate and former director of the Center for Disease Control
and Prevention's National Center for HIV/AIDS, Viral Hepatitis, STD,
and TB Prevention, put it simply: "We want everyone to have their best
sex with the least harm possible." That, said Fenton, is "what sexual
health is all about."[21]

   Stated thus, the agenda seems almost beyond reproach. To be sure,
the phrasing does presuppose a desire to have sex, and therefore, as I
discuss below, it renders invisible (or deems problematic) those who
adopt an identity as asexual: what if your "best sex" is no sex at all?
One might also worry about the ambiguity in the determination of
"harm": Do we mean to the individual? To the society? Who decides
what counts as harmful? Still, the insertion of "their" before "best sex"
relativizes what might be a normative and universalist pronouncement
and appears to grant definitional control to the individual subject.
This is a powerful agenda, especially when advanced, as in Fenton's
case, from the standpoint of social justice and equality and with attention to the social determinants of health. Put more precisely, then, the
goal is to build the social, cultural, political and economic supports,
and tear down the impediments, so as to permit everyone to have their
best sex with the least harm possible. Thus, the goal is not libertarian
individualism but the flourishing of individuals within a society structured to enable Fenton's vision.[22]

The concept of sexual health is ample enough to accommodate this progressive agenda. Yet at the same time, many of the most visible expressions of sexual health seem very well inclined to promote outcomes that exist in tension with this vision and that might be deemed problematic and undesirable. I present these negative outcomes not as inevitabilities—in fact, I want to insist that none of these are *inherent* in the concept or practices of sexual health, precisely because sexual health can be made to mean so many different things. In place of a dark story of domination or a triumphant one of liberation, I call attention to specific problematic tendencies in sexual health as practiced, each of which exists alongside countertendencies and alternative possibilities. My analysis to this point has sufficiently well suggested these potential problems that the list should come as no great surprise. They include using the language of science to reinforce and justify conventional moral distinctions and claims about normality and present them as universals; limiting the range of public discourse and scholarly research with regard to sexuality; treating sex largely in negative terms; and favoring individual solutions to sexual problems over collective ones. Below, I take up each of these concerns in turn, describing both tendencies and countertendencies.

THE SCIENTIZATION OF MORALITY?

In a recent volume, sexuality studies scholars David Halperin and Trevor Hoppe described how the "broad and far-reaching progressive reforms" related to sexuality that have been enacted in recent decades in the United States nonetheless coincide with a "war on sex": "Outside the privileged domain of certain approved, legally permitted, and constitutionally protected sexual practices, sexual freedom has come under sustained attack. There has been a war, in short, on the kinds of sex that are morally disapproved, or that are stigmatized, or that simply fall outside the range of practices currently sanctified by legal guarantees."[23] If this characterization of "warfare" is accurate, where do the allegiances of sexual health promotion lie? To the extent that invoking "health" sanitizes and legitimizes sexuality, then sexual health activities may extend the space of freedom and offer protections to forms of sexual expression that might otherwise be unfairly stigmatized and positioned as vulnerable to attack. Yet to the extent that "health" functions as an engine of normative judgment—simply, yet fatefully, by calling some things normal and others pathological and by drawing a line between the two—then inevitably the discourses and practices of sexual health will be in the business of boundary construction. Moreover, by laying down those boundaries with the apparent imprimatur of science, sexual health may grant an aura of objectivity and naturalness to cultural norms, making it harder to see them as anything but foreordained and inevitable.

As we have seen, definers of sexual health from 1974 onward have struggled with the question of how, or whether, to distinguish visions of health from judgments of what kinds of sex are to be deemed good, right, and proper. The implementation of sexual health initiatives inevitably confronts this question as well. Tools used to diagnose sexual conditions or dysfunctions seem inescapably to characterize some forms of sex as abnormal or unhealthy—although of course, they may thereby provide pathways to treatment that many people desire. Results from sex surveys may be taken up in ways that convert statistical norms into claims about what is normal and thus proper. Campaigns to promote safer sex to prevent HIV infection may, as Halperin has argued elsewhere, adopt psychological speculation that "tends to smuggle into an ostensibly scientific analysis many stealth assumptions about good and bad sex, functional and dysfunctional subjectivity, proper and improper human subjects."[24]

A particular worry in light of these concerns is that sexualities that struggle for legitimacy might be especially inclined to find themselves on the receiving end of negative judgments that equate being different with being unhealthy. Will the practitioner of polyamory be more likely to be diagnosed with "compulsive sexual behavior disorder"? Will the sex worker escape critical judgment of participation in commercial sex? Will the person who refuses to declare allegiance to any of the conventional categories of sexual or gender identity be deemed psychologically immature?

The risks of such distinction making can be further compounded by tendencies to assert normative conclusions in global and sweeping ways. The question of whether sexual health can properly be characterized in universal terms goes back to the earliest discussions of how to define it, but the debate over that issue has been sharpened by the development of powerful and highly mobile tools to operationalize sexual health, such as the diagnostic codes of the ICD. Will the particular norms generated in reference to a given group, situation, country, or time period inevitably be applied universally in the name of health, without regard to cultural differences that matter for how gender, sexuality, rights, pleasures, and health are understood?

It is hard to give a definitive answer to such questions. After all, I have also shown that sexual health diagnoses have changed over time in response to global activist pressures and new conceptions of human rights deriving from various parts of the world, and that survey results can just as easily challenge existing norms as reinforce them. The normal, I have insisted, is in a constant state of transformation. Moreover, the experts doing the judging of sexual normality are an increasingly diverse lot. In fact, I have suggested that while the diversification of sexual health and the proliferation of sexual health expertise in recent decades may increase the inclination to measure people against various norms, it simultaneously expands the range of competing normative judgments. Experts do not speak with equal authority, and some judgments may carry more weight. Yet there is no longer just one "normal," if there ever was. Thus, the simple critique of "normativity" is an inadequate starting point for developing a theory of, or a politics around, the contemporary linkages between sexuality and health.[25]

Which will win out, the tendency or the countertendency? It seems highly unlikely that there can be a general answer to the question, though certain examples may prove instructive.

Perhaps the most interesting test case of the normative adaptability of sexual health is the especially challenging issue of asexuality. If, in the words of the WHO's working definition, "sexual health requires a positive and respectful approach to sexuality and sexual relationships, as well as the possibility of having pleasurable and safe sexual experiences," then it might seem that asexual people cannot be sexually healthy by definition. The sexualities scholar Eunjung Kim has observed critically that "the explicit connection made between sexual activeness and healthiness" seems inevitably and unfairly to construe asexuality "as abnormal and reflective of poor health."[26] Many practitioners in the professional words of sexual health (especially in the field of sexual medicine) remain inclined to describe asexual behavior or feelings as a dysfunction using clinical diagnostic terms, such as "hypoactive sexual desire disorder."[27] (While ostensibly the diagnosis is warranted only when the lack of desire brings distress to the person experiencing it, it is not hard to imagine how the pervasive negative social judgments about asexuality would themselves prompt distress).

Yet in recent years, as asexuality has "come out of the closet," defenders of an asexual identity have organized politically to form a community and challenge authoritative expert definitions; they have insisted there is nothing "wrong with" them or lacking in them. Moreover, and intriguingly, they have argued that asexuality is, in itself, a kind of sexual orientation—"an intrinsic part of who we are, just like other sexual orientations," in the words of the Asexual Visibility and Education Network, the best-known asexuality advocacy group in the United States.[28] Not only is asexuality thereby construed as a certain kind of sexuality (or, increasingly, as a wide range of possible subtypes[29]), but asexual activists have modeled themselves on the earlier depathologizing struggles of LGBT people, and have proposed tacking on an "A" to the ever-expanding acronym denoting varieties of sexual and gender difference. Perhaps, then, asexuality is on the path to incorporation within consensus visions of sexual health. But if, in the words of psychologists Brenna Conley-Fonda and Taylor Leisher, "sexual health does not require sex," then perhaps, this process of inclusion will necessitate a change to the definition itself, as these clinicians have proposed: "The exclusion of asexual people from the working definition demonstrates a lack of understanding and consideration for the wide berth of sexualities. Recognizing that asexual people can maintain a healthy sexual life with or without sexual desire being present allows for a more nuanced and inclusive discussion about the role of sexual desire in sexual health. Ultimately, by providing space for asexual people within the sexual health definition, a community far too often overlooked is able to be recognized and respected."[30]

If this comes to pass—if asexuality is accommodated within mainstream understandings of sexual health—it will prove not that the domain of sexual health is free from the exercise of normative judgment, but that the dividing lines between the normal and the abnormal, and the healthy and the unhealthy, are themselves the ever-shifting product of cultural, political, and medical change. The practitioners of sexual health contribute to such outcomes, but change is also the product of developments that lie well outside their immediate control.

THE CONTRACTION OF DISCURSIVE POSSIBILITIES?

A second concern follows directly from the preceding. To the degree that the institutions and spokespersons of sexual health recode moral and political preferences about "proper" sexuality in the presumably objective languages of health and science, they may constrict the space for substantive public debate about sexual matters. When sexual health is made a scientific concern—when the healthicization of sex also means the expertification of sex—the potential consequences are broad ranging. "Leaving it to the experts" not only may inhibit a democratic process of debating laws, rights, and ideologies related to sexuality but also may stunt people's capacities for expressing or even imagining their own sexual desires.

The healthicization of sexuality also holds important implications for scholarly work. For sexualities scholars, sexual health is truly a double-edged sword. By sanitizing sex and making it seem more respectable as a topic of scholarly inquiry—and by opening floodgates of funding reserved for health-related investigation—sexual health has endowed sexuality studies with powerful resources as well as legitimacy. Yet insofar as healthicization reinforces the idea that the only sexual topics that legitimately merit scholarly investigation are those that can be made to seem relevant to health, the reign of sexual health may also impede the study of sexuality as a genuinely important topic in its own right. For those seeking to promote open academic study of the broadest possible array of sexual issues—including questions that have nothing immediately to do with health and disease—this analysis rightly prompts worries.[31]

Yet for reasons already noted, these concerns need to be qualified. On the one hand, sexuality nowadays is often deemed a matter for the experts, but on the other hand (as discussed in chapter 7), the range of expert voices is broadening. The array of expertise is opening up to incorporate many nonprofessional and noncredentialed authorities whose pathways to sexual health expertise are in some cases quite unconventional and may be linked to social movement activism. As sexual health expertise becomes more diverse, arguably the discourses of sexual health overall become more pervasive—yet also somewhat more flexible, variable, and contestable. So, the effects of expertification are not so easy to predict.

Moreover, the concern that healthicization will constrict sexuality risks making the error of treating "health" as an overpowering constant while imagining that "sexuality" is the variable that is molded by it. If, as I have argued, health and medicine are in turn being sexualized— reshaped and repositioned through the demand that they acknowledge and attend to sexuality—then it is too simple to argue that health and medicine are constraining sexuality. In this story, "sexuality," "health," and "medicine" are all moving targets.

SEX NEGATIVITY?

Sexual health, like health generally, according to the WHO, is "not merely the absence of disease, dysfunction or infirmity." Advocates of sexual health take this injunction of "positivity" seriously—yet sometimes the ritualistic recitation of the mantra makes one wonder whether some advocates might be "protesting too much." As Chris Barcelos has described, too many projects of ostensible sexual health "promotion" direct their attention at what they want to *prevent*, and never seem to get around to any "promoting."[32] Of course, eliminating threats may be a sine qua non of advancing beyond "merely the absence of disease": arguably, one cannot fully enjoy the positives while still suffering from the negatives. Yet in that case, we still might wonder exactly what is entailed in bringing about the "state of physical, emotional, mental and social well-being in relation to sexuality" that the working definition holds out as a tantalizing promise. "Probably our biggest struggle is not letting the disease [approach] overtake all of the other [work]," commented Lynn Barclay, the president and chief executive officer of the American Sexual Health Association. "We get funding to do disease education. Nobody wants us to do pleasure education. Don't I wish!"[33]

Once again, the situation is complicated, with both tendencies and countertendencies on display. As we have seen, two of the most pervasive watchwords of sexual health—and particularly of what I have termed sexual health governance—are "risk" and "responsibility." By this familiar logic, sex is a troublesome and potentially dangerous concern that must be properly "managed." Yet sexual health is also pursued and practiced in the name of rights, and increasingly advocates are identifying one particular right—the right to pleasure—as the component of sexual health practice that demands the most support. (Of course, asexual people might disagree, depending on how pleasure itself is defined.) The recent activities of the WAS to direct attention to sexual pleasure (described in chapter 3) testify to the widespread perception that a discourse of pleasure is precisely what has been underdeveloped in the worlds of sexual health to date. "We had to argue . . . with the human rights lawyers," the former WAS president Eli Coleman explained, describing the complexities of recent discussions promoted by the organization to provide the grounding for a right to pleasure. "We need to push the envelope to . . . have sexual pleasure recognized as part of human rights."[34]

Writing of pleasure generally, the sexualities and STS scholar Kane Race has argued that "pleasure is more or less absent from serious talk within public health, though it is a common enough motive for, and element of, human activity." For Race, the potential disruptiveness of pleasure as a motivator is that it "offsets the actuarial calculation of risks and harms with a more situated inquiry into the terms of everyday life, while evoking a sense of agency and experimentation."[35] To the extent, then, that central figures in the worlds of sexual health prove successful at centering and mainstreaming attention to sexual pleasure, such efforts complicate any simple story of the "negativizing" of sex in the name of health.

However, a central challenge in approaching the issue of sex negativity is the uneven social distribution of risk, responsibility, and pleasure. Who is imagined to pose risk? Who is enjoined to behave responsibly? Who gets to pursue pleasure? As the sociologists Laura Carpenter and Monica Casper have emphasized in a study of sexual health technologies, notions of sexual threat tend especially to cling to the already disadvantaged: "Members of some groups—'fallen' women, racial or ethnic minorities, poor people, people in developing nations— are typically culturally positioned as unhygienic, with toxic bodies and transmissible 'conditions,' and thus in need of containment."[36] (One should certainly add sexual and gender minorities to the list, as the history of the AIDS epidemic, and Carpenter and Casper's own analysis, amply demonstrate.)

Partly in response to such challenges, scholars have emphasized how the struggle to valorize pleasure is intrinsically political and tied to broader analyses of intersecting inequalities. Black feminist scholar Joan Morgan has argued for "recognition of black women's pleasure (sexual and otherwise) as not only an integral part of fully realized humanity, but one that understands that a politics of pleasure is capable of intersecting, challenging, and redefining dominant narratives about race, beauty, health and sex in ways that are generative and necessary."[37] It follows that the pursuit of sexual health is neither automatically sex positive (just because the definition says so) nor inevitably sex negative (in light of the preoccupations with averting harms or controlling "dangerous" populations). A more careful analysis of tendencies and countertendencies would consider how these open possibilities are intertwined with other political concerns and histories of social inequalities that extend beyond the domains of sexual health per se.

THE INDIVIDUALIZATION OF SOCIAL PROBLEMS?

In repeated examples throughout this book (though not in all), the prevailing discourses that surround sexuality and health are those that emphasize the authentic needs of autonomous, expressive individuals—that is, individuals conceived of in isolation, as if they existed apart from the social worlds that shape their sexual and health imaginaries. One key link across chapters in this book is the pervasive, haunting presence of such an imagined individual—simultaneously, an innate possessor of sexual rights and responsibilities, an entrepreneurial consumer who treats health and sexual wellness as lifestyle pursuits and projects of self-making, and a patient whose dissatisfactions can be rated and maladjustments diagnosed. This individual, as we have seen, is someone who may seek to "tell their story"; or who may invoke the evidence of experience alongside or counter to the data of experts, or who may invest in projects of self-improvement and authentic self-expression.

To find this "neoliberal subject" lurking at the heart of sexual health discourses and practices is no particular surprise, and not just because that self-enterprising individual is a key protagonist of the contemporary pursuit of health generally.[38] Empirical studies by scholars of sexuality such as Barry Adam have suggested that even self-styled sexual outlaws who question public health imperatives (such as gay men who reject the norms of safer sex) often justify their oppositional practices "through a rhetoric of individualism, personal responsibility, consenting adults, and contractual interaction."[39] The neoliberal commonsense is omnipresent, and it would be surprising *not* to find it instantiated in contemporary arenas of sexual interaction.

Yet Adam's research interviews were also "filled with evidence that gay and bisexual men, whether single or in couples, high or low risk, do also know and show allegiance to care and community when circumstances permit."[40] Scholars studying other groups, such as gay and bisexual immigrant men in the United States, have also detected complex patterns of reasoning in sexual interactions that stand as alternatives to mainstream individualistic thinking.[41] And the case of sexual communication and risk taking is only one example of how the apparent dominance of the "neoliberal individual" is not an inevitable or intrinsic feature within projects to create sexual health. My discussion of sexual wellness in chapter 8 demonstrated how individualistic consumerism can sometimes coincide with the promotion of feminist values and the ideals of gay liberation. And in particular, chapter 10 furnished examples of political projects—on the Left and on the Right—that seek to enlist individuals and bind them to collective initiatives to build new worlds of sexual health. So, again, what appears to be a strong tendency within sexual health turns out to coexist with countertendencies; and the question of which force will prove stronger is not a question that "sexual health" can answer.

Working "With" and "Beyond" Sexual Health

The concurrence of these various tendencies and countertendencies leads to an indeterminacy that can be both frustrating and liberating. The frustration comes from the fact that the domains of sexual health appear to fuel or enable multiple yet sometimes opposing projects that all proclaim what is true or what is desirable. Moreover, these projects hold different implications for different groups in society, meaning that troubling questions surface about how sexual health initiatives can be made consistent with the goals of equity and social justice. The freedom, I believe, comes from the resulting opportunities to work both "with" sexual health and "beyond" it.

This brings us back to the fundamental question of how sexual health is best pursued and apprehended. The point is that sexual health is not an "outcome" in the way we routinely talk about other health outcomes: it is not an end goal, or destination, engineered by science and delivered to us by proper treatment. Kevin Fenton's formulation—the best sex, with the least harm possible—is not bad as a gloss, but even that fails to capture the pliability and ingenuity of sexual health initiatives. Suspending the inclination to measure health endeavors strictly by their outcomes, we might instead conceive of the worlds of sexual health in terms of processes—or as a diverse collection of tools that can be put to myriad uses.[42]

One virtue of this fecundity is an open-endedness of interpretation. The web of meanings and potpourri of programs springing forth from the different worlds of sexual health resist "epistemic closure": they give rise to a wide array of sexual truths, but—perhaps for the better—they do not converge on "Truth" with a capital "T." Similarly, these projects do not offer "normative closure": they cannot tell us what to value, or how to be, though they propose numerous rival possibilities. Nor do they give us "political closure": sometimes claiming to be apolitical and "merely" scientific, and sometimes aligning themselves with distinctive agendas for social change, sexual health initiatives present us in the end with the same range of political choices already found competing all around us, without providing independent means to adjudicate among them. Sexual health, as I proposed in the introduction, raises vital questions about what it means to live as a good and proper subject of a modern world. But sexual health does not answer these questions—or it provides many different answers. We should lower our expectations about what the discourses and practices of sexual health can give us—and look elsewhere for additional clues to advance matters of truth, values, and politics.

This is not a call to abandon the projects of sexual health. Nor is it a call to stand "against" sexual health. In discussing this book during various stages of its development, I have sometimes been asked, If so many people are promoting sexual health, who, then, opposes it? That's a reasonable question, given the popularity of the term and concept. Generally speaking, because sexual health can be made to mean so many different things, people are "for" sexual health—though always in the particular sense in which *they* mean the term. But in theory one could be "against" sexual health in a more thoroughgoing way: one might on principle oppose *any* alignment of sexuality with health, on the grounds that it is inherently problematic to subject sexuality to the normative diagnoses and prescriptive expectations that come with the territory of health, whatever form those diagnoses and prescriptions might take. Yet effecting a divorce of sexuality from health (or a divorce of either one from norms) is problematic, and not only because it would deny medical treatments to sufferers and health promotion to communities in need. As I have already suggested, I am ultimately unpersuaded by the politics of blanket anti-normativity: it seems not only to pose an unrealizable (if romantic) goal for sexual liberation but also to evade the critical, on-the-ground political questions about which norms, values, and beliefs actually seem worth fighting for.[43]

I would propose instead, as I have suggested, to work "with" sexual health and simultaneously "beyond" it. To work "with" sexual health is to commit to taking stands within the messy array of meanings and values that define the field. One could commit, for example, to strengthening the voices most at risk of being silenced. The sexual health of people with physical and intellectual disabilities is a good case in point: while scholars and activists have done important work to theorize and defend the sexual rights and prerogatives of disabled people, the issue remains largely marginalized within sexual health discourses generally.[44] The voices of sex workers are also mostly absent from discourses of sexual health, even when new technological possibilities, such as the rise of the "camming" industry, have provided workers with new means to negotiate health and safety.[45] Those whose practices or identities do not fit the gender binary are often literally rendered invisible by the operationalizing of sexual health: surveys, sexual dysfunction scales, and instructions for sexual history taking that presume the existence of two and only two genders cause many people to fall by the wayside.[46] Another topic that gets far less attention than it merits, given the salience of the issue of incarceration rates in the United States, is sexual health in prison. As the psychologist James Horley has written: "Loss of freedom alone is challenging and punishing enough for many prison inmates. Compounded with unrelenting worry about such experiences as sexual assault and STDs, especially debilitating or life-threatening diseases, the personal impacts can produce lethal outcomes."[47]

Being receptive to amplifying important but subordinated voices and issues also means attending particularly to the sexual health needs of those, such as young queer people of color, who confront multiple, intersecting structures of social oppression.[48] And it may take the form of defending against the erasures of identities and perspectives in global contexts. In 2019, for example, a United Nations–sponsored global summit on sexual and reproductive health, held in Nairobi to mark the twenty-fifth anniversary of the famous International Conference on Population and Development (the "Cairo Conference"), brought together more than 9,500 participants from 173 countries. However, LGBT delegates complained that the voices and specific concerns of sexual and gender minorities were substantially absent from the sessions. The limited mention of their sexual health needs seemed particularly to avoid the challenges posed in the many countries where gay sex remains illegal.[49]

Finally, working "with" sexual health might involve reclaiming and highlighting important histories that stand at risk of being forgotten. Productive strategies for confronting the HIV/AIDS epidemic and preventing its spread owe an immeasurable debt to activists of different stripes, around the world, who have pioneered novel approaches over nearly four decades.[50] As insights and approaches such as these are mainstreamed and incorporated, it is easy for their oppositional and grassroots origins to be obscured, and for the critical analyses of health and sexuality that animated them to be ironed away. Recalling these histories and their implications is important intellectual and political work.

These are examples of orientations and dispositions for working "with" sexual health—and thereby joining the fray of the broader politics implicated by sexual health projects. Yet arguably, such goals would be furthered by simultaneously working "beyond" sexual health. This notion of "beyond" rejects the idea of sexual health as mere outcome or clear destination, gesturing instead at alternative terrains.

For example, drawing on scholarship on the oppositional "counterpublics" that form as alternatives to a larger public sphere, Kane Race has described an intriguing (if somewhat elusive) construct called "counterpublic health." Race takes as his model "the remarkably effective and innovative collective strategies of subordinate groups . . . trying to ensure their own health and survival in the context of threats such as HIV/AIDS"—initiatives that join strategies of individual survival to engaged critiques of social and political systems that put communities at risk. Counterpublic health projects of this sort promote health indirectly, by way of "grasp[ing] the sociopolitical conditions in which certain dangers materialize." The pursuit of counterpublic health is an oppositional practice but is not, according to Race, opposed to health as such, nor is it "an investment in transgression for its own sake." Rather, the idea is to open a new space of possibilities by foregrounding an analysis of power and inequality from the standpoint of subordinated communities.[51]

Drawing on the concepts I introduced in chapter 9, we might say that projects of counterpublic health are workshops for elaborating new modes of "biosexual citizenship"—new ways of imagining the active engagement of individuals and groups in ventures of collective self-determination in relation to bodies, pleasures, and health institutions.[52] Bringing this idea together with my analysis in chapter 7, we can say that such projects may often generate and benefit from community-based lay expertise, rooted in social movements around sexual freedom, feminism, and racial justice, that relies on hybrid ways of knowing—blending academic and technical knowledge with knowledge that is vernacular and experience-based. Scholars have only begun the work of identifying pathways for the development of counterpublic health initiatives of this sort. In one recent description of what she calls "counterpublic sexual health," Kath Albury examines young people's use of social media platforms to "undertake peer-to-peer practices of intimacy, knowledge exchange and community-formation" in ways that reject moralistic and medicalized approaches to pleasure and health, including through the exchange of sexually explicit material. Albury asks whether such young people might participate in building a counterpublic "as experts, partners, policy-makers and/or researchers, rather than simply as clients, research subjects or 'target populations.'"[53]

Perhaps, as concepts such as these suggest, it is possible to refigure sexual health by rethinking the premises, purposes, and manner of bringing the two terms into relation. Corrêa, Petchesky, and Parker, for example, propose to locate sexuality in relation to health but also in relation to justice, broadly construed: "A sex worker's struggle against poverty, police brutality, HIV, and moral stigma is a multi-pronged struggle for a whole and dignified life. A transgender or intersex person's capacity to be who she/he is, in public without shame, or to access necessary health and prenatal care, is inseparable from her/his ability to find work in an environment free of discrimination and harassment."[54]

For these authors, the error begins with the starting assumption that bodies and lives can be extracted from their social and political context—and that "erotic justice" and "social justice" can be achieved independently of one another.[55] Recent work by Chris Barcelos that rethinks sexual health proceeds similarly by seeking to "[reimagine] what health promotion would look like through the lens of reproductive justice."[56] For Barcelos, the key goals include foregrounding desire, pleasure, and consent; "fostering the conditions under which people can exercise a full range of reproductive options"; and favoring structural approaches over remedies aimed at individuals, by enhancing people's "ability to have the economic, social, and political power and resources to make decisions about their bodies, sexuality and reproduction."[57]

Again, going beyond sexual health does not mean seeking to overthrow sexual health, and therefore it may go hand in hand with what I have called working "with" sexual health. But it might mean questioning an implicit presumption that fusing sexual and health concerns is the best path to individual fulfillment and social improvement. People care about many things. The stories told in these pages concern a plethora of animating motivations, including justice, equity, autonomy, community, freedom, pleasure, spirituality, self-improvement, and caretaking. While, as I have shown, it is more than possible to position "health" or "sexuality" as a gateway to any or all of these, there is no necessity to presume that either term should always bear special status as a master value, or even to assume an intrinsic connection between sexual health and any of these ultimate ends. Challenging the primacy of sexual health as the path to addressing a host of social issues would not mean denying its significance in any way. But it would disrupt the romance of health and sexuality just enough to permit each to seek out other company and new associations.

Acknowledgments

Books live and contend in a space of ideas, but they are products of substance that depend on concrete support and the possibilities thereby unleashed. The earliest glimmers of the idea behind this book came my way while in residence as a fellow at the Center for Advanced Study in the Behavioral Sciences at Stanford University. Programs like CASBS are special because they create the space and intellectual companionship for such sparks to ignite. Later, a John Simon Guggenheim Fellowship, combined with a visiting scholar appointment in the Sociology Department at Harvard University, gave me the time and freedom to map out the project and provided me with many interlocutors, especially from the intellectual communities surrounding both Michèle Lamont and Sheila Jasanoff. Later still, as the Mildred Londa Weisman Fellow at the Radcliffe Institute for Advanced Study, I benefited not only from the time afforded me to draft chapters but also from the warm and generative interdisciplinary environment nurtured by Lizabeth Cohen and the unique Judy Vichniac (d. 2019).

Meanwhile, throughout, I received many forms of support from my home institution, Northwestern University, including funding from the Sexualities Project at Northwestern and a faculty fellowship at the Alice Kaplan Institute for the Humanities. Northwestern proved the perfect home base to complete this work, and the end result owes much to the intellectual climate of its distinctive Sociology Department, Gender & Sexuality Studies Program, and program in Science in Human Culture. I have also learned more from my graduate students than they may realize, and I concluded sessions of seminars on the "politics of knowledge" and the "sociology of health and biomedicine" anxious to jot down new insights into my work.

Early in the process of writing this book, I collaborated with Laura Mamo. She and I were each in the nascent stages of a book project on topics related to health and sexuality; we agreed to join forces to think about those projects, craft some articles, and then go our own ways for the eventual books. It proved a dynamic model for promoting good scholarship, as well as an especially enjoyable one. I'm grateful to Laura for her clear judgment and her insights, as well as her enthusiasm and friendship. Chapter 2 draws substantially on an article we coauthored.

I am fortunate to have benefited from the work of a number of research assistants at different stages of this project—particularly Joseph Guisti, Gemma Mangione, Alka Menon, and Kellie Owens, as well as Aaron Benavides. Several individuals—Héctor Carrillo, Jonathan Rabinovitz, and Stefan Timmermans—were kind enough to read draft chapters and provide thoughtful advice, and Richard Parker, Jennifer Reich, and an anonymous reviewer offered incisive feedback on the entire manuscript. Others commented on drafts of related talks in their roles as discussants: Dani Filc, Theo Leenman, Anat Leibler, Michelle Murphy, and Eve Shapiro. Finally, I owe a special debt to those individuals who agreed to be interviewed. I'm truly grateful to them for their time and their thoughtful engagement.

I have lived with this book for a very long time, and I have discussed its contents and themes with many dozens of colleagues and friends, all of whom made helpful suggestions, and some of whom grasped the goals more precisely than I myself was able to convey. I also presented my ideas in raw and half-baked form as talks and learned from the questions and comments of attendees. My incomplete list of those to whom I am especially grateful includes Ken Alder, Rene Almeling, Robby Aronowitz, Bart Bonikowski, Charles Bosk (d. 2020), Geof Bowker, Allan Brandt, Phil Brown, Alberto Cambrosio, Chas Camic, Bruce Carruthers, Adele Clarke, Peter Conrad, Nancy Cott, Alice Dreger, Nina Eliasoph, Richard Elovich, Wendy Espeland, Ulrike Felt, John Gagnon (1931–2016), Cathy Gere, Ilana Gershon, Alain Giami, Tom Gieryn, Jeremy Greene, Carol Heimer, Steve Hilgartner, Jennifer Hirsch, Sheila Jasanoff, Anna Kirkland, David Kirp, Andy Lakoff, Michèle Lamont, Kirsten Leng, AJ Lewis, Margaret Lock, Heather Love, Alyssa Lynne, Jal Mehta, Beth Mertz, Chandra Mukerji, Brian Mustanski, Dan Navon, Aaron Norton, Richard Parker, Shobita Parthasarathy, Scott Pytluk, Paul Ramirez, David Ribes, Dorothy Roberts, Sarah Rodriguez, Charles Rosenberg, Leslie Salzinger, Theo Sandfort, Thomas Schlich, Steve Shapin, Arlene Stein, Charlie Thorpe, Marcia Tiede, Helen Tilley, Stefan Timmermans, Henry Turner, Tom Waidzunas, Keith Wailoo, Jeff Weintraub (who suggested the book's title), George Weisz, and Daniel Wolfe.

Publishing this book has given me the opportunity to continue a happy relationship with the University of Chicago Press, where the remarkable Doug Mitchell (1943–2019), who edited a previous book of mine, offered me encouragement on this project at an early stage. I am grateful to my terrific editor, the wise, sensible, and supportive Karen Darling, who provided invaluable help and shepherded the project with insight and efficiency, as well as to her omnicompetent assistant, Tristan Bates. As the project moved toward completion, Elizabeth Ellingboe oversaw production, Katherine Faydash edited the manuscript with precision and good judgment, and Deirdre Kennedy managed all promotional aspects.

Some of the material in chapter 2 appeared previously in different form as Steven Epstein and Laura Mamo, "The Proliferation of Sexual Health: Diverse Social Problems and the Legitimation of Sexuality," *Social Science & Medicine* 188 (2017): 176–90. Much of the material in chapter 5 appeared with a different framing argument as "Cultivated Co-Production: Sexual Health, Human Rights, and the Revision of the ICD," *Social Studies of Science*, advance online publication, 30 April 2021, https://journals.sagepub.com/doi/10.1177/03063127211014283. Portions of the material in chapter 9 appeared in different form as Steven Epstein, "Governing Sexual Health: Bridging Biocitizenship and Sexual Citizenship," in *Biocitizenship: The Politics of Bodies, Governance, and Power*, ed. Kelly Happe, Jenell Johnson, and Marina Levina (New York: NYU Press, 2018), 21–50.

I am thankful for supportive friends, including Sarita Groisser, who carefully applied her eyes and ears to the task of reviewing the page proofs for errors. In all aspects of the work that led to this book, I am grateful to my family for their support, including Elvira Carrillo, whose company, Exactos Servicios, carefully prepared the graphs and tables. It is impossible to overstate how much I owe to Héctor Carrillo, my life partner and one of my favorite sociologists.

Notes

A complete, alphabetized bibliography, with clickable hyperlinks, can be downloaded from the University of Chicago Press page for this book, https://press.uchicago.edu/sites/epstein/.

INTRODUCTION

1. The descriptions in these pages are from my field notes from attending the conference, 10–12 July 2019, in Chicago, as well as from the conference program and information and materials available on the conference website, at https://sexualhealth2019.org/ (accessed 14 July 2019 but no longer accessible).
2. Margaret Atwood, *The Handmaid's Tale* (Toronto: McClelland and Stewart, 1985).
3. "Wondrous Vulva Puppet," Dorrie Lane's Wondrous Vulva Puppet Shop, https://www.vulvapuppet.com.
4. The planning organizations included the American Sexual Health Association, the American Sexually Transmitted Diseases Association, the Center for Sexual Health Promotion at Indiana University's School of Public Health, the National Coalition for Sexual Health, the Denver Prevention Training Center, and the National Alliance of State and Territorial AIDS Directors.
5. 2019 National Sexual Health Conference, Sponsor and Exhibor Prospectus (PDF booklet downloaded 18 July 2019 from the conference website but no longer accessible), 3.
6. Ibid., 4.
7. When registrants were asked to indicate up to two areas of focus, 52 percent of them chose "HIV/AIDS" as one of the two, and 42 percent chose sexually transmitted diseases. Ibid.
8. Ibid., 1.

9. *Defining Sexual Health: Report of a Technical Consultation on Sexual Health, 28–31 January 2002, Geneva* (Geneva: World Health Organization, 2006), 5. I discuss the history of definitions in chapters 1 and 3.

10. Anna Kirkland, "What Is Wellness Now?," *Journal of Health Politics, Policy & Law* 39, no. 5 (2014): 957–70; Anna Kirkland, "Critical Perspectives on Wellness," *Journal of Health Politics, Policy and Law* 39, no. 5 (2014): 971–88; Carl Cederström and André Spicer, *The Wellness Syndrome* (Cambridge, UK: Polity, 2015).

11. Peter Greenhouse, "A Definition of Sexual Health," *BMJ* 310 (1995): 1468–69.

12. From the results of a Google search for "sexual health" (with the phrase in quotation marks) conducted on 21 June 2019.

13. "Sexual Health Certificate Program," University of Michigan School of Social Work, https://ssw.umich.edu/offices/continuing-education/certificate-courses/sexual-health.

14. "Chair in Sexual Health," University of Minnesota Program in Human Sexuality, https://www.sexualhealth.umn.edu/about/chair-sexual-health; "Joycelyn Elders Chair in Sexual Health Education," University of Minnesota Program in Human Sexuality, https://www.sexualhealth.umn.edu/about/joycelyn-elders-chair-sexual-health-education.

15. See also the discussion of "ownership" in chapter 8.

16. "World Sexual Health Day," World Health Organization, https://www.who.int/news-room/events/detail/2021/09/04/default-calendar/world-sexual-health-day. See the discussion in chapter 3.

17. "ICD-11 for Morbidity and Mortality Statistics," World Health Organization, https://icd.who.int/browse11/l-m/en. See the discussion in chapter 5.

18. See the discussion in chapter 9.

19. Michel Foucault, *The History of Sexuality, Volume 1: An Introduction*, trans. Robert Hurley (New York: Vintage Books, 1980), 8.

20. Andrea Swartzendruber and Jonathan M. Zenilman, "A National Strategy to Improve Sexual Health," *Journal of the American Medical Association* 304, no. 9 (2010): 1005–6, esp. 1005.

21. "Sexual Health MeSH Descriptor Data 2021," National Library of Medicine, https://meshb.nlm.nih.gov/record/ui?ui=D000074384. From 2013 to 2018, "sexual health" was an alternative search term falling under the subject heading of "reproductive health."

22. I borrow this formulation from Marie Murphy's analysis of a related arena: sex education in medical schools. Marie Murphy, "Everywhere and Nowhere Simultaneously: The 'Absent Presence' of Sexuality in Medical Education," *Sexualities* 22, no. 1–2 (2019): 203–23.

23. Emily Pollack, "1 Million People Infected with Curable Sexually Transmitted Diseases Each Day," *Nation's Health* 49, no. 6 (2019): 22; Liam Stack, "Sexually Transmitted Disease Cases Rise to Record High, C.D.C. Says,"

New York Times, 8 October 2019, A19; Ann M. Starrs et al., "Accelerate Progress—Sexual and Reproductive Health and Rights for All: Report of the Guttmacher–Lancet Commission," *Lancet* 391 (2018): 2642–92, esp. 2642; Adrienne O'Neil et al., "The #MeToo Movement: An Opportunity in Public Health?," *Lancet* 391 (2018): 2587–89; "Birth Control Gets Caught Up in the Abortion Wars" (editorial), *New York Times*, 26 February 2019, A24; Sophie Cousins, "Abortion: US Global Gag Rule Is Having 'Chilling Effect' on Sexual Health Service Providers," *BMJ* 363 (2018): k4886; "Global $108 Billion Sexual Wellness Industry Outlook 2020–2027: Rise in Millennial Population, Surge in Disposable Income," *Cision PR Newswire*, 2 September 2020, https://www.prnewswire.com/news-releases/global -108-billion-sexual-wellness-industry-outlook-2020-2027-rise-in-millen nial-population-surge-in-disposable-income-301123244.html.

24. Although the analogy is imperfect, my conceptualization of "catching" is influenced by R. P. McDermott's essay on "the acquisition of a child by a learning disability." (I am grateful to Ilana Gershon for suggesting the connection.) R. P. McDermott, "The Acquisition of a Child by a Learning Disability," in *Understanding Practice: Perspectives on Activity and Context*, ed. Seth Chaiklin and Jean Lave (Cambridge: Cambridge University Press, 1993), 269–305.

25. On the study of conjoined terms, see Jennifer Reardon's discussion of the emergence of "science and justice" as an example of what, following Donna Haraway, she describes as a "conjugation." Jenny Reardon, "On the Emergence of Science and Justice," *Science, Technology & Human Values* 38, no. 2 (2013): 176–200.

26. Gayle S. Rubin, "Thinking Sex: Notes for a Radical Theory of the Politics of Sexuality," in *Pleasure and Danger: Exploring Female Sexuality*, ed. Carole S Vance (New York: Routledge, 1984), 267–318; John D'Emilio and Estelle B. Freedman, *Intimate Matters: A History of Sexuality in America* (New York: Harper & Row, 1988); Gilbert H. Herdt, ed. *Moral Panics, Sex Panics: Fear and the Fight over Sexual Rights* (New York: NYU Press, 2009); Roger N. Lancaster, *Sex Panic and the Punitive State* (Berkeley: University of California Press, 2011); Janice M. Irvine, "The Other Sex Work: Stigma in Sexuality Research," *Social Currents* 2, no. 2 (2015): 116–25.

27. These may include, for example, sexualities that are non-heteronormative, non-monogamous, non-procreative, or commercial, or that transgress boundaries of race, social class, or age.

28. Peter Conrad and Joseph W. Schneider, *Deviance and Medicalization: From Badness to Sickness* (St. Louis, MO: C. V. Mosby, 1980); Peter Conrad, *The Medicalization of Society* (Baltimore, MD: Johns Hopkins University Press, 2007).

29. Peter Conrad, "The Shifting Engines of Medicalization," *Journal of Health and Social Behavior* 46, no. 1 (2005): 3–14. A related literature is that on

"pharmaceuticalization"; see John Abraham, "Pharmaceuticalization of Society in Context: Theoretical, Empirical and Health Dimensions," *Sociology* 44, no. 4 (2010): 603–22; Susan E. Bell and Anne E. Figert, "Medicalization and Pharmaceuticalization at the Intersections: Looking Backward, Sideways and Forward," *Social Science & Medicine* 75 (2012): 775–83; Laura Mamo and Steven Epstein, "The Pharmaceuticalization of Sexual Risk: Vaccine Development and the New Politics of Cancer Prevention," *Social Science & Medicine* 101 (2013): 155–65.

30.   Adele E. Clarke et al., "Biomedicalization: Technoscientific Transformations of Health, Illness, and U.S. Biomedicine," *American Sociological Review* 68, no. 2 (2003): 161–94; Adele E. Clarke et al., eds., *Biomedicalization: Technoscience, Health, and Illness in the US* (Durham, NC: Duke University Press, 2010).

31.   Drew Halfmann, "Recognizing Medicalization and Demedicalization: Discourses, Practices, and Identities," *Health* 16, no. 2 (2011): 186–207.

32.   On medicalization and sexuality, see Leonore Tiefer, "The Medicalization of Impotence: Normalizing Phallocentrism," *Gender & Society* 8, no. 3 (1994): 363–77; Steven Epstein, "Sexualizing Governance and Medicalizing Identities: The Emergence of 'State-Centered' LGBT Health Politics in the United States," *Sexualities* 6, no. 2 (2003): 131–71; Jennifer R. Fishman, "The Making of Viagra: The Biomedicalization of Sexual Dysfunction," in *Biomedicalization: Technoscience, Health, and Illness in the US*, ed. Adele E. Clarke et al. (Durham, NC: Duke University Press, 2010), 289–306; Thea Cacchioni and Leonore Tiefer, "Why Medicalization? Introduction to the Special Issue on the Medicalization of Sex," *Journal of Sex Research* 49, no. 4 (2012): 307–10; Janine Farrell and Thea Cacchioni, "The Medicalization of Women's Sexual Pain," *Journal of Sex Research* 49, no. 4 (2012): 328–36; Alain Giami and Christopher Perrey, "Transformations in the Medicalization of Sex: HIV Prevention between Discipline and Biopolitics," *Journal of Sex Research* 49, no. 4 (2012): 353–61; Leonore Tiefer, "Medicalizations and Demedicalizations of Sexuality Therapies," *Journal of Sex Research* 49, no. 4 (2012): 311–18; Aaron T. Norton, "Surveying Risk Subjects: Public Health Surveys as Instruments of Biomedicalization," *BioSocieties* 8 (2013): 265–88; Alyson K. Spurgas, *Diagnosing Desire: Biopolitics and Femininity into the Twenty-First Century* (Columbus: Ohio State University Press, 2020).

33.   Foucault, *History of Sexuality*; Allan M. Brandt, *No Magic Bullet: A Social History of Venereal Disease in the United States since 1880* (New York: Oxford University Press, 1985); Peter Lewis Allen, *The Wages of Sin: Sex and Disease, Past and Present* (Chicago: University of Chicago Press, 2000); Arnold I. Davidson, *The Emergence of Sexuality: Historical Epistemology and the Formation of Concepts* (Cambridge, MA: Harvard University Press, 2001).

34.   Nikolas Rose, "Beyond Medicalisation," in *The Social Medicine Reader, Volume 2: Differences and Inequalities*, ed. Jonathan Oberlander et al., 3rd ed.

(Durham, NC: Duke University Press, 2019), 31–36, esp. 35. See also Half-mann, "Recognizing Medicalization and Demedicalization." On the heterogeneity and disunity of modern medicine, see Annemarie Mol and Marc Berg, "Differences in Medicine: An Introduction," in *Differences in Medicine: Unraveling Practices, Techniques, and Bodies*, ed. Marc Berg and Annemarie Mol (Durham, NC: Duke University Press, 1998), 1–12.

35. Stephen J. Collier and Andrew Lakoff, "On Regimes of Living," in *Global Assemblages: Technology, Politics, and Ethics as Anthropological Problems*, ed. Aihwa Ong and Stephen J. Collier (Malden, MA: Blackwell, 2005), 22–39, esp. 23.

36. Sexual health, therefore, is an aspect of the "vital politics" that, in Nikolas Rose's formulation, situate human "life itself" as the target and stakes. Nikolas Rose, *The Politics of Life Itself: Biomedicine, Power, and Subjectivity in the Twenty-First Century* (Princeton, NJ: Princeton University Press, 2006).

37. See Steven Epstein and Laura Mamo, "The Proliferation of Sexual Health: Diverse Social Problems and the Legitimation of Sexuality," *Social Science & Medicine* 188 (2017): 176–90. On healthicization and healthism (and their contested connections with [bio]medicalization), see also Robert Crawford, "Healthism and the Medicalization of Everyday Life," *International Journal of Health Services* 10, no. 3 (1980): 365–88; Deborah Lupton, *The Imperative of Health: Public Health and the Regulated Body* (London: Sage, 1995), esp. 131–57; Martin O'Brien, "Health and Lifestyle: A Critical Mess? Notes on the Dedifferentiation of Health," in *The Sociology of Health Promotion: Critical Analyses of Consumption, Lifestyle and Risk*, ed. Robin Bunton, Sarah Nettleton, and Roger Burrows (London: Routledge, 1995), 191–205; Clarke et al., "Biomedicalization," 171–72; Robert Crawford, "Health as a Meaningful Social Practice," *Health* 10, no. 4 (2006): 401–20; Jonathan M. Metzl and Anna Kirkland, eds., *Against Health: How Health Became the New Morality* (New York: NYU Press, 2010); Alan Petersen, Mark Davis, Suzanne Fraser, and Jo Lindsay, "Healthy Living and Citizenship: An Overview," *Critical Public Health* 20, no. 4 (2010): 391–400; Kristin K. Barker, "Mindfulness Meditation: Do-It-Yourself Medicalization of Every Moment," *Social Science & Medicine* 106 (2014): 168–76; Christopher Mayes, *The Biopolitics of Lifestyle: Foucault, Ethics and Healthy Choices* (London: Routledge, 2016); Gemma Mangione, "The Art and Nature of Health: A Study of Therapeutic Practice in Museums," *Sociology of Health & Illness* 40, no. 2 (2018): 283–96.

38. Metzl and Kirkland, *Against Health*.

39. On changing conceptions of normality in the nineteenth and twentieth centuries (and the crucial place of both sexuality and health in that evolution), see Peter Cryle and Elizabeth Stephens, *Normality: A Critical Genealogy* (Chicago: University of Chicago Press, 2017).

40. Orlando Patterson, *Freedom: Volume 1, Freedom in the Making of Western Culture* (New York: Basic Books, 1991), ix. I am grateful to Orlando Patterson for pointing out this connection to me.

41.   Theo Sandfort and Anke Ehrhardt, "Sexual Health: A Useful Public Health Paradigm or a Moral Imperative?," *Archives of Sexual Behavior* 33, no. 3 (2004): 181–87, esp. 184.

42.   I take up this question in chapter 7.

43.   Cryle and Stephens, *Normality*, 359. On the remaking of the normal and the pathological in modern biomedicine, see Daniel Navon, *Mobilizing Mutations: Human Genetics in the Age of Patient Advocacy* (Chicago: University of Chicago Press, 2019), ch. 7.

44.   Put in the language of social science, the problematic assumption is that sexuality is necessarily the dependent variable in the relation between sexuality and health.

45.   The sociologist Celia Roberts is certainly correct to say that "sex and sexuality . . . are not 'natural' objects worked on or taken up by medicine, but are produced" in social interactions involving medical professionals, scientists, patients, and many others. But we might also flip it around: "health" and "biomedicine" are likewise produced in social interactions involving a wide array of actors invested in sexual matters, including experts, professionals, and social movements. Celia Roberts, "Medicine and the Making of a Sexual Body," in *Handbook of the New Sexuality Studies*, ed. Steven Seidman, Nancy L. Fischer, and Chet Meeks (Abingdon, UK: Routledge, 2006), 81–89, esp. 81.

46.   I am indebted here to Judy Segal, whose article "reverses the key terms of . . . the medicalization of sex to talk about the sexualization of the medical." Judy Z. Segal, "The Sexualization of the Medical," *Journal of Sex Research* 49, no. 4 (2012): 369–78, esp. 369. See also Gary Dowsett's observation that the "shift from the taxonomic preoccupation of early-modernity and its pathologisation of sexual deviance to the sexualisation of healthy living has been a dramatic achievement." Gary W. Dowsett, "'And Next, Just for Your Enjoyment!': Sex, Technology and the Constitution of Desire," *Culture, Health & Sexuality* 17, no. 4 (2015): 527–39, esp. 536.

47.   Peter Conrad and Deborah Potter, "Human Growth Hormone and the Temptations of Biomedical Enhancement," *Sociology of Health & Illness* 26, no. 2 (2004): 184–215.

48.   Steven Epstein, *Impure Science: AIDS, Activism, and the Politics of Knowledge* (Berkeley: University of California Press, 1996); Epstein, "Sexualizing Governance"; Steven Epstein, *Inclusion: The Politics of Difference in Medical Research* (Chicago: University of Chicago Press, 2007); Keith Wailoo, Julie Livingston, Steven Epstein, and Robert Aronowitz, eds., *Three Shots at Prevention: The HPV Vaccine and the Politics of Medicine's Simple Solutions* (Baltimore: Johns Hopkins University Press, 2010).

49.   These are among various subsets of "Health" that have their own Medical Subject Headings (MeSH) in the tree structure of the National Library of

Medicine. See "Population Health MeSH Descriptor Data 2021,"
National Library of Medicine, https://meshb.nlm.nih.gov/record/ui?ui
=D000075485.

50.   It also has features of what Scott Frickel and Neil Gross call a "scientific/
intellectual movement." Scott Frickel and Neil Gross, "A General Theory of
Scientific/Intellectual Movements," *American Sociological Review* 70, no. 2
(2005): 204–32.

51.   For a critical and practical discussion, see the chapter "What Is This a
Case of, Anyway?," in Kristin Luker, *Salsa Dancing into the Social Sciences:
Research in an Age of Info-Glut* (Cambridge, MA: Harvard University Press,
2008), 51–75.

52.   As the sociologist Andrew Abbott has proposed, perhaps "we should not
look for boundaries of things but things of boundaries." Andrew Abbott,
"Things of Boundaries," *Social Research* 62 (1995): 857–82, esp. 857.

53.   Foucault, *History of Sexuality*, 17, 34.

54.   Ibid., 103.

55.   I address these topics in chapter 2.

56.   On intersectional approaches to sexuality, see Joane Nagel, "Ethnicity
and Sexuality," *Annual Review of Sociology* 26 (2000): 107–33; Siobhan B.
Somerville, *Queering the Color Line: Race and the Invention of Homosexuality in
American Culture* (Durham, NC: Duke University Press, 2000); Roderick A.
Ferguson, *Aberrations in Black: Toward a Queer of Color Critique* (Minneapolis:
University of Minnesota Press, 2004); Lisa Bowleg, "When Black + Lesbian + Woman ≠ Black Lesbian Woman: The Methodological Challenges
of Qualitative and Quantitative Intersectionality Research," *Sex Roles* 59,
no. 5 (2008): 312–25; Patrick R. Grzanka, ed. *Intersectionality: Foundations
and Frontiers*, 2nd ed. (New York: Routledge, 2019); Ghassan Moussawi and
Salvador Vidal-Ortiz, "A Queer Sociology: On Power, Race, and Decenter-
ing Whiteness," *Sociological Forum* 35, no. 4 (2020): 1272–89.

57.   Subsequent scholars have sought to build on Foucault's work by develop-
ing the intersections. See, for example, Irene Diamond and Lee Quinby,
eds., *Feminism & Foucault: Reflections on Resistance* (Boston: Northeastern
University Press, 1988); Ann Laura Stoler, *Race and the Education of Desire:
Foucault's History of Sexuality and the Colonial Order of Things* (Durham, NC:
Duke University Press, 1995).

58.   While relying on Foucault's insights throughout, I return in chapters 2
and 7 to a consideration of difficulties in applying his analysis to an understanding of sexual health.

59.   Ken Plummer, "Critical Sexuality Studies," in *The Wiley-Blackwell Companion to Sociology*, ed. George Ritzer (West Sussex, UK: Blackwell, 2012),
243–68; Gary W. Dowsett, "The Price of Pulchritude, the Cost of Concupis-
cence: How to Have Sex in Late Modernity," *Culture, Health & Sexuality* 17,

suppl. 1 (2015): 5–19; Breanne Fahs and Sara I. McClelland, "When Sex and Power Collide: An Argument for Critical Sexuality Studies," *Journal of Sex Research* 53, nos. 4–5 (2016): 392–416.

60.   Plummer, "Critical Sexuality Studies," 250.

61.   While the proponents of "critical sexuality studies" that I cite are social scientists, I see affinities and points of connection with much work in the humanities. See Laura L. Doan, *Disturbing Practices: History, Sexuality, and Women's Experience of Modern War* (Chicago: University of Chicago Press, 2013); Heather Love, "Reading the Social: Erving Goffman and Sexuality Studies," in *Theory Aside*, ed. Jason Potts and Daniel Stout (Durham, NC: Duke University Press, 2014), 237–60; Valerie Traub, *Thinking Sex with the Early Moderns* (Philadelphia: University of Pennsylvania Press, 2016).

62.   William Simon and John H. Gagnon, "Sexual Scripts," *Society* 22, no. 1 (1984): 53–60.

63.   Sonia Corrêa, Rosalind Petchesky, and Richard Parker, *Sexuality, Health and Human Rights* (London: Routledge, 2008); Eve Kosofsky Sedgwick, *Epistemology of the Closet* (Berkeley: University of California Press, 1990); Moussawi and Vidal-Ortiz, "Queer Sociology." On the various aspects of applying a queer lens to empirical inquiry in the social sciences, see D'Lane Compton, Tey Meadow, and Kristen Schilt, eds., *Other, Please Specify: Queer Methods in Sociology* (Oakland: University of California Press, 2018); Amin Ghaziani and Matt Brim, *Imagining Queer Methods: Four Provocations for an Emerging Field* (New York: NYU Press, 2019).

64.   Héctor Carrillo, *Pathways of Desire: The Sexual Migration of Mexican Gay Men* (Chicago: University of Chicago Press, 2017), 9.

65.   On sexuality and the state, as well as the concept of sexual citizenship, see the discussion and notes in chapter 9.

66.   Inderpal Grewal and Caren Kaplan, "Global Identities: Theorizing Transnational Studies of Sexuality," *GLQ* 7, no. 4 (2001): 663–79; Martin F. Manalansan, IV, *Global Divas: Filipino Gay Men in the Diaspora* (Durham, NC: Duke University Press, 2003); Carrillo, *Pathways of Desire*; Ghassan Moussawi, "Queer Exceptionalism and Exclusion: Cosmopolitanism and Inequalities in 'Gay-Friendly' Beirut," *Sociological Review* 66, no. 1 (2018): 174–90; Zowie Davy et al., eds., *The Sage Handbook of Global Sexualities* (London: Sage, 2020); Vrushali Patil and Jyoti Puri, "Postcolonial Sexualities," in *Companion to Sexuality Studies*, ed. Nancy A. Naples (Hoboken, NJ: Wiley, 2020), 61–78; Evren Savci, *Queer in Translation: Sexual Politics under Neoliberal Islam* (Durham, NC: Duke University Press, 2021).

67.   On sexuality and passion, see Héctor Carrillo, *The Night Is Young: Sexuality in Mexico in the Time of AIDS* (Chicago: University of Chicago Press, 2002), 180–208, 255–87; Carrillo, *Pathways of Desire*, 216–56. On sexuality and pleasure, see Carole S. Vance, ed. *Pleasure and Danger: Exploring Female Sexu-*

ality (Boston: Routledge & Kegan Paul, 1984); Michelle Fine and Sara I. McClelland, "Sexuality Education and Desire: Still Missing after All These Years," *Harvard Educational Review* 76, no. 3 (2006): 297–338; Kelsy Burke, *Christians under Covers: Evangelicals and Sexual Pleasure on the Internet* (Berkeley: University of California Press, 2016); Kane Race, "Reluctant Objects: Sexual Pleasure as a Problem for HIV Biomedical Prevention," *GLQ* 22, no. 1 (2016): 1–31; Angela Jones, "Sex Is Not a Problem: The Erasure of Pleasure in Sexual Science Research," *Sexualities* 22, no. 4 (2019): 643–68; Angela Jones, *Camming: Money, Power, and Pleasure in the Sex Work Industry* (New York: NYU Press, 2020). On sexuality and carnality, see Jason Orne, *Boystown: Sex and Community in Chicago* (Chicago: University of Chicago Press, 2017), esp. 12–13. On corporeal experiences and desire, see Juana María Rodríguez, *Sexual Futures, Queer Gestures, and Other Latina Longings* (New York: NYU Press, 2014), 99–138.

68. On intersectional approaches to sexuality, see *supra* note 56.

69. Matthew Gutmann, "Men's Sexual Health and Destiny," in *Handbook on Gender and Health*, ed. Jasmine Gideon (Cheltenham, UK: Edward Elgar, 2016), 457–73.

70. On gender binarism, see Anne Fausto-Sterling, "The Five Sexes, Revisited," *The Sciences*, July–August 2000, 19–23; Sharon Elaine Preves, "Negotiating the Constraints of Gender Binarism: Intersexuals' Challenge to Gender Categorization," *Current Sociology* 48, no. 3 (2000): 27–50; Georgiann Davis, *Contesting Intersex: The Dubious Diagnosis* (New York: NYU Press, 2015); J. E. Sumerau, Lain A. B. Mathers, and Dawne Moon, "Foreclosing Fluidity at the Intersection of Gender and Sexual Normativities," *Symbolic Interaction* 43, no. 2 (2019): 205–34. On the assumption of the normality of cisgender experience (or cisnormativity), see B. Aultman, "Cisgender," *TSQ: Transgender Studies Quarterly* 1, no. 1–2 (2014): 61–62. On heterosexism and heteronormativity, see Michael Warner, introduction to *Fear of a Queer Planet: Queer Politics and Social Theory*, ed. Michael Warner (Minneapolis: University of Minnesota Press, 1993), vii–xxxi; Stevi Jackson, "Gender, Sexuality and Heterosexuality: The Complexity (and Limits) of Heteronormativity," *Feminist Theory* 7, no. 1 (2006): 105–21; Jane Ward and Beth Schneider, "The Reaches of Heteronormativity: An Introduction," *Gender & Society* 23, no. 4 (2009): 433–39.

71. Moussawi and Vidal-Ortiz, "Queer Sociology." See also Ferguson, *Aberrations in Black*.

72. Chris A. Barcelos, *Distributing Condoms and Hope: The Racialized Politics of Youth Sexual Health* (Berkeley: University of California Press, 2020). On the racial aspects of what sorts of bodies are deemed healthy, see also Sabrina Strings, *Fearing the Black Body: The Racial Origins of Fat Phobia* (New York: NYU Press, 2019).

73. As Julian Carter has described, "racial and sexual meanings directly produce one another: their relationship is not analogical but mutually constitutive." Julian B. Carter, *The Heart of Whiteness: Normal Sexuality and Race
in America, 1880–1940* (Durham, NC: Duke University Press, 2007), 159.
See also Nagel, "Ethnicity and Sexuality"; Somerville, *Queering the Color
Line*; Ferguson, *Aberrations in Black*; Mignon R. Moore, *Invisible Families: Gay
Identities, Relationships, and Motherhood among Black Women* (Berkeley: University of California Press, 2011); Salvador Vidal-Ortiz, Brandon Andrew
Robinson, and Christina Khan, *Race and Sexuality* (Cambridge, UK: Polity,
2018); Moussawi and Vidal-Ortiz, "Queer Sociology."

74. David J. Hess, *Science Studies: An Advanced Introduction* (New York: NYU
Press, 1997); Sergio Sismondo, *An Introduction to Science and Technology
Studies* (Malden, MA: Blackwell, 2004).

75. For a broad introduction to the field, see Ulrike Felt, Rayvon Fouché, Clark A.
Miller, and Laurel Smith-Doerr, eds., *The Handbook of Science and Technology Studies*, 4th ed. (Cambridge, MA: MIT Press, 2016).

76. On bodies in relation to health and biomedicine, see, for example, Stefan
Hirschauer, "The Manufacture of Bodies in Surgery," *Social Studies of Sci-
ence* 21, no. 2 (1991): 279–319; Nelly Oudshoorn, *Beyond the Natural Body:
An Archeology of Sex Hormones* (London: Routledge, 1994); Margaret Lock,
"Anomalous Ageing: Managing the Postmenopausal Body," *Body & Society*
4, no. 1 (1998): 35–61; Annemarie Mol, *The Body Multiple: Ontology in Medi-
cal Practice* (Durham, NC: Duke University Press, 2002); Steven Epstein,
"Bodily Differences and Collective Identities: The Politics of Gender and
Race in Biomedical Research in the United States," *Body and Society* 10,
nos. 2–3 (2004): 183–203; Didier Fassin and Estelle D'Halluin, "The Truth
from the Body: Medical Certificates as Ultimate Evidence for Asylum
Seekers," *American Anthropologist* 107, no. 4 (2005): 597–608.

77. Mol and Berg, "Differences in Medicine," 3.

78. Peter Keating and Alberto Cambrosio, "From Screening to Clinical Research: The Cure of Leukemia and the Early Development of the Cooperative Oncology Groups, 1955–1966," *Bulletin of History of Medicine* 76, no. 2
(2002): 299–334, esp. 300; Clarke et al., "Biomedicalization," 162.

79. See the discussion in chapter 9.

80. Stephen Molldrem and Mitali Thakor, "Genealogies and Futures of Queer
STS: Issues in Theory, Method, and Institutionalization," *Catalyst: Feminism, Theory, Technoscience* 3, no. 1 (2017): 1–15.

81. Jennifer R. Fishman, Laura Mamo, and Patrick R. Grzanka, "Sex, Gender,
and Sexuality in Biomedicine," in *The Handbook of Science and Technology
Studies*, 4th ed., ed. Ulrike Felt, et al. (Cambridge, MA: MIT Press, 2017),
379–405.

82. Ibid., 382.

83. Ibid., 379.

84. Alain Giami, "Sexual Health: The Emergence, Development, and Diversity of a Concept," *Annual Review of Sex Research* 13 (2002): 1–35; Sandfort and Ehrhardt, "Sexual Health"; Weston M. Edwards and Eli Coleman, "Defining Sexual Health: A Descriptive Overview," *Archives of Sexual Behavior* 33, no. 3 (2004): 189–95; Richard Parker et al., "Global Transformations and Intimate Relations in the 21st Century: Social Science Research on Sexuality and the Emergence of *Sexual Health* and *Sexual Rights* Frameworks," *Annual Review of Sex Research* 15 (2004): 362–98; Laura M. Carpenter, "Sexual Health," in *Blackwell Encyclopedia of Sociology*, ed. George Ritzer (London: Blackwell, 2007), https://onlinelibrary.wiley.com/doi/abs/10.1002/9781405165518.wbeoss093.

85. In addition, I have benefited substantially from how other scholars have conceptualized research on other "compound" entities of contemporary salience—for example, Didier Fassin, "That Obscure Object of Global Health," in *Medical Anthropology at the Intersections: Histories, Activisms, and Futures*, ed. Marcia C. Inhorn and Emily A. Wentzell (Durham, NC: Duke University Press, 2012), 95–115.

86. By "discourse," Bernstein means "a constellation of words, materialities, and practices as they coalesce in historically and culturally situated ways, constructing the empirical object under consideration and the social locations to which it is manifest." Elizabeth Bernstein, *Brokered Subjects: Sex, Trafficking, and the Politics of Freedom* (Chicago: University of Chicago Press, 2018), 25. See also David Valentine, *Imagining Transgender: An Ethnography of a Category* (Durham, NC: Duke University Press, 2007).

87. Reiner Keller, "The Sociology of Knowledge Approach to Discourse (SKAD)," *Human Studies* 34 (2011): 43–65, esp. 48.

88. See the article itself for a more detailed explanation of the methodology. Epstein and Mamo, "Proliferation," 179.

89. "Google Books Ngram Viewer," Google, https://books.google.com/ngrams.

90. "Google Books Ngram Viewer: What Does the Ngram Viewer Do?," Google, https://books.google.com/ngrams/info.

91. While Ngrams have become a popular illustrative tool, I believe that scholars should use them with some caution, not only because of potential limitations but also because Google does not make the details of their proprietary algorithm available for scrutiny. See Sarah Zhang, "The Pitfalls of Using Google Ngram to Study Language," *Wired*, 12 October 2015, https://www.wired.com/2015/10/pitfalls-of-studying-language-with-google-ngram/.

92. Karin Knorr Cetina, *Epistemic Cultures: How the Sciences Make Knowledge* (Cambridge, MA: Harvard University Press, 1999), 24.

93. More precisely, I have adapted the methodological prescription of actor-network theory to "follow the actors." Bruno Latour, *Science in Action: How to Follow Scientists and Engineers through Society* (Cambridge, MA: Harvard

University Press, 1987). In this case I have followed "the actors as they use the term."

94. Stefan Helmreich and Sophia Roosth, "Life Forms: A Keywords Entry," *Representations* 112 (2010): 27–53, esp. 29.

95. Larissa Buchholz, "What Is a Global Field? Theorizing Fields Beyond the Nation-State," *Sociological Review Monographs* 64, no. 2 (2016): 31–60; Andreas Wimmer, "Domains of Diffusion: How Culture and Institutions Travel around the World and with What Consequences," *American Journal of Sociology* 126, no. 6 (2021): 1389–1438. On the characteristically global nature of present-day regulation of health and biomedicine, see Carol A. Heimer, JuLeigh C. Petty, and Rebecca J. Culyba, "Risk and Rules: The 'Legalization' of Medicine," in *Organizational Encounters with Risk*, ed. Bridget Hutter and Michael Power (Cambridge: Cambridge University Press, 2005), 92–131; Alberto Cambrosio, Peter Keating, Thomas Schlich, and George Weisz, "Regulatory Objectivity and the Generation and Management of Evidence in Medicine," *Social Science & Medicine* 63 (2006): 189–99.

96. On the nation-state's "continuing influence in the realm of forces and connections" even within global processes, see Michael Burawoy, "Introduction: Reading for the Global," in *Global Ethnography: Forces, Connections, and Imaginations in a Postmodern World*, ed. Michael Burawoy et al. (Berkeley: University of California Press, 2000), 1–35, esp. 35. For a strong argument in favor of keeping the nation-state central when we study culturally distinctive "ways of knowing" (or "civic epistemologies"), see Sheila Jasanoff, *Designs on Nature: Science and Democracy in Europe and the United States* (Princeton, NJ: Princeton University Press, 2005).

97. In these ways, my work is in conversation with the emergent subfield of the "sociology of global health." See Joseph Harris and Alexandre White, "The Sociology of Global Health," *Sociology of Development* 5, no. 1 (2019): 9–30. On the WHO in particular, see Nitsan Chorev, *The World Health Organization between North and South* (Ithaca, NY: Cornell University Press, 2012).

CHAPTER ONE

1. Elizabeth Daley, "Happy Birthday, Sexual Health: Planned Parenthood Is 100 Years Old," *The Advocate*, 16 October 2016, https://www.advocate.com /health/2016/10/16/happy-birthday-sexual-health-planned-parenthood -100-years-old.

2. "Planned Parenthood," Wikipedia, accessed 19 February 2021, https://en .wikipedia.org/wiki/Planned_Parenthood.

3. Peter Lewis Allen, *The Wages of Sin: Sex and Disease, Past and Present* (Chicago: University of Chicago Press, 2000); Arnold I. Davidson, *The Emergence of Sexuality: Historical Epistemology and the Formation of Concepts* (Cambridge, MA: Harvard University Press, 2001).

4. Thoughtful and informative articles on these events (and their precur-
    sors and sequelae) have been published by people who have had at least
    one foot inside the worlds they analyze. See Alain Giami, "Sexual Health:
    The Emergence, Development, and Diversity of a Concept," *Annual Review
    of Sex Research* 13 (2002): 1–35; Theo Sandfort and Anke Ehrhardt, "Sexual
    Health: A Useful Public Health Paradigm or a Moral Imperative?," *Archives
    of Sexual Behavior* 33, no. 3 (2004): 181–87; Weston M. Edwards and Eli
    Coleman, "Defining Sexual Health: A Descriptive Overview," *Archives of
    Sexual Behavior* 33, no. 3 (2004): 189–95; Eli Coleman, "From Sexology to
    Sexual Health," in *Routledge Handbook of Sexuality, Health, and Rights*,
    ed. Peter Aggleton and Richard Parker (London: Routledge, 2010), 135–44.
5. Lorraine Daston, "Introduction: The Coming into Being of Scientific Ob-
    jects," in *Biographies of Scientific Objects*, ed. Lorraine Daston (Chicago: Uni-
    versity of Chicago Press, 2000), 1–14, esp. 3.
6. See, for example, Nancy Fraser and Linda Gordon, "A Genealogy of Depen-
    dency: Tracing a Keyword of the U.S. Welfare State," *Signs* 19, no. 2 (1994):
    309–36; Chandra Mukerji, "Cultural Genealogy: Method for a Historical
    Sociology of Culture or Cultural Sociology of History," *Cultural Sociology* 1,
    no. 1 (2007): 49–71; David Armstrong, "Origins of the Problem of Health-
    Related Behaviors: A Genealogical Study," *Social Studies of Science* 39, no. 6
    (2009): 909–26; Tom Boellstorff, "But Do Not Identify as Gay: A Proleptic
    Genealogy of the MSM Category," *Cultural Anthropology* 26, no. 2 (2011):
    287–312; Cécile Stephanie Stehrenberger and Svenja Goltermann, "Disas-
    ter Medicine: Genealogy of a Concept," *Social Science & Medicine* 120 (2014):
    317–24.
7. Michel Foucault, *Language, Counter-Memory, Practice: Selected Essays and
    Interviews* (Ithaca, NY: Cornell University Press, 1977). For a recent socio-
    logical approach to similar questions, see Gabriel Abend, "Making Things
    Possible," *Sociological Methods and Research*, advance online publication,
    10 July 2020, https://doi.org/10.1177/0049124120926204.
8. Ian Hacking, *Historical Ontology* (Cambridge, MA: Harvard University
    Press, 2002), 23. While the language of "ontology" has become well en-
    trenched in science studies, I am sympathetic to the impulse behind
    Michael Lynch's proposed alternative of "ontography." See Michael Lynch,
    "Ontography: Investigating the Production of Things, Deflating Ontology,"
    Social Studies of Science 43, no. 3 (2013): 444–62. On the similar method of
    "historical epistemology," see Arnold I. Davidson, *The Emergence of Sexual-
    ity: Historical Epistemology and the Formation of Concepts* (Cambridge, MA:
    Harvard University Press, 2001), xiii, 32, 180–82; Giami, "Sexual Health,"
    2–3. Alternatively, Lorraine Daston has proposed the term "applied meta-
    physics" to describe the study of how phenomena "come into being and
    pass away as objects of scientific inquiry." Daston, "Introduction," 1. On
    tracing the development of an "epistemic object," see also Hans-Jörg

Rheinberger, "Cytoplasmic Particles: The Trajectory of a Scientific Object," in *Biographies of Scientific Objects*, ed. Lorraine Daston (Chicago: University of Chicago Press, 2000), 270–94, esp. 274.

9.   David Ribes and Jessica Beth Polk, "Organizing for Ontological Change: The Kernel of an AIDS Research Infrastructure," *Social Studies of Science* 45 (2015): 214–41.

10. Evelyn Fox Keller and Elisabeth A. Lloyd, introduction to *Keywords in Evolutionary Biology*, ed. Evelyn Fox Keller and Elisabeth A. Lloyd (Cambridge, MA: Harvard University Press, 1992), 1–6, esp. 1–2.

11. Medical advice about sexuality formed a part of the circulation of medical advice generally at this time. See Paul Starr, *The Social Transformation of American Medicine* (New York: Basic Books, 1982), esp. 127.

12. Henry G. Hanchett, *Sexual Health: A Plan and Practical Guide for the People in All Matters Concerning the Organs of Reproduction of Both Sexes and All Ages* (New York: Charles T. Hurlburt, 1887).

13. Ibid., 4. In this discussion I emphasize medical advice related to sexuality and leave aside the development of medical specialty areas devoted to reproductive health and reproductive science. See Adele Clarke, *Disciplining Reproduction: Modernity, American Life Sciences, and "the Problems of Sex"* (Berkeley: University of California Press, 1998); Rene Almeling, *GUYnecology: The Missing Science of How Men's Health Matters for Reproduction* (Berkeley: University of California Press, 2020). On medical sex advice during this period, see also M. E. Melody and Linda M. Peterson, *Teaching America about Sex: Marriage Guides and Sex Manuals from the Late Victorians to Dr. Ruth* (New York: NYU Press, 1999).

14. Helen Lefkowitz Horowitz, *Rereading Sex: Battles over Sexual Knowledge and Suppression in Nineteenth-Century America* (New York: Knopf, 2002), 3–4.

15. Ibid., 6.

16. Ibid., 7. On the "masturbation scare," see 86–122.

17. Charles E. Rosenberg, "At the Boundaries of Transgression: F.C. Hollick, Invisible Bestseller" (unpublished ms., Cambridge, MA, 2016). I am grateful to Charles Rosenberg for sharing with me, and permitting me to cite, his unpublished work.

18. Ibid., 16.

19. Jessamyn Neuhaus, "The Importance of Being Orgasmic: Sexuality, Gender, and Marital Sex Manuals in the United States, 1920–1963," *Journal of the History of Sexuality* 9, no. 4 (2000): 447–73, esp. 448.

20. Ibid., 447.

21. Annamarie Jagose, *Orgasmology* (Durham, NC: Duke University Press, 2013), 41–73.

22. Jane Ward, *The Tragedy of Heterosexuality* (New York: NYU Press, 2020), 40–48, esp. 47.

23. Peter Cryle and Elizabeth Stephens, *Normality: A Critical Genealogy* (Chicago: University of Chicago Press, 2017), 164.

24. Julian B. Carter, *The Heart of Whiteness: Normal Sexuality and Race in America, 1880–1940* (Durham, NC: Duke University Press, 2007), 2.

25. Roy Porter and Lesley Hall, *The Facts of Life: The Creation of Sexual Knowledge in Britain, 1650–1950* (New Haven, CT: Yale University Press, 1995), 208–9, 218. See also Laura Doan, "Marie Stopes's Wonderful Rhythm Charts: Normalizing the Natural," *Journal of the History of Ideas* 78, no. 4 (2017): 595–620.

26. Neuhaus, "Importance," 454.

27. Theodoor Hendrik van de Velde, *Ideal Marriage: Its Philosophy and Techniques*, trans. Stella Brown (New York: Civici Friede, 1938), title page.

28. On the birth of sexology, see Erwin J. Haeberle, *The Birth of Sexology: A Brief History in Documents* (Washington, DC: World Association for Sexology, 1983); Gert Hekma, "A History of Sexology: Social and Historical Aspects of Sexuality," in *From Sappho to de Sade: Moments in the History of Sexuality*, ed. Jan Bremmer (Milton Park, UK: Routledge, 1989), 173–93; Porter and Hall, *Facts of Life*, 155–77; Janice M. Irvine, *Disorders of Desire: Sexuality and Gender in Modern American Sexology* (Philadelphia: Temple University Press, 2005), 5–6.

29. Chris Waters, "Sexology," in *Palgrave Advances in the Modern History of Sexuality*, ed. H. G. Cocks and Matt Houlbrook (Houndmills, UK: Palgrave Macmillan, 2006), 41–63, esp. 45.

30. Jeffrey Weeks, *Sexuality and Its Discontents: Meanings, Myths and Modern Sexualities* (London: Routledge & Kegan Paul, 1985), 69.

31 Hekma, "History of Sexology," 176–81.

32. Haeberle, *Birth of Sexology*, 4; Waters, "Sexology," 42.

33. Coleman, "From Sexology," 135.

34. Kirsten Leng, *Sexual Politics and Feminist Science: Women Sexologists in Germany, 1900–1933* (Ithaca, NY: Cornell University Press, 2018). On these points, as well as the vexed question of the boundaries of sexology as a field of knowledge production and dissemination, see also Laura Doan, "Troubling Popularisation: On the Gendered Circuits of a 'Scientific' Knowledge of Sex," *Gender & History* 31, no. 2 (2019): 1–15.

35. Leng, *Sexual Politics*, 19. See also Irvine, *Disorders of Desire*, 2.

36. Waters, "Sexology," 46.

37. Veronika Fuechtner, Douglas E. Haynes, and Ryan M. Jones, "Introduction: Toward a Global History of Sexual Science: Movements, Networks, and Deployments," in *A Global History of Sexual Science, 1880–1960*, ed. Veronika Fuechtner, Douglas E. Haynes, and Ryan M. Jones (Oakland: University of California Press, 2018), 1–25. See also Alain Giami and Jane Russo, "The Diversity of Sexologies in Latin America: Emergence, Development, and

Diversification," *International Journal of Sexual Health* 25, no. 1 (2013): 1–12; Benjamin Kahan, "Conjectures on the Sexual World-System," *GLQ* 23, no. 3 (2017): 327–57.

38. Fuechtner et al., "Introduction," 3.
39. Ibid., 9.
40. Haeberle, *Birth of Sexology*, 8–9.
41. Hekma, "History of Sexology," 185.
42. Ibid; Leng, *Sexual Politics*. On the complex interconnections of sexological thinking with contemporaneous notions of racial difference and sameness, see Siobhan B. Somerville, *Queering the Color Line: Race and the Invention of Homosexuality in American Culture* (Durham, NC: Duke University Press, 2000), 15–38; Marlon B. Ross, "Beyond the Closet as Raceless Paradigm," in *Black Queer Studies: A Critical Anthology*, ed. E. Patrick Johnson and Mae G. Henderson (Durham, NC: Duke University Press, 2005), 161–89, esp. 167–68.
43. Sigmund Freud, *Three Essays on the Theory of Sexuality* (New York: Basic Books, 1962).
44. Alfred C. Kinsey, Wardell B. Pomeroy, and Clyde E. Martin, *Sexual Behavior in the Human Male* (Philadelphia: W. B. Saunders, 1948); Alfred C. Kinsey, *Sexual Behavior in the Human Female* (Philadelphia: W. B. Saunders, 1953); Haeberle, *Birth of Sexology*, 10; Hekma, "History of Sexology," 186; Irvine, *Disorders of Desire*, 31–66.
45. Haeberle, *Birth of Sexology*, 11; Irvine, *Disorders of Desire*, 67–94, 187–227.
46. Fuechtner et al., "Introduction," 21.
47. Waters, "Sexology," 49–50.
48. Fuechtner et al., "Introduction," 21. Because the time period covered by this edited collection ends in 1960, the authors do not discuss the formal involvement of present-day sexologists in activities under the banner of sexual health (including the rebranding of the World Association of Sexology as the World Association for Sexual Health), and the term "sexual health" does not appear in the volume's index. I discuss these later developments in chapter 3.
49. Irvine, *Disorders of Desire*, 153–86.
50. Dagmar Herzog, *Sexuality in Europe: A Twentieth-Century History* (Cambridge: Cambridge University Press, 2011), 2.
51. Michel Foucault, *The History of Sexuality, Volume 1: An Introduction*, trans. Robert Hurley (New York: Vintage Books, 1980), 101.
52. Herzog, *Sexuality in Europe*, 2.
53. Weeks, *Sexuality and Its Discontents*, 244.
54. Waters, "Sexology," 55; Leng, *Sexual Politics*, 24–25.
55. Sandfort and Ehrhardt, "Sexual Health," 182.
56. Kristin Luker, "Sex, Social Hygiene, and the State: The Double-Edged Sword of Social Reform," *Theory and Society* 27, no. 5 (1998): 601–34, esp. 606.

57. Ibid., 611. See also Allan M. Brandt, *No Magic Bullet: A Social History of Venereal Disease in the United States since 1880* (New York: Oxford University Press, 1985), 46.

58. Kristin Luker, *When Sex Goes to School: Warring Views on Sex—and Sex Education—since the Sixties* (New York: W. W. Norton, 2006), 38–39.

59. Brandt, *No Magic Bullet*, 5. See also John D'Emilio and Estelle B. Freedman, *Intimate Matters: A History of Sexuality in America* (New York: Harper & Row, 1988), 203–8.

60. Brandt, *No Magic Bullet*, 7.

61. R. Danielle Egan and Gail Hawkes, "Childhood Sexuality, Normalization and the Social Hygiene Movement in the Anglophone West, 1900–1935," *Social History of Medicine* 23, no. 1 (2009): 56–78, esp. 57. See also Nicola Kay Beisel, *Imperiled Innocents: Anthony Comstock and Family Reproduction in Victorian America* (Princeton, NJ: Princeton University Press, 1997); Jeffrey P. Moran, *Teaching Sex: The Shaping of Adolescence in the 20th Century* (Cambridge, MA: Harvard University Press, 2000), 23.

62. D'Emilio and Freedman, *Intimate Matters*, 205.

63. Moran, *Teaching Sex*, 35.

64. Brandt, *No Magic Bullet*, 37; Luker, "Sex, Social Hygiene," 610.

65. Luker, "Sex, Social Hygiene," 612.

66. Brandt, *No Magic Bullet*, 36; Luker, "Sex, Social Hygiene," 614, 624.

67. George Chauncey Jr., *Gay New York: Gender, Urban Culture, and the Making of the Gay Male World, 1890–1940* (New York: Basic Books, 1994), 143–45.

68. Many states enacted their own versions of the Comstock Act, in some cases effectively criminalizing contraception. Tambra K. Cain, "Comstock Laws," in *Encyclopedia of Women's Health*, ed. Sana Loue and Martha Sajatovic (Boston: Springer, 2004), https://doi.org/10.1007/978-0-306 48113 -0_101.

69. Brandt, *No Magic Bullet*, 59.

70. Ibid., 73.

71. Luker, "Sex, Social Hygiene," 619.

72. Brandt, *No Magic Bullet*, 168–73.

73. Melody and Peterson, *Teaching America*.

74. On this point, see also Giami, "Sexual Health," 7; Edwards and Coleman, "Defining Sexual Health," 189.

75. Elizabeth Siegel Watkins, *On the Pill: A Social History of Oral Contraceptives, 1950–1970* (Baltimore: Johns Hopkins University Press, 1998).

76. Jeffrey Escoffier, ed., *Sexual Revolution* (New York: Thunder's Mouth Press, 2003).

77. Barry D. Adam, Jan Willem Duyvendak, and André Krouwel, *The Global Emergence of Gay and Lesbian Politics: National Imprints of a Worldwide Movement* (Philadelphia: Temple University Press, 1999); Bonnie G. Smith, *Global Feminisms since 1945* (London: Routledge, 2000); Myra Marx Ferree

and Aili Mari Tripp, *Global Feminism: Transnational Women's Activism, Organizing, and Human Rights* (New York: NYU Press, 2006).

78.   Janice M. Irvine, "Shame Comes Out of the Closet," *Sexuality Research and Social Policy* 6, no. 1 (2009): 70–79.

79.   Michelle Murphy, *Seizing the Means of Reproduction: Entanglements of Feminism, Health, and Technoscience* (Durham, NC: Duke University Press, 2012), 8.

80.   Murphy, *Seizing the Means*; Michelle Murphy, "Reproduction," in *Marxism and Feminism*, ed. Shahrzad Mojab (London: Zed Books, 2015), 287–304.

81.   Murphy, *Seizing the Means*, 16–17; Murphy, "Reproduction."

82.   Mary S. Calderone, "Sexual Health and Family Planning: The Seventh Annual Bronfman Lecture," *American Journal of Public Health* 58, no. 2 (1968): 223–31. Sandfort and Ehrhardt identify Calderone's article as one of the earliest references to sexual health obtained in their search of the Medline and PsycINFO databases. Sandfort and Ehrhardt, "Sexual Health," 182. SIECUS has gone through several name changes and is now known as SIECUS: Sex Ed for Social Change.

83.   Calderone, "Sexual Health," 228, 230.

84.   My research assistant Joseph Guisti combed through successive editions of multiple popular medical dictionaries to trace the entry of the term "sexual health." See chapter 3 for further discussion.

85.   Nitsan Chorev, *The World Health Organization between North and South* (Ithaca, NY: Cornell University Press, 2012), 2–3.

86.   Ibid.

87.   Daniel Callahan, *The Roots of Bioethics: Health, Progress, Technology, Death* (Oxford: Oxford University Press, 2012), 63, 69.

88.   Mary S. Calderone, "Education in Human Sexuality for Health Professionals," *American Review of World Health*, Winter–Summer 1970, 25–29, esp. 25 (emphasis in the original).

89.   However, as noted in the introduction, the National Library of Medicine did not create a Medical Subject Heading for sexual health until 2018. For these various codes and their histories, see "Population Health MeSH Descriptor Data 2021," National Library of Medicine, https://meshb.nlm.nih.gov/record/ui?ui=D000075485. I am grateful to Kellie Owens for tracing this history.

90.   I am grateful to Marcia Tiede at the Northwestern University Library for tracking down this information for me.

91.   Linna M. Anderson, "Early History of ASHA," in *Creating a Sexually Healthy Nation: Celebrating 100 Years of the American Sexual Health Association*, ed. Martha Kempner (Research Triangle Park, NC: American Sexual Health Association, 2014), n.p. See also "Who We Are," American Sexual Health Association, http://www.ashasexualhealth.org/who-we-are/.

92.   "Mental Health MeSH Descriptor Data 2021," National Library of Medicine, https://meshb.nlm.nih.gov/record/ui?ui=D008603. I am grateful

to Charles Rosenberg for suggesting this point. "Hygiene" nowadays often serves very specific euphemistic functions, such as in the phrase "feminine hygiene products."

93. Giami, "Sexual Health," 9–14; Coleman, "From Sexology," 136.

94. Giami, "Sexual Health," 10.

95. Coleman, "From Sexology," 136. On attempts in recent decades to professionalize sexology and establish its legitimacy, see Irvine, *Disorders of Desire*.

96. Coleman, "From Sexology," 135.

97. World Health Organization, *Education and Treatment in Human Sexuality: The Training of Health Professionals, Report of a WHO Meeting* [Held in Geneva from 6 to 12 February 1974], Technical Report Series No. 572 (Geneva: World Health Organization, 1975), http://www.who.int/iris/handle/10665/38247.

98. Ibid., 5. A report from the 1972 meeting was published as D. R. Mace, R. H. O. Bannerman, and J. Burton, *The Teaching of Human Sexuality in Schools for Health Professionals*, Public Health Paper No. 57 (Geneva: World Health Organization, 1974), http://apps.who.int/iris/handle/10665/37441. On the 1972 meeting, see also Giami, "Sexual Health," 9.

99. WHO, *Education and Treatment*, 5–6.

100. Ibid.

101. For example, Edwards and Coleman, "Defining Sexual Health," 191.

102. WHO, *Education and Treatment*, title page.

103. "Sexual Health," World Health Organization, https://www.who.int/reproductivehealth/topics/sexual_health/sh_definitions/en/.

104. Eli Coleman, interviewed by author, 11 July 2019.

105. WHO, *Education and Treatment*, 26–27.

106. Ibid., 28–29.

107. Ibid., 6.

108. Ibid. (my emphasis).

109. Ibid.

110. Richard Parker et al., "Global Transformations and Intimate Relations in the 21st Century: Social Science Research on Sexuality and the Emergence of *Sexual Health* and *Sexual Rights* Frameworks," *Annual Review of Sex Research* 15 (2004): 362–98; Richard Parker, "Critical Intersections and Engagements: Gender, Sexuality, Health, and Rights in Medical Anthropology," in *Medical Anthropology at the Intersections: Histories, Activisms, and Futures*, ed. Marcia C. Inhorn and Emily A. Wentzell (Durham, NC: Duke University Press, 2012), 206–37.

111. WHO, *Education and Treatment*, 19.

112. Ibid., 7.

113. Steven Epstein and Stefan Timmermans, "From Medicine to Health: The Proliferation and Diversification of Cultural Authority," *Journal of Health and Social Behavior* 62, no. 3 (2021): 240–54.

114. "Iris," World Health Organization, http://apps.who.int/iris/simple-search ?query=.

115. Leonore Tiefer, "Medicalizations and Demedicalizations of Sexuality Therapies," *Journal of Sex Research* 49, no. 4 (2012): 311–18, esp. 312.

116. I thank Nina Eliasoph for pointing me to the question of how global bureaucracies negotiate the meanings of intangible cultural phenomena.

117. The origin of the terms "sex positive" and "sex negative" is often attributed to the midcentury writings of Wilhelm Reich. See Chad M. Mosher, "Historical Perspectives on Sex Positivity: Contributing to a New Paradigm within Counseling Psychology," *Counseling Psychologist* 45, no. 4 (2017): 487–503.

118. Gayle S. Rubin, "Thinking Sex: Notes for a Radical Theory of the Politics of Sexuality," in *Pleasure and Danger: Exploring Female Sexuality*, ed. Carole S. Vance (New York: Routledge, 1984), 267–318.

119. The report from the 1972 meeting (published in 1974) had made one reference to sexual health, characterizing it as consisting of three "basic elements": "a capacity to enjoy and control sexual and reproductive behaviour"; "freedom from fear, shame, guilt, false beliefs, and other psychological factors"; and "freedom from organic disorders, diseases, and deficiencies." Mace et al., *Teaching of Human Sexuality*, 10.

120. Calderone, "Education," 25. However, in that article, Calderone did proceed to describe differences between men and women with regard to their sexual natures.

121. However, the question of whether it was even possible to define sexual health in a culturally neutral way would become an explicit topic of debate among experts and professionals in subsequent years, as I describe in chapter 3.

122. WHO, *Education and Treatment*, 9.

123. Ibid., 10.

124. Ibid., 17–18.

125. Laura Carpenter has observed how this definition of sexual health, in its breadth, prefigured subsequent ones: "Pleasure, agency, and freedom from physiological and psychological disorders have been central components of all subsequent major definitions of sexual health." Laura M. Carpenter, "Sexual Health," in *Blackwell Encyclopedia of Sociology*, ed. George Ritzer (London: Blackwell, 2007), https://onlinelibrary.wiley.com/doi/abs/10 .1002/9781405165518.wbeoss093.

126. I discuss the relation between sexual health and sexual rights in chapters 2 and 3.

CHAPTER TWO

1. "#Sexualhealth," Twitter, https://twitter.com/hashtag/sexualhealth ?src=hash&f=live (these particular examples retrieved 15 February 2020).

2. For details on the selection of articles from medical journals and newspaper, see *infra* note 8. The count of appearances in Google Books was performed at https://books.google.com/ngrams. Information on NIH grants was obtained from the NIH Freedom of Information Office. Research assistants Joseph Guisti, Gemma Mangione, Kellie Owens, and Aaron Benavidez assisted with various aspects of the analysis presented in this chapter.

3. An article on sexual health by Sandfort and Ehrhardt from 2004 detected a similar upsurge in academic publications on sexual health, also beginning in the early 1990s. Their analysis, which ended in 2002, used the Medline and PsycINFO databases. Theo Sandfort and Anke Ehrhardt, "Sexual Health: A Useful Public Health Paradigm or a Moral Imperative?," *Archives of Sexual Behavior* 33, no. 3 (2004): 181–87, esp. 182. As shown more clearly in my figure 3, occurrences of sexual health in Google Books (as a proportion of all two-word phrases) have leveled off, starting in 2008. In contrast, the numbers of PubMed articles with "sexual health" in the titles (as a proportion of all PubMed articles in a given year) has continued to rise sharply. See https://pubmed.ncbi.nlm.nih.gov/?term=%22sexual +health%22%5BTitle%5D&sort= (searched 8 February 2021).

4. An alternative approach to my analysis would be to begin with the presumption that "the singularity of objects, so often presupposed, turns out to be an accomplishment." The empirical philosopher Annemarie Mol has helpfully proposed that objects that appear singular can in fact be ontologically multiple, and therefore the discovery of multiplicity need elicit no great surprise. However, while I find her approach generative, I think that Mol's analysis is best suited to identifiable objects that are manipulated in practical ways and therefore can be studied "praxiographically," as she proposes—entities such as bodies and diseases, in her study, or testosterone, in a recent study by Rebecca Jordan-Young and Katrina Karkazis. The kind of multiplicity that characterizes a discursively rich, semantically flexible, transdisciplinary assemblage like sexual health is of a somewhat different sort. See Annemarie Mol, *The Body Multiple: Ontology in Medical Practice* (Durham, NC: Duke University Press, 2002), 119; Rebecca M. Jordan-Young and Katrina Karkazis, *Testosterone: An Unauthorized Biography* (Cambridge, MA: Harvard University Press, 2019), 24–34.

5. Paul J. DiMaggio and Walter W. Powell, "The Iron Cage Revisited: Institutional Isomorphism and Collective Rationality in Organizational Fields," *American Sociological Review* 48, no. 2 (1983): 147–60.

6. Although specialization in medicine is not new, the historian of medicine George Weisz has described "the explosion of new specialist categories that have emerged continuously since the 1960s" in many countries, owing both to "innovations produced by the academic research sector" and to "what are perceived as new social needs." George Weisz, *Divide and Conquer:*

A Comparative History of Medical Specialization (Oxford: Oxford University Press, 2006), 231.

7.   I take my cues here, in part, from the anthropologist Didier Fassin's discussion of a similarly concatenated (and even more ubiquitous) term, "global health." In an article dissecting that topic, Fassin attended to the semiotic richness of the term, the network of associations within which it can be encountered, and its various real-world effects. Didier Fassin, "That Obscure Object of Global Health," in *Medical Anthropology at the Intersections: Histories, Activisms, and Futures*, ed. Marcia C. Inhorn and Emily A. Wentzell (Durham, NC: Duke University Press, 2012), 95–115.

8.   As described more fully in Epstein and Mamo, "Proliferation," our analysis focused primarily on three kinds of data that were designed to tap into both expert or professional and nonexpert or public worlds. First, beginning with the 1,587 medical and health-related journal articles published in the PubMed database (https://www.ncbi.nlm.nih.gov/pubmed/) through 2013 that used the phrase "sexual health" as part of the article title (excluding letters, to ensure a more consistent sample), we assembled a data set consisting of the abstracts of the subset of 1,173 scientific articles that contained abstracts. Second, we compiled a data set of the 485 articles (excluding letters and ads) published in the *New York Times*, the *Los Angeles Times*, and the *Washington Post* through 2013 that used the phrase "sexual health" (anywhere in the body of the article). Finally and less systematically, we conducted online searches to locate webpages devoted substantially to sexual health, including those belonging to journals, organizations, foundations, private companies, advocacy groups, religious organizations, and government agencies. (It was beyond the scope of this analysis to consider translated terms that are in lesser use, such as *salud sexual, santé sexuelle*, and so on.)

9.   Initial results from this coding focused our attention on the kinds of practical activity enjoined by the term "sexual health." We therefore proceeded to break down the invocations of sexual health according to the forms of behavior modification or targeted action that they seemed to call for. Through this process, which brought us to see how sexual health operates as a series of "solutions," we then generated inductively our list of social problem frames within which these discussions of sexual health appeared to cluster.

10.   In the article with Laura Mamo, we described these social problem areas as "niches." In retrospect, "niche" appears to suggest a location in geographic or social space, which may not be the best way of characterizing the phenomenon in all six instances. On the construction and framing of social problems, see Joel Best, ed., *Images of Issues: Typifying Contemporary Social Problems* (New York: Aldine de Gruyter, 1989). My approach to framing draws on the discursive and semiotic conception of it described in

Marc W. Steinberg, "Tilting the Frame: Considerations on Collective Action Framing from a Discursive Turn," *Theory and Society* 27 (1998): 845–72.

11. See the article for a longer discussion. On the study of social problems, see Stephen Hilgartner and Charles L. Bosk, "The Rise and Fall of Social Problems: A Public Arenas Model," *American Journal of Sociology* 94, no. 1 (1988): 53–78; Best, *Images of Issues*; Joel Best, "Introduction: The Diffusion of Social Problems," in *How Claims Spread: The Cross-National Diffusion of Social Problems*, ed. Joel Best (New York: Walter de Gruyter, 2001), 1–18.

12. On the sociological use of ideal types for analytical and explanatory purposes, see Max Weber, *The Methodology of the Social Sciences* (New York: Free Press, 1949), 89–112.

13. Keith Wailoo, Julie Livingston, Steven Epstein, and Robert Aronowitz, eds., *Three Shots at Prevention: The HPV Vaccine and the Politics of Medicine's Simple Solutions* (Baltimore: Johns Hopkins University Press, 2010); Laura Mamo and Steven Epstein, "The Pharmaceuticalization of Sexual Risk: Vaccine Development and the New Politics of Cancer Prevention," *Social Science & Medicine* 101 (2013): 155–65; Laura Mamo and Steven Epstein, "The New Sexual Politics of Cancer: Oncoviruses, Disease Prevention, and Sexual Health Promotion," *BioSocieties* 12 (2016): 367–91.

14. Sten H. Vermund, Amy B. Geller, and Jeffrey S. Crowley, *Sexually Transmitted Infections: Adopting a Sexual Health Paradigm* (Washington, DC: National Academies Press, 2021), xvi.

15. Exemplars include the International Society for Sexual Medicine (ISSM) and its *Journal of Sexual Medicine*, as well as the International Society for the Study of Women's Sexual Health (ISSWSH). Sue W. Goldstein, "History of the International Society for the Study of Women's Sexual Health," in *Women's Sexual Function and Dysfunction: Study, Diagnosis and Treatment*, ed. Irwin Goldstein et al. (London: Taylor & Francis, 2006), 11–18; Ronald Lewis and Gorm Wagner, "History of the International Society of Sexual Medicine (ISSM)—the Beginnings," *Journal of Sexual Medicine* 5 (2008): 740–45. On the history of sexual medicine as a medical subfield, see John Bancroft, "A History of Sexual Medicine in the United Kingdom," *Journal of Sexual Medicine* 2, no. 4 (2005): 569–74; Linda J. Rosen and Raymond C. Rosen, "Fifty Years of Female Sexual Dysfunction Research and Concepts: From Kinsey to the Present," in *Women's Sexual Function and Dysfunction: Study, Diagnosis and Treatment*, ed. Irwin Goldstein et al. (London: Taylor & Francis, 2006), 3–10; Alan Riley, "The Birth and Development of Sexual Medicine: Reflections of My Personal Journey," *Journal of Sexual Medicine* 4, no. 3 (2007): 815–19; Dirk Schultheiss and Sidney Glina, "Highlights from the History of Sexual Medicine," *Journal of Sexual Medicine* 7 (2010): 2031–43. For a critical take, see Leonore Tiefer, "Beneath the Veneer: The Troubled Past and Future of Sexual Medicine," *Journal of Sex & Marital Therapy* 33, no. 5 (2007): 473–77.

16.   "Aims and Scope," *Journal of Sexual Medicine*, https://www.jsm.jsexmed.org /content/aims?code=jsxm-site.

17.   On Viagra and related drugs ("sexuopharmaceuticals"), see Laura Mamo and Jennifer R. Fishman, "Potency in All the Right Places: Viagra as a Gendered Technology of the Body," *Body & Society* 7, no. 4 (2001): 13–35; Barbara L. Marshall and Stephen Katz, "Forever Functional: Sexual Fitness and the Ageing Male Body," *Body & Society* 8, no. 4 (2002): 43–70; Meika Loe, *The Rise of Viagra: How the Little Blue Pill Changed Sex in America* (New York: NYU Press, 2004); Annie Potts, "Deleuze on Viagra (or, What Can a 'Viagra-Body' Do?)," *Body & Society* 10, no. 1 (2004): 17–36; Barbara L. Marshall, "Sexual Medicine, Sexual Bodies and the 'Pharmaceutical Imagination,'" *Science as Culture* 18, no. 2 (2009): 133–49; Jennifer R. Fishman, "The Making of Viagra: The Biomedicalization of Sexual Dysfunction," in *Biomedicalization: Technoscience, Health, and Illness in the U.S.*, ed. Adele E. Clarke et al. (Durham, NC: Duke University Press, 2010), 289–306; Emily Wentzell, "How Did Erectile Dysfunction Become 'Natural'? A Review of the Critical Social Scientific Literature on Medical Treatment for Male Sexual Dysfunction," *Journal of Sex Research* 54 (2017): 486–506. On non-Western contexts of use, see Emily Wentzell, "Making Male Sexuality: Hybrid Medical Knowledge and Erectile Dysfunction in Mexico," in *Gender and the Science of Difference: Cultural Politics of Contemporary Science and Medicine*, ed. Jill A. Fisher (New Brunswick, NJ: Rutgers University Press, 2011), 224–38; Everett Zhang, *The Impotence Epidemic: Men's Medicine and Sexual Desire in Contemporary China* (Durham, NC: Duke University Press, 2015).

18.   From Joseph Guisti's field notes at the World Meeting on Sexual Medicine, Chicago, 26–30 August 2012, and a follow-up email conversation between Guisti and Sue Goldstein, also in 2012.

19.   Jane Cottingham, "Sexual and Reproductive: Connections and Disconnections in Public Health," in *Routledge Handbook of Sexuality, Health, and Rights*, ed. Peter Aggleton and Richard Parker (London: Routledge, 2010), 145–52.

20.   "Reproductive Health," Wikipedia, accessed 19 February 2021, http://en .wikipedia.org/wiki/Sexual_health.

21.   Laura Mamo, "Queering the Fertility Clinic," *Journal of Medical Humanities* 34 (2013): 227–39.

22.   Rosalind P. Petchesky, "Sexual Rights: Inventing a Concept, Mapping an International Practice," in *Framing the Sexual Subject: The Politics of Gender, Sexuality, and Power*, ed. Richard Parker, Regina Maria Barbosa, and Peter Aggleton (Berkeley: University of California Press, 2000), 81–103. On sexual rights, see also Alice M. Miller and Carole S. Vance, "Sexuality, Human Rights, and Health," *Health and Human Rights* 7, no. 2 (2004): 5–15; Richard Parker et al., "Global Transformations and Intimate Relations in the 21st Century: Social Science Research on Sexuality and the Emergence of

Sexual Health and *Sexual Rights* Frameworks," *Annual Review of Sex Research* 15 (2004): 362–98; Sonia Corrêa and Cymene Howe, "Global Perspectives on Sexual Rights," in *21st Century Sexualities: Contemporary Issues in Health, Education, and Rights*, ed. Gilbert Herdt and Cymene Howe (London: Routledge, 2007), 170–73; Sonia Corrêa, Rosalind Petchesky, and Richard Parker, *Sexuality, Health and Human Rights* (London: Routledge, 2008); Mario Pecheny, "Political Agents or Vulnerable Victims? Framing Sexual Rights as Sexual Health in Argentina," in *Routledge Handbook of Sexuality, Health, and Rights*, ed. Peter Aggleton and Richard Parker (London: Routledge, 2010), 359–69; Ilsa L. Lottes, "Sexual Rights: Meanings, Controversies, and Sexual Health Promotion," *Journal of Sex Research* 50, no. 3–4 (2013): 367–91; Eszter Kismödi, Jane Cottingham, Sofia Gruskin, and Alice M. Miller, "Advancing Sexual Health through Human Rights: The Role of the Law," *Global Public Health* 10, no. 2 (2015): 252–67; Alice M. Miller, Eszter Kismödi, Jane Cottingham, and Sofia Gruskin, "Sexual Rights as Human Rights: A Guide to Authoritative Sources and Principles for Applying Human Rights to Sexuality and Sexual Health," *Reproductive Health Matters* 23, no. 46 (2015): 16–30. Because sexual rights have often been tied to reproductive rights, this sexual health frame sometimes intersects in practice with the preceding one. In chapter 3, I discuss explicit attempts to join the two sets of concerns under the banner of "sexual and reproductive health and rights."

23. Lottes, "Sexual Rights"; Parker et al., "Global Transformations."
24. Parker et al., "Global Transformations," 367.
25. Shirin Heidari and Claudia García Moreno, "Gender-Based Violence: A Barrier to Sexual and Reproductive Health and Rights," *Reproductive Health Matters* 24 (2016): 1–4.
26. Didier Fassin and Estelle D'Halluin, "The Truth from the Body: Medical Certificates as Ultimate Evidence for Asylum Seekers," *American Anthropologist* 107, no. 4 (2005): 597–608; Miriam Ticktin, "The Gendered Human of Humanitarianism: Medicalising and Politicising Sexual Violence," *Gender & History* 23, no. 2 (2011): 250–65; Jaimie Morse, "Legal Mobilization in Medicine: Nurses, Rape Kits, and the Emergence of Forensic Nursing in the United States since the 1970s," *Social Science & Medicine* 222 (2019): 323–34.
27. Parker et al., "Global Transformations"; Laura M. Carpenter, "Sexual Health," in *Blackwell Encyclopedia of Sociology*, ed. George Ritzer (London: Blackwell, 2007), https://onlinelibrary.wiley.com/doi/abs/10.1002/9781405165518.wbeoss093; Richard G. Parker, "Sexuality, Health, and Human Rights," *American Journal of Public Health* 97, no. 6 (2007): 972–73; Lottes, "Sexual Rights." That this may be a widespread phenomenon is suggested by Pecheny's discussion of "framing sexual rights as sexual health in Argentina" and, more generally in the Latin American context, by his references to

the recent "widespread use of health discourse as a vehicle for the promotion of human rights." Pecheny, "Political Agents," 360.

28. Kristina Gupta, "'Screw Health': Representations of Sex as a Health-Promoting Activity in Medical and Popular Literature," *Journal of Medical Humanities* 32 (2011): 127–40, esp. 129. Such repackaging speaks to the culture wars that continue to swirl around sex education and that pit abstinence-only approaches against more sex-positive forms. On sex education, see Jeffrey P. Moran, *Teaching Sex: The Shaping of Adolescence in the 20th Century* (Cambridge, MA: Harvard University Press, 2000); Janice M. Irvine, *Talk about Sex: The Battles over Sex Education in the United States* (Berkeley: University of California Press, 2002); Kristin Luker, *When Sex Goes to School: Warring Views on Sex—and Sex Education—since the Sixties* (New York: W. W. Norton, 2006); Jessica Fields, *Risky Lessons: Sex Education and Social Inequality* (New Brunswick, NJ: Rutgers University Press, 2008); Nancy Kendall, *The Sex Education Debates* (Chicago: University of Chicago Press, 2013).

29. For example, as I discuss in chapter 10, in recent years the conservative Christian organization Focus on the Family has dubbed one of its employees a "sexual health analyst."

30. Lexie Pitzen, "Mosaic Sexual Health Clinic Aims to Be Alternative to Planned Parenthood," *Tallahassee Reports*, 19 February 2021, https://talla hasseereports.com/2021/02/19/mosaic-sexual-health-clinic-aims-to-be -alternative-to-planned-parenthood/.

31. See the discussion in chapter 5.

32. This statistic appeared on the organization's website, http://www.sash .net/, when I accessed it on 18 July 2013, but it is no longer found there.

33. See Janice M. Irvine, "Reinventing Perversion: Sex Addiction and Cultural Anxieties," *Journal of the History of Sexuality* 5, no. 3 (1995): 429–50.

34. For an example, see Bill Herring, "How the Society for the Advancement of Sexual Health Advances Sexual Health," *Sexual Addiction & Compulsivity* 21, no. 1 (2013): 39–41.

35. "Sexual Health," CVS Pharmacy, https://www.cvs.com/shop/sexual-health. The eVitamins page was labeled "Sexual Health" in 2017 but is now called "Intimate Products"; however, "sexual health" remains in the URL: "Intimate Products," eVitamins, http://www.evitamins.com/sexual-health.

36. Dennis Altman, "Globalization, Political Economy, and HIV/AIDS," *Theory and Society* 28, no. 4 (1999): 559–84; Parker et al., "Global Transformations," 365.

37. These differences in the conceptualizing of sexuality in different contexts are consistent with Stefan Vogler's finding that understandings of sexuality vary across organization settings according to the reigning "epistemic logics"—the "institutionalized ways of knowing that guide action in orga-

nizational settings and vary based on institutional, cultural, and political factors." Stefan Vogler, *Sorting Sexualities: Expertise and the Politics of Legal Classification* (Chicago: University of Chicago Press, 2021), 10.

38. On the ISSWSH, see Goldstein, "History of the ISSWSH." On the WAS, see World Association for Sexual Health, *Sexual Health for the Millennium: A Declaration and Technical Document* (Minneapolis: World Association for Sexual Health, 2008), https://worldsexualhealth.net/wp-content/up loads/2013/08/millennium-declaration-english.pdf, 146–47; Eli Coleman, "From Sexology to Sexual Health," in *Routledge Handbook of Sexuality, Health, and Rights*, ed. Peter Aggleton and Richard Parker (London: Routledge, 2010), 135–44. On the Society for the Advancement of Sexual Health, see "National Council on Sexual Addiction and Compulsivity," World Heritage Encyclopedia, http://self.gutenberg.org/articles/national _council_on_sexual_addiction_and_compulsivity. On the *International Journal of Sexual Health*, see "Publication History," International Journal of Sexual Health, https://www.tandfonline.com/loi/wijs20. In another instance of rebranding, noted in chapter 1, the American Social Health Association became the American Sexual Health Association in 2012.

39. "Health Department Announces Historic Expansion of HIV and STI Services at Sexual Health Clinics," NYC Health, https://www1.nyc.gov/site /doh/about/press/pr2017/pr003-17.page.

40. A version of this search conducted on an earlier date is depicted in Epstein and Mamo, "Proliferation," 184.

41. Michael R. Kauth, "Introduction to Special Issue on Veteran's Sexual Health and Functioning," *International Journal of Sexual Health* 24 (2012): 1–5; Christine M. Markham et al., "Behavioral and Psychosocial Effects of Two Middle School Sexual Health Education Programs at Tenth-Grade Follow-Up," *Journal of Adolescent Health* 54, no. 2 (2014): 151–59; Zhuoyan Li et al., "Sexual Health in Hematopoietic Stem Cell Transplant Recipients," *Cancer* (2015): 4124–31; Rowan Oliver, "Contraceptive and Sexual Health Care Issues in Women with Schizophrenia," *Journal of Family Planning and Reproductive Health Care* 39, no. 4 (2013): 289–91; Kurt C. Organista et al., "Sexual Health of Latino Migrant Day Labourers under Conditions of Structural Vulnerability," *Culture, Health & Sexuality* 15, no. 1 (2013): 58–72; Zhang Youchun et al., "Sexual Health Knowledge and Health Practices of Female Sex Workers in Liuzhou, China, Differ by Size of Venue," *AIDS and Behavior* 18, suppl. 2 (2014): 162–70; Lesław Rusiecki et al., "Sexual Health in Polish Elderly Men with Coronary Artery Disease: Importance, Expectations, and Reality," *Asian Journal of Andrology* 22, no. 5 (2020): 526–31; Erica Heiman, Sharon Haynes, and Michael McKee, "Sexual Health Behaviors of Deaf American Sign Language (ASL) Users," *Disability and Health Journal* 8 (2015): 579–85; Sinead N. Younge, Maya A. Corneille, Miriam Lyde, and Jessica Cannady,

"The Paradox of Risk: Historically Black College/University Students and Sexual Health," *Journal of American College Health* 61, no. 5 (2013): 254–62.

42. "National CLAS Standards," US Department of Health and Human Services, https://www.thinkculturalhealth.hhs.gov/clas; Steven Epstein, *Inclusion: The Politics of Difference in Medical Research* (Chicago: University of Chicago Press, 2007).

43. Home page of the Association of Black Sexologists and Clinicians, http://www.theabsc.com/; "About Us," Association of Black Sexologists and Clinicians, http://www.theabsc.com/about-us/.

44. Cindy Patton, *Sex and Germs: The Politics of AIDS* (Boston: South End Press, 1985); Dennis Altman, *AIDS in the Mind of America* (Garden City, NJ: Anchor Press, 1986).

45. Héctor Carrillo, *Pathways of Desire: The Sexual Migration of Mexican Gay Men* (Chicago: University of Chicago Press, 2017), 271.

46. Laura M. Carpenter and Monica J. Casper, "A Tale of Two Technologies: HPV Vaccination, Male Circumcision, and Sexual Health," *Gender & Society* 23, no. 6 (2009): 790–816, esp. 809; Sonja Mackenzie, *Structural Intimacies: Sexual Stories in the Black AIDS Epidemic* (New Brunswick, NJ: Rutgers University Press, 2013), 41–71.

47. I write at a moment when stylistic norms concerning capitalization of racial groups are in flux and the different options reflect diverging assessments of the political implications of capitalization. My practice in this book is to capitalize the names of all racial groups, including "White," generally for the reasons described in Kwame Anthony Appiah, "Time to Capitalize 'Black'—and 'White,'" *The Atlantic*, 18 June 2020, https://www.theatlantic.com/ideas/archive/2020/06/time-to-capitalize-blackand-white/613159/.

48. On the nondevelopment of andrology, see Rene Almeling, *GUYnecology: The Missing Science of How Men's Health Matters for Reproduction* (Berkeley: University of California Press, 2020). However, on the treatment of male infertility, see Liberty Walther Barnes, *Conceiving Masculinity: Male Infertility, Medicine, and Identity* (Philadelphia: Temple University Press, 2014).

49. Michelle Murphy, *Seizing the Means of Reproduction: Entanglements of Feminism, Health, and Technoscience* (Durham, NC: Duke University Press, 2012), 16–17; Alexandra Minna Stern, *Eugenic Nation: Faults and Frontiers of Better Breeding in Modern America* (Oakland: University of California Press, 2016), 4.

50. Chris A. Barcelos, *Distributing Condoms and Hope: The Racialized Politics of Youth Sexual Health* (Berkeley: University of California Press, 2020); Dorothy Roberts, *Killing the Black Body: Race, Reproduction, and the Meaning of Liberty*, 2nd ed. (New York: Vintage, 2017), xvi.

51. Jenny Dyck Brian, Patrick R. Grzanka, and Emily S. Mann, "The Age of LARC: Making Sexual Citizens on the Frontiers of Technoscientific Healthism," *Health Sociology Review* 29, no. 3 (2020), 312–28, esp. 316. Chris Barcelos

has analyzed how these tropes infuse youth sexual health promotion campaigns. Barcelos, *Distributing Condoms*, 53, 145.

52. Barcelos, *Distributing Condoms*.

53. This critique was presented at the session "Sexual Health and Persons with Disabilities," chaired by Samantha Crane, Leigh Ann Davis, and Beverly Franz at the National Sexual Health Conference, Chicago, 11 July 2019 (author's field notes). On disability, sexuality, and sexual health, see Robert McRuer, *Crip Theory: Cultural Signs of Queerness and Disability* (New York: NYU Press, 2006); Michael Gill, *Already Doing It: Intellectual Disability and Sexual Agency* (Minneapolis: University of Minnesota Press, 2015); Don Kulick, *Loneliness and Its Opposite: Sex, Disability, and the Ethics of Engagement* (Durham, NC: Duke University Press, 2015); Kyle Callen, "Disabled Sexualities: A Theoretical Review of Sociological Approaches and a Call to Problematize the Normative/Non-Normative Dialectic," *Sexualities*, advance online publication, 19 November 2020, https://doi.org/10.1177/1363460720973892.

54. My research assistant Aaron Benavidez obtained contact data for the authors of articles in the PubMed database, either through information published in PubMed or by examining articles. The trend over time is fairly consistent, except that gradually the quantity of North American authorship has caught up with that from Europe.

55. As Andreas Wimmer has proposed, an adequate theory of global diffusion must be "unapologetically nonreductionist," conceiving of the global networks of diffusion as "a polycentric structure with a diverse set of channels that proliferate like the roots of mushrooms, rather than a more monopolistic, starlike structure connecting a single center to its peripheries." Andreas Wimmer, "Domains of Diffusion: How Culture and Institutions Travel around the World and with What Consequences," *American Journal of Sociology* 126, no. 6 (2021): 1389–1438, esp. 1391, 1436. This point is consistent with the literature on sexuality and cultural globalization, which suggests the complex, back-and-forth relationship between "local" and "global" meanings, practices, and identities. For an overview, see Carrillo, *Pathways of Desire*.

56. To obtain data on web searches, I used the Google Trends tool (https://trends.google.com/trends/) on 30 April 2020. Google Trends graphs depict interest in a term by region over a specified time period, drawing from raw data taken from "an unbiased sample" of Google search data. Interest in a term is expressed as a fraction of the total number of searches conducted in that region during that time period. In other words, a higher rank indicates that searches for "sexual health" constituted a higher proportion of all searches in that region, not a higher absolute number of searches. See "FAQ about Google Trends Data," Google, https://support.google.com/trends/answer/4365533?hl=en&ref_topic=6248052. Like

other data visualization tools provided by Google, this one should be used with caution in light of the relatively sparse information provided by the company about how the algorithm operates.

57.   I believe that the explanation for why "sexual health" is especially salient as a Google search term in the United Kingdom is that attention to sexual health is well integrated into the formal operation of the National Health Service in addition to local, regional, and national government health agencies and advocacy groups. See chapter 9.

58.   Lucila Soriano Flores and Rinna Riesenfeld Robinson, *Formación inicial como promotoras/es en salud sexual bajo los principios de la declaración ministerial* (Initial training as sexual health promoters under the principles of the ministerial statement) (Mexico City: Federación Mexicana de Educación Sexual y Sexología, 2012).

59.   On moral panics in relation to sexuality, see Gayle S. Rubin, "Thinking Sex: Notes for a Radical Theory of the Politics of Sexuality," in *Pleasure and Danger: Exploring Female Sexuality*, ed. Carole S. Vance (New York: Routledge, 1984), 267–318; Gilbert H. Herdt, ed. *Moral Panics, Sex Panics: Fear and the Fight over Sexual Rights* (New York: NYU Press, 2009); Roger N. Lancaster, *Sex Panic and the Punitive State* (Berkeley: University of California Press, 2011).

60.   However, there are also contrary cases in which individuals and groups use the language of sexual health as a strategy of *repoliticization*: they draw on the connection to science and expertise in order to make new political claims about sexual matters. I develop this argument in chapter 10.

61.   Carpenter, "Sexual Health." See also Jamie O'Quinn and Jessica Fields, "The Future of Evidence: Queerness in Progressive Visions of Sexuality Education," *Sexuality Research & Social Policy* 17 (2020): 175–87.

62.   "Erobotics, a Solution for the Sexual Health and Well-Being of Astronauts," Yahoo News, n.d., https://news.yahoo.com/erobotics-solution-sexual -health-well-being-astronauts-105022166.html.

63.   Parker et al., "Global Transformations"; Allan M. Brandt, "How AIDS Invented Global Health," *New England Journal of Medicine* 368 (2013): 2149–52; Andrew Lakoff, *Unprepared: Global Health in a Time of Emergency* (Oakland: University of California Press, 2017), 5, 76. Previous commentators on the rise of sexual health have all made reference to the important place of the HIV/AIDS epidemic. See Alain Giami, "Sexual Health: The Emergence, Development, and Diversity of a Concept," *Annual Review of Sex Research* 13 (2002): 1–35, esp. 2; Weston M. Edwards and Eli Coleman, "Defining Sexual Health: A Descriptive Overview," *Archives of Sexual Behavior* 33, no. 3 (2004): 189–95, esp. 189; Parker et al., "Global Transformations," 365; Carpenter, "Sexual Health"; Coleman, "From Sexology," 138. On some of the international dimensions of the role of the HIV/AIDS epidemic in tethering sexual and health discourses, see also Stacy Leigh Pigg, "Expecting the

Epidemic: A Social History of the Representation of Sexual Risk in Nepal,"
Feminist Media Studies 2, no. 1 (2002): 97–125, esp. 113.

64. Altman, *AIDS in the Mind of America*; Cindy Patton, *Inventing AIDS* (New
York: Routledge, 1990); Steven Epstein, *Impure Science: AIDS, Activism, and
the Politics of Knowledge* (Berkeley: University of California Press, 1996);
Jennifer Brier, *Infectious Ideas: U.S. Political Responses to the AIDS Crisis*
(Chapel Hill: University of North Carolina Press, 2009).

65. Rosalind Petchesky, Sonia Corrêa, and Richard Parker, "Reaffirming Pleasures in a World of Dangers," in *Routledge Handbook of Sexuality, Health, and
Rights*, ed. Peter Aggleton and Richard Parker (London: Routledge, 2010),
401–11, esp. 403.

66. Dagmar Herzog, *Sexuality in Europe: A Twentieth-Century History* (Cambridge:
Cambridge University Press, 2011), 182.

67. Patton, *Sex and Germs*; Altman, *AIDS in the Mind of America*.

68. Peter Lewis Allen, *The Wages of Sin: Sex and Disease, Past and Present* (Chicago: University of Chicago Press, 2000), 135.

69. Ibid., 137.

70. Robert D. McFadden, "Judge Overturns U.S. Rule Blocking 'Offensive' Educational Material on AIDS," *New York Times*, 12 May 1992, B3; Allen, *The
Wages of Sin*, 138.

71. Steven Epstein, "The New Attack on Sexuality Research: Morality and the
Politics of Knowledge Production," *Sexuality Research and Social Policy* 3,
no. 1 (2006): 1–12, esp. 1.

72. Ashley Currier and Tara McKay, "Pursuing Social Justice through Public
Health: Gender and Sexual Diversity Activism in Malawi," *Critical African
Studies* 9, no. 1 (2017): 71–90, esp. 76, 86.

73. Sandfort and Ehrhardt, "Sexual Health," 182.

74. Cottingham, "Sexual and Reproductive." On the ICPD, see also Saul E. Hal-
fon, *The Cairo Consensus: Demographic Surveys, Women's Empowerment, and
Regime Change in Population Policy* (Lanham, MD: Lexington Books, 2007).

75. Cottingham, "Sexual and Reproductive," 145.

76. Parker et al., "Global Transformations," 368. See also Petchesky, "Sexual
Rights."

77. *Report of the International Conference on Population and Development: Cairo,
5–13 September 1994* (A/CONF.171/13) (New York: United Nations, 18 October
1995), 40, https://www.un.org/development/desa/pd/sites/www.un.org
.development.desa.pd/files/icpd_en.pdf. Overall, the report makes use of a
number of wordings, including "sexual health," "sexual and reproductive health,"
"reproductive and sexual health," and "family planning and sexual health."

78. Cottingham, "Sexual and Reproductive," 150 (emphasis in the original).

79. On "the inseparability of 'viral' discourses in the 1990s," see Cait Mc-
Kinney and Dylan Mulvin, "Bugs: Rethinking the History of Computing,"
Communication, Culture and Critique 12 (2019): 476–98.

80.   See Mark Davis, "After the Clinic? Researching Sexual Health Technology in Context," *Culture, Health & Sexuality* 17, no. 4 (2015): 398–411; Gary W. Dowsett, "'And Next, Just for Your Enjoyment!': Sex, Technology and the Constitution of Desire," *Culture, Health & Sexuality* 17, no. 4 (2015): 527–39; Deborah Lupton, "Quantified Sex: A Critical Analysis of Sexual and Reproductive Self-Tracking Using Apps," *Culture, Health & Sexuality* 17, no. 4 (2015): 440–53; Renee Marie Shelby, "Techno-Physical Feminism: Anti-Rape Technology, Gender, and Corporeal Surveillance," *Feminist Media Studies* 20, no. 8 (2020): 1088–1109.

81.   Peter Conrad, *The Medicalization of Society* (Baltimore: Johns Hopkins University Press, 2007).

82.   See *supra* note 17.

83.   Adele E. Clarke et al., "Biomedicalization: Technoscientific Transformations of Health, Illness, and U.S. Biomedicine," *American Sociological Review* 68, no. 2 (2003): 161–94. On risk and medicine, see also David Armstrong, "The Rise of Surveillance Medicine," *Sociology of Health & Illness* 17, no. 3 (1995): 393–404; Alan Petersen, "Risk, Governance and the New Public Health," in *Foucault, Health and Medicine*, ed. Robin Bunton and Alan R. Petersen (Florence, KY: Routledge, 1997), 189–206; Nikolas Rose, *The Politics of Life Itself: Biomedicine, Power, and Subjectivity in the Twenty-First Century* (Princeton, NJ: Princeton University Press, 2006); Robert Aronowitz, *Risky Medicine: Our Quest to Cure Fear and Uncertainty* (Chicago: University of Chicago Press, 2015).

84.   Laura Mamo, Amber Nelson, and Aleia Clark, "Producing and Protecting Risky Girlhoods," in *Three Shots at Prevention: The HPV Vaccine and the Politics of Medicine's Simple Solutions*, ed. Keith Wailoo et al. (Baltimore: Johns Hopkins University Press, 2010), 121–45; Robert Aronowitz, "Gardasil: A Vaccine against Cancer and a Drug to Reduce Risk," in *Three Shots at Prevention: The HPV Vaccine and the Politics of Medicine's Simple Solutions*, ed. Keith Wailoo et al. (Baltimore: Johns Hopkins University Press, 2010), 21–38.

85.   Steven Epstein and Stefan Timmermans, "From Medicine to Health: The Proliferation and Diversification of Cultural Authority," *Journal of Health and Social Behavior* 62, no. 3 (2021): 240–54.

86.   Anna Kirkland, "What Is Wellness Now?," *Journal of Health Politics, Policy & Law* 39, no. 5 (2014): 957–70; Justin Lee, "Investigating the Hybridity of 'Wellness' Practices," e-Scholarship, UCLA Department of Sociology, Theory and Research in Comparative Social Analysis, 2005, https://escholarship.org/uc/item/88c4t567.

87.   Expanding on Paul Starr's discussion of the cultural authority of medicine, our characterization of "cultural authority" in the health domain refers to what Starr called "the probability that particular definitions of reality and judgments of meaning and value will prevail as valid and

true"—or more specifically, the ability to interpret symptoms, diagnose, and prognosticate, and define the parameters of health, disease, treatment, and wellness. Paul Starr, *The Social Transformation of American Medicine* (New York: Basic Books, 1982), 13; Epstein and Timmermans, "From Medicine to Health."

88. I return to this theme in chapter 7, where I discuss the diverse character of sexual health expertise, and in chapter 8, where I examine manifestations of the present-day injunction to live a sexually healthy lifestyle.

89. See the discussion in the introduction.

90. Steven Epstein and Laura Mamo, "Toward Buzzword Studies: Sexual Health and the Power of Buzz" (paper presented at the ESOCITE/4S Conference, Buenos Aires, Argentina, 22 August 2014).

91. For some examples, see Rogers Brubaker, "The 'Diaspora' Diaspora," *Ethnic and Racial Studies* 28, no. 1 (2005): 1–19; Peer C. Fiss and Paul M. Hirsch, "The Discourse of Globalization: Framing and Sensemaking of an Emerging Concept," *American Sociological Review* 70, no. 1 (2005): 29–52; Leslie McCall, "The Complexity of Intersectionality," *Signs* 30, no. 3 (2005): 1771–1800; Gilbert Rist, "Development as Buzzword," *Development in Practice* 17, nos. 4–5 (2007): 485–91; Ian Scoones, "Sustainability," *Development in Practice* 17, nos. 4–5 (2007): 589–96; Kathy Davis, "Intersectionality as Buzzword: A Sociology of Science Perspective on What Makes a Feminist Theory Successful," *Feminist Theory* 9, no. 1 (2008): 67–85; Jerry A. Jacobs and Scott Frickel, "Interdisciplinarity: A Critical Assessment," *Annual Review of Sociology* 35 (2009): 43–65; Kevin Grove, *Resilience* (London: Routledge, 2018); Michael Penkler, Kay Felder, and Ulrike Felt, "Challenging Diversity: Steering Effects of Buzzwords in Projectified Health Care," *Science, Technology & Human Values* 45, no. 1 (2020): 138–63. Although not all authors of these articles have characterized their object as a buzzword, all of them have pointed to buzzword-like qualities that are, in at least some respects, reminiscent of sexual health. For example, Rogers Brubaker, writing about "diaspora," has observed: "As the term has proliferated, its meaning has been stretched to accommodate the various intellectual, cultural and political agendas in the service of which it has been enlisted. This has resulted in what one might call a "'diaspora' diaspora'—a dispersion of the meanings of the term in semantic, conceptual, and disciplinary space." Brubaker, "'Diaspora' Diaspora," 1.

92. On the sensorial and social dimensions of "buzz," see Lisa Jean Moore and Mary Kosut, *Buzz: Urban Beekeeping and the Power of the Bee* (New York: NYU Press, 2013).

93. While I do not develop the point further, I thank Trevor Pinch for suggesting that buzzwords might profitably be investigated from the standpoint of their sonic properties.

94.   Appeared at https://goodvibesblog.com/ (accessed 9 November 2014; no longer accessible). The buzzing nature of sex toys is also suggested in the title of Hallie Lieberman, *Buzz* (New York: Pegasus, 2017).

95.   On keywords, see Raymond Williams, *Keywords* (New York: Oxford University Press, 1983). On brands, see Celia Lury, *Brands: The Logos of the Global Economy* (London: Routledge, 2004). On sticky ideas, see Chip Heath and Dan Heath, *Made to Stick: Why Some Ideas Survive and Others Die* (New York: Random House, 2007). I am grateful to my research assistant Alka Menon for researching these associated terms.

96.   I am grateful to Ulrike Felt for suggesting this point. On the "mediatization" of discourse, see Maarten A. Hajer, *Authoritative Governance: Policy-Making in the Age of Mediatization* (Oxford: Oxford University Press, 2009).

97.   Adam M. Hedgecoe, "Terminology and the Construction of Scientific Disciplines: The Case of Pharmacogenomics," *Science, Technology & Human Values* 28, no. 4 (2003): 513–37. On hype and expectations and their relation to the advance of science and technology, see Jon Guice, "Designing the Future: The Culture of New Trends in Science and Technology," *Research Policy* 28, no. 1 (1999): 81–98; Mads Borup, Nik Brown, Kornelia Konrad, and Harro Van Lente, "The Sociology of Expectations in Science and Technology," *Technology Analysis & Strategic Management* 18, nos. 3–4 (2006): 285–98.

98.   Bernadette Bensaude Vincent, "The Politics of Buzzwords at the Interface of Technoscience, Market and Society: The Case of 'Public Engagement in Science,'" *Public Understanding of Science* 23, no. 3 (2014): 238–53, esp. 238–39.

99.   "Buzzword," Merriam-Webster Dictionary, https://www.merriam-webster .com/dictionary/buzzword.

100.   Renée Dye, "The Buzz on Buzz," *Harvard Business Review*, November– December 2000, 139–46, esp. 140.

101.   Bensaude Vincent, "Politics of Buzzwords," 239, 245. Bensaude Vincent is one of the few scholars who have sought to analyze the buzzword phenomenon in general (and not just a specific buzzword). Others include Andrea Cornwall and Karen Brock, "What Do Buzzwords Do for Development Policy? A Critical Look at 'Participation,' 'Empowerment' and 'Poverty Reduction,'" *Third World Quarterly* 26, no. 7 (2005): 1043–60; Andrea Cornwall, "Buzzwords and Fuzzwords: Deconstructing Development Discourse," *Development in Practice* 17, nos. 4–5 (2007): 471–84; Yair Neuman, Ophir Nave, and Eran Dolev, "Buzzwords on Their Way to a Tipping-Point: A View from the Blogosphere," *Complexity* 16, no. 4 (2010): 58–68.

102.   Lars Grönvik, "The Fuzzy Buzz Word: Conceptualisations of Disability in Disability Research Classics," *Sociology of Health & Illness* 29, no. 5 (2007): 750–66.

103. Davis, "Intersectionality as Buzzword," 69. Davis invokes the earlier work of Murray S. Davis, who, she says, argued that "successful theories thrive on ambiguity and incompleteness."

104. While those who are suspicious of the malleability of buzzwords might deem them "empty signifiers" in the theorist Ernesto Laclau's terms—as "a signifier without a signified"—they might better be considered what Laclau called "equivocal signifiers," or those signifiers that are ambiguous or floating and take on meaning according to context. Ernesto Laclau, *Emancipation(s)* (London: Verso, 1996), 36.

105. Much academic work has examined the generative character of ambiguity (or of polysemy, multivocality, or "productive instability"). See Wendy Griswold, "The Fabrication of Meaning: Literary Interpretation in the United States, Great Britain, and the West Indies," *American Journal of Sociology* 92, no. 5 (1987): 1077–1117; Ann Mische, "Cross-Talk in Movements: Reconceiving the Culture-Network Link," in *Social Movements and Networks: Relational Approaches to Collective Action*, ed. Mario Diani and Doug McAdam (Oxford: Oxford University Press, 2003), 258–80; Francesca Polletta, *It Was Like a Fever: Storytelling in Protest and Politics* (Chicago: University of Chicago Press, 2006), 172; Iddo Tavory and Ann Swidler, "Condom Semiotics: Meaning and Condom Use in Rural Malawi," *American Sociological Review* 74 (2009): 171–89; James Mahoney and Kathleen Ann Thelen, *Explaining Institutional Change: Ambiguity, Agency, and Power* (Cambridge: Cambridge University Press, 2010), xi; David Lewis and Mark Schuller, "Engagements with a Productively Unstable Category: Anthropologists and Nongovernmental Organizations," *Current Anthropology* 58, no. 5 (2017): 634–51. On the utility of ambiguity in scientific knowledge-making in particular, see Aaron Panofsky and Catherine Bliss, "Ambiguity and Scientific Authority: Population Classification in Genomic Science," *American Sociological Review* 82, no. 1 (2017): 59–87.

106. Tarleton Gillespie, "The Politics of 'Platforms,'" *New Media & Society* 12, no. 3 (2010): 347–64, esp. 349.

107. Jeremy A. Greene, "Making Medicines Essential: The Emergent Centrality of Pharmaceuticals in Global Health," *BioSocieties* 6 (2011): 10–33, esp. 28. A number of scholars have proposed alternative labels (other than "buzzword," that is) to characterize those terms that successfully thrive on ambiguity. These include Bonnie Urciuoli's "strategically deployable shifters," Jan Surman and coauthors' "nomadic concepts," and what Jane Jenson, drawing on the work of Paul Bernard, calls the "quasi-concepts" used in policy making. Bonnie Urciuoli, "Neoliberal Education: Preparing the Student for the New Workplace," in *Ethnographies of Neoliberalism*, ed. Carol Greenhouse (Philadelphia: University of Pennsylvania Press, 2011), 162–76; Jan Surman, Katalin Stráner, and Peter Haslinger, "Nomadic Concepts

in the History of Biology," *Studies in History and Philosophy of Biological and Biomedical Sciences* 48 (2014): 127–29; Jane Jenson, "Modernising the European Social Paradigm: Social Investments and Social Entrepreneurs," *Journal of Social Policy* 46 (2016): 31–47, esp. 33–34.

108.   Ilana Löwy, "The Strength of Loose Concepts—Boundary Concepts, Federative Experimental Strategies and Disciplinary Growth: The Case of Immunology," *History of Science* 30, no. 4 (1992): 371–96. Somewhat similarly, the historian of science Peter Galison has described forms of communication—"pidgins" and "creoles"—associated with the so-called trading zones that link scientific specialty areas. Peter Galison, "Trading Zone: Coordinating Action and Belief," in *The Science Studies Reader*, ed. Mario Biagioli (New York: Routledge, 1999), 137–60.

109.   Susan Leigh Star and James R. Griesemer, "Institutional Ecology, 'Translations' and Boundary Objects: Amateurs and Professionals in Berkeley's Museum of Vertebrate Zoology, 1907–39," *Social Studies of Science* 19, no. 3 (1989): 387–420, esp. 393.

110.   Bensaude Vincent also suggested this similarity. Bensaude Vincent, "Politics of Buzzwords," 246.

111.   For example, Peer Fiss and Paul Hirsch, in their analysis of "globalization," hypothesized "that the more heterogeneous the communities that employ 'globalization' as an explanation, the more we should observe contention in framing by the actors in these fields." Fiss and Hirsch, "Discourse of Globalization," 34. On symbolic power and symbolic violence, see Pierre Bourdieu, "Symbolic Power," *Critique of Anthropology* 4 (Summer 1979): 77–85.

112.   W. B. Gallie, "Essentially Contested Concepts," *Proceedings of the Aristotelian Society* 56 (1955–56): 167–98, esp. 169.

113.   On bandwagons, see Joan H. Fujimura, "The Molecular Biological Bandwagon in Cancer Research: Where Social Worlds Meet," *Social Problems* 35, no. 3 (1988): 261–83. On the steering functions of buzzwords, see Penkler et al., "Challenging Diversity."

114.   Penkler et al., "Challenging Diversity."

115.   Susan Leigh Star raised somewhat similar questions about the "growth and death of boundary objects." Susan Leigh Star, "This Is Not a Boundary Object: Reflections on the Origin of a Concept," *Science, Technology & Human Values* 35, no. 5 (2010): 601–17, esp. 613–14.

CHAPTER THREE

1.   A sign posted at registration for the Congress attributed the characterization of attendees as being either "Prescribers" or "Non-prescribers" to the Brazilian Health Surveillance Agency's Regulation 96/08, which governs the advertising and promotion of medications. The comments that follow

are drawn from my field notes from the Twenty-First Congress of the World Association for Sexual Health ("Sexual Issues Straight from the Heart"), Porto Alegre, Brazil, 21–24 September 2013.

2. Eli Coleman, "From Sexology to Sexual Health," in *Routledge Handbook of Sexuality, Health, and Rights*, ed. Peter Aggleton and Richard Parker (London: Routledge, 2010), 135–44, esp. 141.

3. A slide shown at the WAS Congress in 2013 cited this quote as Eusebio Rubio-Aurioles (2005), "The WAS changes its name to World Association for Sexual Health." I have been unable to locate the original source.

4. Eli Coleman, interviewed by author, 11 July 2019.

5. To be sure, such successes can be attributed not only to organizational work but also to the efforts of energetic and well-connected leaders, such as Coleman, who have helped to promote a unified vision of sexual health.

6. "History of World Sexual Health Day," World Association for Sexual Health, https://worldsexualhealth.net/organization/world-sexual-health-day/.

7. World Association for Sexual Health, *Sexual Health for the Millennium: A Declaration and Technical Document* (Minneapolis: World Association for Sexual Health, 2008), https://worldsexualhealth.net/wp-content/up loads/2013/08/millennium-declaration-english.pdf, 2–8, 18.

8. See the discussion in chapter 1.

9. Home page, World Association for Sexual Health, http://www.worldsexol ogy.org; "Declaration of Sexual Rights," World Association for Sexual Health, last modified March 2014, https://worldsexualhealth.net/wp-content /uploads/2013/08/Declaration-of-Sexual-Rights-2014-plain-text.pdf.

10. World Health Organization, *The Work of WHO 1975: Annual Report of the Director-General to the World Health Assembly and the United Nations* (Geneva: World Health Organization, 1976), 43. In addition, the global burden of STIs is discussed at p. 70.

11. Susan Leigh Star and James R. Griesemer, "Institutional Ecology, 'Translations' and Boundary Objects: Amateurs and Professionals in Berkeley's Museum of Vertebrate Zoology, 1907–39," *Social Studies of Science* 19, no. 3 (1989): 387–420.

12. Nitsan Chorev, *The World Health Organization between North and South* (Ithaca, NY: Cornell University Press, 2012), 13.

13. WHO Regional Office for Europe, *Concepts of Sexual Health: Report on a Working Group* (Copenhagen: World Health Organization, 1987), 2–3. See also Alain Giami, "Sexual Health: The Emergence, Development, and Diversity of a Concept," *Annual Review of Sex Research* 13 (2002): 1–35, esp. 14–16; Weston M. Edwards and Eli Coleman, "Defining Sexual Health: A Descriptive Overview," *Archives of Sexual Behavior* 33, no. 3 (2004): 189–95, esp. 191–92.

14. Coleman, "From Sexology," 137. Coleman's response is to argue that, by the same reasoning, one would be forced to abandon any attempt to define "health" altogether. Coleman, interview.

15. WHO Regional Office for Europe, *Concepts of Sexual Health*, 1, 4–5. See also
     the discussion in Giami, "Sexual Health," 14–15; and in Edwards and Cole-
     man, "Defining Sexual Health," 191. On symbolic power and symbolic vio-
     lence, see Pierre Bourdieu, "Symbolic Power," *Critique of Anthropology* 4
     (Summer 1979): 77–85.

16. WHO Regional Office for Europe, *Concepts of Sexual Health*, 18.

17. Ibid., 4.

18. On cultural authority in health and medicine, see Paul Starr, *The Social
     Transformation of American Medicine* (New York: Basic Books, 1982), 13–15;
     Steven Epstein and Stefan Timmermans, "From Medicine to Health: The
     Proliferation and Diversification of Cultural Authority," *Journal of Health
     and Social Behavior* 62, no. 3 (2021): 240–54.

19. Ken Plummer, "The Social Reality of Sexual Rights," in *Routledge Handbook
     of Sexuality, Health, and Rights*, ed. Peter Aggleton and Richard Parker (Lon-
     don: Routledge, 2010), 45–55, esp. 47–48.

20. See Dennis Altman, "AIDS and the Globalization of Sexuality," *Social Iden-
     tities* 14, no. 2 (2008): 145–60; Sonia Corrêa, Rosalind Petchesky, and Rich-
     ard Parker, *Sexuality, Health and Human Rights* (London: Routledge, 2008).
     On sexual rights, see also chapter 2, note 22.

21. Nancy F. Cott, *The Grounding of Modern Feminism* (New Haven, CT: Yale Uni-
     versity Press, 1987), 42.

22. Carmen Barroso, "From Reproductive to Sexual Rights," in *Routledge Hand-
     book of Sexuality, Health, and Rights*, ed. Peter Aggleton and Richard Parker
     (London: Routledge, 2010), 379–88, esp. 382. On the crucial place of sexu-
     ality within the ideological concerns of US radical feminists of the 1970s,
     see also Alice Echols, *Daring to Be Bad: Radical Feminism in America, 1967–
     1975* (Minneapolis: University of Minnesota Press, 1989).

23. Barry D. Adam, Jan Willem Duyvendak, and André Krouwel, *The Global
     Emergence of Gay and Lesbian Politics: National Imprints of a Worldwide Move-
     ment* (Philadelphia: Temple University Press, 1999); Dennis Altman, *Global
     Sex* (Chicago: University of Chicago Press, 2001).

24. Altman, "AIDS and Globalization"; Richard Parker, "Critical Intersections
     and Engagements: Gender, Sexuality, Health, and Rights in Medical An-
     thropology," in *Medical Anthropology at the Intersections: Histories, Activisms,
     and Futures*, ed. Marcia C. Inhorn and Emily A. Wentzell (Durham, NC:
     Duke University Press, 2012), 206–37.

25. Dennis Altman, *AIDS in the Mind of America* (Garden City, NJ: Anchor Press,
     1986); Cindy Patton, *Inventing AIDS* (New York: Routledge, 1990); Steven
     Epstein, *Impure Science: AIDS, Activism, and the Politics of Knowledge* (Berke-
     ley: University of California Press, 1996); Jennifer Brier, *Infectious Ideas:
     U.S. Political Responses to the AIDS Crisis* (Chapel Hill: University of North
     Carolina Press, 2009).

26. On AIDS activism, see the preceding note. See also Cathy J. Cohen, *The Boundaries of Blackness: AIDS and the Breakdown of Black Politics* (Chicago: University of Chicago Press, 1999); Paula A. Treichler, *How to Have Theory in an Epidemic: Cultural Chronicles of AIDS* (Durham, NC: Duke University Press, 1999); Deborah B. Gould, *Moving Politics: Emotion and ACT UP's Fight against AIDS* (Chicago: University of Chicago Press, 2009); Celeste Watkins-Hayes, *Remaking a Life: How Women Living with HIV/AIDS Confront Inequality* (Berkeley: University of California Press, 2019); Christophe Broqua, *Action = Vie: A History of AIDS Activism and Gay Politics in France* (Philadelphia: Temple University Press, 2020).

27. Richard Parker et al., "Global Transformations and Intimate Relations in the 21st Century: Social Science Research on Sexuality and the Emergence of *Sexual Health* and *Sexual Rights* Frameworks," *Annual Review of Sex Research* 15 (2004): 362–98, esp. 367.

28. Altman, "AIDS and Globalization," 156.

29. Corrêa et al., *Sexuality, Health*, 173. See also Altman, "AIDS and Globalization," 155–58. For examples of various declarations and itemizations of sexual rights that have been put forward by different organizations, see the appendixes to Ilsa L. Lottes, "Sexual Rights: Meanings, Controversies, and Sexual Health Promotion," *Journal of Sex Research* 50, nos. 3–4 (2013): 367–91.

30. Lottes, "Sexual Rights," 367.

31. Alice M. Miller, "Sexual but Not Reproductive: Exploring the Junction and Disjunction of Sexual and Reproductive Rights," *Health and Human Rights* 4, no. 2 (2000): 68–109, esp. 77–78.

32. Ilsa Lottes, "New Perspectives on Sexual Health," in *New Views on Sexual Health: The Case of Finland*, ed. Ilsa Lottes and Osmo Kontula (Helsinki: Population Research Institute, Family Federation of Finland, 2000), 7–28, esp. 7; Rosalind P. Petchesky, "Sexual Rights: Inventing a Concept, Mapping an International Practice," in *Framing the Sexual Subject: The Politics of Gender, Sexuality, and Power*, ed. Richard Parker, Regina Maria Barbosa, and Peter Aggleton (Berkeley: University of California Press, 2000), 81–103; Parker et al., "Global Transformations."

33. Sonia Corrêa, "From Reproductive Health to Sexual Rights: Achievements and Future Challenges," *Reproductive Health Matters* 10 (1997): 107–16; Lottes, "Sexual Rights," 372.

34. At the same time, the Platform for Action's language put forward what Corrêa, Petchesky, and Parker have called "a mixed and ambiguous message, as important for its silences as for its newly crafted statement of women's sexual rights." Corrêa et al., *Sexuality, Health*, 170. See also Corrêa, "From Reproductive Health"; Barroso, "From Reproductive," 381–82.

35. Alice M. Miller, Eszter Kismödi, Jane Cottingham, and Sofia Gruskin, "Sexual Rights as Human Rights: A Guide to Authoritative Sources and

Principles for Applying Human Rights to Sexuality and Sexual Health," *Reproductive Health Matters* 23, no. 46 (2015): 16–30.

36. Corrêa et al., *Sexuality, Health*, 164.
37. Alice M. Miller and Carole S. Vance, "Sexuality, Human Rights, and Health," *Health and Human Rights* 7, no. 2 (2004): 5–15; Sonia Corrêa and Cymene Howe, "Global Perspectives on Sexual Rights," in *21st Century Sexualities: Contemporary Issues in Health, Education, and Rights*, ed. Gilbert Herdt and Cymene Howe (London: Routledge, 2007), 170–73; Eszter Kismödi, Jane Cottingham, Sofia Gruskin, and Alice M. Miller, "Advancing Sexual Health through Human Rights: The Role of the Law," *Global Public Health* 10, no. 2 (2015): 252–67.
38. Alicia Ely Yamin and Vanessa M. Boulanger, "Why Global Goals and Indicators Matter: The Experience of Sexual and Reproductive Health and Rights in the Millenium Development Goals," *Journal of Human Development and Capabilities* 15, no. 2–3 (2014): 218–31, esp. 221.
39. World Health Organization, *Sexual Health, Human Rights and the Law* (Geneva: World Health Organization, June 2015), http://www.who.int/reproductive health/publications/sexual_health/sexual-health-human-rights-law/en/.
40. Pan American Health Organization (PAHO) and World Health Organization, *Promotion of Sexual Health: Recommendations for Action* (Report of Meeting Held May 19–22) (Antigua, Guatemala: Pan American Health Organization and World Health Organization, 2000).
41. Giami, "Sexual Health," 16.
42. PAHO and WHO, *Promotion of Sexual Health*, 2–3.
43. Ibid., 5.
44. Ibid., 1–2.
45. Ibid., 6.
46. Ibid. (emphasis in the original).
47. World Health Organization, *Education and Treatment in Human Sexuality: The Training of Health Professionals, Report of a WHO Meeting [Held in Geneva from 6 to 12 February 1974]*, Technical Report Series No. 572 (Geneva: World Health Organization, 1975), 6, http://www.who.int/iris/handle/10665 /38247. See chapter 1 for discussion.
48. PAHO and WHO, *Promotion of Sexual Health*, 11, 38; WAS, "Declaration of Sexual Rights."
49. PAHO and WHO, *Promotion of Sexual Health*, 34.
50. Ibid., 10.
51. Ibid. The example provided by the working group was that of female genital mutilation.
52. Ibid., 13.
53. For discussion and analysis relevant to these debates, see Diane Richardson, *Sexuality and Citizenship* (Cambridge, England: Polity Press, 2018), 49–72.

54. Chandan Reddy, "Asian Diasporas, Neoliberalism, and Family: Reviewing the Case for Homosexual Asylum in the Context of Family Rights," *Social Text* 23, no. 3–4 (2005): 101–19; Eric Fassin, "National Identities and Transnational Intimacies: Sexual Democracy and the Politics of Immigration in Europe," *Public Culture* 22, no. 3 (2010): 507–29; Ghassan Moussawi, "Queer Exceptionalism and Exclusion: Cosmopolitanism and Inequalities in 'Gay-Friendly' Beirut," *Sociological Review* 66, no. 1 (2018): 174–90; Stephen D. Seely, "Queer Theory from the South: A Contribution to the Critique of Sexual Democracy," *Sexualities* 23, no. 7 (2020): 1228–47.

55. Seely, "Queer Theory from the South," 1229.

56. Fassin, "National Identities."

57. Moussawi, "Queer Exceptionalism," 9.

58. Corrêa, "From Reproductive Health," 109–10.

59. "The Yogyakarta Principles: Principles on the Application of International Human Rights Law in Relation to Sexual Orientation and Gender Identity" (Yogyakarta, Indonesia, March 2007), 6, http://yogyakartaprinciples .org/principles-en/official-versions-pdf/; Carsten Balzer and Carla Lagata, "Human Rights," *TSQ: Transgender Studies Quarterly* 1, no. 1–2 (2014): 99– 103. The Yogyakarta Principles are not without their critics, however, and Matthew Waites has argued that they "privilege a binary model of gender, and sexual behaviours, identities and desires that are defined exclusively in relation to a single gender within this binary." Matthew Waites, "Critique of 'Sexual Orientation' and 'Gender Identity' in Human Rights Discourse: Global Queer Politics beyond the Yogyakarta Principles," *Contemporary Politics* 15, no. 1 (2009): 137–56, esp. 138. I thank Alyssa Lynne for discussion of the Yogyakarta Principles, to which I return in chapter 5 in my analysis of human rights and the ICD.

60. On "articulations," see Ernesto Laclau and Chantal Mouffe, *Hegemony and Socialist Strategy: Towards a Radical Democratic Politics* (London: Verso, 1985), 112–13.

61. Richard G. Parker, "Sexuality, Health, and Human Rights," *American Journal of Public Health* 97, no. 6 (2007): 972–73; Petchesky, "Sexual Rights," 91.

62. "Sexual Health and Rights," American Jewish World Service, https://ajws .org/what-we-do/sexual-health-and-rights/.

63. "Sexual Rights," Family Watch International, https://familywatch.org /resources/family-policy-resource-center/#PRC-sexual-rights.

64. World Health Organization, *Defining Sexual Health: Report of a Technical Consultation on Sexual Health, 28–31 January 2002, Geneva* (Geneva: World Health Organization, 2006).

65. Ibid., 2.

66. Ibid., 5.

67. Ibid.

68. On the involvement of the WAS here, see Edwards and Coleman, "Defining Sexual Health," 193–94. According to Coleman, it was squeamishness about associating itself publicly with "rights" as much as with "sexuality" that led to the WHO's long delay in publishing the report from the conference. Coleman, interview.

69. WHO, *Defining Sexual Health*, ch. 3.

70. Theo Sandfort and Anke Ehrhardt, "Sexual Health: A Useful Public Health Paradigm or a Moral Imperative?," *Archives of Sexual Behavior* 33, no. 3 (2004): 181–87, esp. 183.

71. WHO, *Defining Sexual Health*, 6.

72. Ibid.

73. Ibid., 21.

74. In the interim, as I discuss in detail in chapter 9, the US Surgeon General had issued a call for "action to promote sexual health and responsible sexual behavior."

75. WHO, *Defining Sexual Health*, 1.

76. World Health Organization, *Measuring Sexual Health: Conceptual and Practical Considerations and Related Indicators*, report WHO/RHR/10.12 (Geneva: World Health Organization, 2010), 3.

77. The expert panel also considered the possible alternative of "sexual well-being," yet immediately flagged the problem that any definition or understanding of "well-being" is "likely to be culture- and context-specific." Ibid., 4.

78. For simplicity, I abbreviate the department's name as SRH even when describing events before "Sexual" became part of its name. The department includes the UNDP-UNFPA-UNICEF-WHO-World Bank Special Programme of Research, Development and Research Training in Human Reproduction.

79. For a list of donors in 2018, see WHO Department of Reproductive Health and Research, *HRP Annual Report 2018*, report WHO/RHR/HRP/19.3 (Geneva: World Health Organization, 2019), 44.

80. Lianne Gonsalves, interviewed by author, 22 July 2019. The views expressed by Dr. Gonsalves (here and elsewhere in this chapter) are her own and do not represent the official policies or positions of the WHO.

81. WHO Department of Reproductive Health and Research, "Sexual Health—a New Focus for WHO," *Progress in Reproductive Health Research*, no. 67 (2004): 1–7; WHO Department of Reproductive Health and Research, *Sexual and Reproductive Health: Laying the Foundation for a More Just World through Research and Action (Biennial Report 2004–2005)* (Geneva: World Health Organization, 2006); WHO Department of Reproductive Health and Research, *Developing Sexual Health Programmes: A Framework for Action*, report WHO/RHR/HRP/10.22 (Geneva: World Health Organization, 2010).

82. "WHO and HRP Celebrate World Sexual Health Day," World Health Organization, last modified 4 September 2017, http://www.who.int/reproductivehealth/topics/sexual_health/sexual-health-day/en/. I return to the idea of "operationalizing" sexual health in part 2.

83. Lianne Gonsalves, *Sexual Health and Its Linkages to Reproductive Health: An Operational Approach* (Geneva: World Health Organization, 2017), https://www.who.int/reproductivehealth/publications/sexual_health/sh-linkages-rh/en/, 4–5; Rob Stephenson, Lianne Gonsalves, Ian Askew, and Lale Say, "Detangling and Detailing Sexual Health in the SDG Era," *Lancet* 390 (2017): 1014–15.

84. Stephenson et al., "Detangling and Detailing." A recent volume by Tony Sandset and coauthors, published as I was in the final stages of revising this manuscript, offers a broad investigation of sexual health as a global construct in the era of the SDGs. Tony Sandset, Eivind Engebretsen, and Kristin Heggen, *Sustainable Sexual Health: Analyzing the Implementation of the SDGs* (Oxford, UK: Routledge, 2020).

85. Gonsalves, *Sexual Health and Linkages*, 3.

86. Gonsalves, interview.

87. The three indicators are total fertility rate, contraceptive prevalence rate, and met demand for family planning. "Indicators and a Monitoring Framework," Sustainable Development Solutions Network, http://indicators.report/targets/3-7/.

88. Gonsalves, *Sexual Health and Linkages*, 10.

89. Laura M. Carpenter, "Sexual Health," in *Blackwell Encyclopedia of Sociology*, ed. George Ritzer (London: Blackwell, 2007), https://onlinelibrary.wiley.com/doi/abs/10.1002/9781405165518.wbeoss093.

90. Wendy Kline, *Bodies of Knowledge: Sexuality, Reproduction, and Women's Health in the Second Wave* (Chicago: University of Chicago Press, 2010); Sarah Jacoby, "We Asked 5 Sexual Health Experts What Made 'Our Bodies, Ourselves' Such a Revolutionary Resource," *Self*, 11 April 2018, https://www.self.com/story/our-bodies-ourselves-sexual-health-experts.

91. Katie Batza, *Before AIDS: Gay Health Politics in the 1970s* (Philadelphia: University of Pennsylvania Press, 2018), 5–6. Batza found much less evidence from the time of equivalent forms of lesbian health activism (p. 7). See also Michael Brown and Larry Knopp, "The Birth of the (Gay) Clinic," *Health & Place* 28 (2014): 99–108.

92. Brier, *Infectious Ideas*, 15–19.

93. National Coalition of Gay Sexually Transmitted Disease Services, "Guidelines and Recommendations for Healthful Sexual Activity (4th Rev.)," *Official Newsletter of the National Coalition of Gay STD Services* 2, no. 3 (1981): 14–16, esp. 14, http://chodarr.org/sites/default/files/chodarr2870.pdf; Thomas R. Blair, "Safe Sex in the 1970s: Community Practitioners on the Eve of AIDS," *American Journal of Public Health* 107, no. 6 (2017): 872–79,

esp. 873–74. I am indebted to Cindy Patton and the late Eric Rofes for discussion of these general issues.

94. Blair, "Safe Sex," 875.

95. Coleman, interview.

96. Clayton L. Thomas, ed., *Taber's Cyclopedic Medical Dictionary*, 16th ed. (Philadelphia: F. A. Davis, 1989); Walter Glanze and Lois E. Anderson, eds., *Mosby's Medical Dictionary*, 4th ed. (St. Louis, MO: Mosby, 1994). It should be noted that not all medical dictionaries have created entries for sexual health. I am grateful to my research assistant Joseph Guisti for performing this analysis.

97. This explanation appeared on the ASHA website but is no longer accessible, at http://www.ashasexualhealth.org/who-we-are/312-2/ (accessed 22 August 2018).

98. Lynn Barclay, interviewed by author, 22 July 2019; "Our Focus," American Sexual Health Association, http://www.ashasexualhealth.org/who-we-are /what-we-do/.

99. "What Is Sexual Health?," American Sexual Health Association, http:// www.ashasexualhealth.org/sexual-health/.

100. See Marleen Temmerman, Rajat Khosla, and Lale Say, "Sexual and Reproductive Health and Rights: A Global Development, Health, and Human Rights Priority," *Lancet* 384 (2014): e30–e31; "Sexual and Reproductive Health and Rights," Dutch Research Council, https://www.nwo.nl/en /researchprogrammes/sexual-and-reproductive-health-and-rights-srhr; African Union Commission, Maputo Plan of Action on Sexual and Reproductive Health and Rights, n.d., https://www.ippf.org/sites/default/files /maputo_plan_of_action.pdf.

101. "Sexual and Reproductive Health and Rights," Wikipedia, accessed 28 February 2021, https://en.wikipedia.org/wiki/Sexual_and_reproductive _health_and_rights.

102. WHO Department of Reproductive Health and Research, *HRP Annual Report 2018*.

103. See Margaret E. Keck and Kathryn Sikkink, "Transnational Advocacy Networks in International and Regional Politics," *International Social Science Journal* 51, no. 159 (1999): 89–101.

104. From a web page no longer available on the Ford Foundation website, accessed 27 September 2011.

105. "Sexual Health and Rights," Open Society Foundation, https://www.open societyfoundations.org/reports/sexual-health-and-rights-sex-workers -transgender-people-men-who-have-sex-men-thailand.

106. Barroso, "From Reproductive," 385–86.

107. International Planned Parenthood Federation, *IPPF Charter Guidelines on Sexual and Reproductive Rights* (1997; London: International Planned Par-

enthood Federation, 2003); International Planned Parenthood Federation, *Sexual Rights: An IPPF Declaration* (London: International Planned Parenthood Federation, October 2008); Barroso, "From Reproductive," 385–86.

108. "About Us," Guttmacher Institute, https://www.guttmacher.org/about.

109. "Guttmacher-Lancet Commission Proposes a Bold, New Agenda for Sexual and Reproductive Health and Rights," Guttmacher Institute, last modified 9 May 2018, https://www.guttmacher.org/news-release/2018/guttmacher -lancet-commission-proposes-bold-new-agenda-sexual-and-reproductive.

110. Ann M. Starrs et al., "Accelerate Progress—Sexual and Reproductive Health and Rights for All: Report of the Guttmacher-Lancet Commission," *Lancet* 391 (2018): 2642–92, esp. 2642.

111. "Aims and Scope," Sexual and Reproductive Health Matters, https://www .tandfonline.com/action/journalInformation?show=aimsScope&journal Code=zrhm21.

112. Jane Cottingham, Eszter Kismödi, and Julia Hussein, "*Sexual* and Reproductive Health Matters—What's in a Name?," *Sexual and Reproductive Health Matters* 27, no. 1 (2019): 1–3.

113. Gerda Larsson, "The Importance of Sexual Pleasure: A New Declaration," *Medium.com*, 18 October 2019, https://medium.com/the-case-for-her -sexual-pleasure/the-importance-of-sexual-pleasure-a-new-declaration -60db5cb0f0f6.

114. At the WAS Congress, Philpott and Singh delivered the John Money Lecture, entitled "Placing Pleasure into the Tired Narratives of Danger, Death, Disease in Sexual Health Promotion." Alain Giami, "Abstracts for the 24th Congress of the World Association for Sexual Health (WAS)," *International Journal of Sexual Health* 31, suppl. 1 (2019): A1–A627, esp. A6. On the Pleasure Project, "a guerrilla girls activist collective putting the sexy back into safe sex," see "About Us," Pleasure Project, http://thepleasureproject .org/about-us/who-we-are/.

115. "Declaration on Sexual Pleasure," World Association for Sexual Health, last modified 15 October 2019, https://worldsexualhealth.net/declaration -on-sexual-pleasure/. The declaration developed out of a longer series of conversations among academics and sexual health advocates (including Philpott, Eli Coleman, Eszter Kismödi, and various other experts associated with the WAS) who (as Coleman described) identified pleasure as the missing piece of the broader discussion around sexual health and rights (Coleman, interview). See Jessie V. Ford et al., "Why Pleasure Matters: Its Global Relevance for Sexual Health, Sexual Rights and Wellbeing," *International Journal of Sexual Health* 31, no. 3 (2019): 217–30.

116. "Training Toolkit," Global Advisory Board for Sexual Health and Wellbeing, https://www.gab-shw.org/our-work/training-toolkit/; "Who We Are," Global Advisory Board for Sexual Health and Wellbeing, https://www.gab

-shw.org/about/who-we-are/; Sofia Gruskin et al., "Sexual Health, Sexual Rights and Sexual Pleasure: Meaningfully Engaging the Perfect Triangle," *Sexual and Reproductive Health Matters* 27 (2019): 29–40.

117. WAS, "Declaration on Sexual Pleasure."

118. Coleman, interview. On consent and #MeToo, see chapter 10.

119. WAS, "Declaration on Sexual Pleasure."

120. Larsson, "Importance of Sexual Pleasure."

121. On people with disability and sexual health, see chapter 2, note 53. On people who identify as asexual, see the discussion in the conclusion to this book.

122. Steven Hobaica, Kyle Schofield, and Paul Kwon, "'Here's Your Anatomy . . . Good Luck': Transgender Individuals in Cisnormative Sex Education," *American Journal of Sexuality Education* 14, no. 3 (2019): 358–87. See also Nik M. Lampe and Alexandra C.H. Nowakowski, "New Horizons in Trans and Non-Binary Health Care: Bridging Identity Affirmation with Chronicity Management in Sexual and Reproductive Services," *International Journal of Transgender Health* 22, nos. 1–2 (2021): 141–53.

123. Christian Klesse, "Theorizing Multi-Partner Relationships and Sexualities: Recent Work on Non-Monogamy and Polyamory," *Sexualities* 21, no. 7 (2018): 1109–24; Mimi Schippers, *Polyamory, Monogamy, and American Dreams: The Stories We Tell about Poly Lives and the Cultural Production of Inequality* (London: Routledge, 2019).

124. Peter Conrad and Joseph W. Schneider, *Deviance and Medicalization: From Badness to Sickness* (St. Louis, MO: C. V. Mosby, 1980).

125. Trevor Hoppe, *Punishing Disease: HIV and the Criminalization of Sickness* (Berkeley: University of California Press, 2018). See also Steven Thrasher, "A Black Body on Trial: The Conviction of HIV-Positive 'Tiger Mandingo,'" *BuzzFeed News*, 30 November 2015, https://www.buzzfeednews.com/arti cle/steventhrasher/a-black-body-on-trial-the-conviction-of-hiv-positive -tiger-m.

126. Stefan Vogler, *Sorting Sexualities: Expertise and the Politics of Legal Classification* (Chicago: University of Chicago Press, 2021); Scott De Orio, "The Creation of the Modern Sex Offender," in *The War on Sex*, ed. David M. Halperin and Trevor Hoppe (Durham, NC: Duke University Press, 2017), 247–67.

127. Dorothy Roberts, *Killing the Black Body: Race, Reproduction, and the Meaning of Liberty*, 2nd ed. (New York: Vintage, 2017).

128. David M. Halperin and Trevor Hoppe, eds., *The War on Sex* (Durham, NC: Duke University Press, 2017). I discuss sexual citizenship more fully in chapter 9. On the complex relation between sexual citizenship and carceral management, see also Sarah Lamble, "Queer Investments in Punitiveness: Sexual Citizenship, Social Movements and the Expanding

Carceral State," in *Queer Necropolitics*, ed. Jin Haritaworn, Adi Kuntsman, and Sylvia Posocco (Oxford: Routledge, 2014), 151–71.

129. Alexandra Minna Stern, *Eugenic Nation: Faults and Frontiers of Better Breeding in Modern America* (Oakland: University of California Press, 2016).

130. Chris A. Barcelos, *Distributing Condoms and Hope: The Racialized Politics of Youth Sexual Health* (Berkeley: University of California Press, 2020), 53. See also Jenny Dyck Brian, Patrick R. Grzanka, and Emily S. Mann, "The Age of LARC: Making Sexual Citizens on the Frontiers of Technoscientific Healthism," *Health Sociology Review* 29, no. 3 (2020): 312–28; Roberts, *Killing the Black Body*, xx.

131. Roberts, *Killing the Black Body*, esp. xx.

CHAPTER FOUR

1. Stanley E. Althof, Raymond C. Rosen, Michael A. Perelman, and Eusebio Rubio-Aurioles, "Standard Operating Procedures for Taking a Sexual History," *Journal of Sexual Medicine* 10 (2012): 26–35, esp. 27.

2. E. D. Moreira et al., "Help-Seeking Behaviour for Sexual Problems: The Global Study of Sexual Attitudes and Behaviors," *International Journal of Clinical Practice* 59, no. 1 (2005): 6–16.

3. As noted previously, my conception of the sexualization of health draws loosely on Judy Z. Segal, "The Sexualization of the Medical," *Journal of Sex Research* 49, no. 4 (2012): 369–78.

4. N. S. Korse et al., "Discussing Sexual Health in Spinal Care," *European Spine Journal* 25 (2016): 766–73.

5. "Cancer Survivorship," Sexual Medicine Society of North America, https://www.smsna.org/about/committees-sig/cancer-survivorship; "Cancer Is a 'Relationship Disease,'" Sexual Medicine Society of North America, https://www.smsna.org/patients/did-you-know/cancer-is-a-relationship -disease.

6. Segal, "Sexualization of the Medical," 371.

7. Marie Murphy, "Everywhere and Nowhere Simultaneously: The 'Absent Presence' of Sexuality in Medical Education," *Sexualities* 22, nos. 1–2 (2019): 203–23, esp. 205. See also Eli Coleman, "Editor's Note: A Crisis in Medical School Education in Sexual Health," *International Journal of Sexual Health* 24 (2012): 237–38; Marie Murphy, "Hiding in Plain Sight: The Production of Heteronormativity in Medical Education," *Journal of Contemporary Ethnography* 45, no. 3 (2016): 256–89; Marie Murphy, "Teaching and Learning about Sexual Diversity within Medical Education: The Promises and Pitfalls of the Informal Curriculum," *Sexuality Research & Social Policy* 16, no. 1 (2019): 84–99; Emmanuele A. Jannini and Yacov Reisman, "Medicine without Sexual Medicine Is Not Medicine: An MJCSM and ESSM Petition

on Sexual Health to the Political and University Authorities," *Journal of Sexual Medicine* 16, no. 6 (2019): 943–45.

8. Murphy, "Hiding in Plain Sight," 259. As Murphy observed, the heteronormative assumptions of medical school weighed especially heavily on LGBT medical students.

9. Jannini and Reisman, "Medicine without Sexual Medicine," 944.

10. Terri Wilder, "Sexual Health Literacy for Providers Is Crucial to Ending the HIV Epidemic," *TheBodyPro*, 18 May 2021, https://www.thebodypro .com/article/sexual-health-literacy-providers-ending-HIV-epidemic.

11. Amy Fenton, "Abandoning Medical Authority: When Medical Professionals Confront Stigmatized Adolescent Sex and the Human Papillomavirus (HPV) Vaccine," *Journal of Health and Social Behavior* 60, no. 2 (2019): 240–56.

12. Althof et al., "Standard Operating Procedures," 27.

13. Merryn Gott, Sharron Hinchliff, and Elisabeth Galena, "General Practitioner Attitudes to Discussing Sexual Health Issues with Older People," *Social Science & Medicine* 58 (2004): 2093–2103; Timothy Joseph Sowicz and Christine K. Bradway, "Factors Affecting Sexual History Taking in a Health Center Serving Homeless Persons," *Qualitative Health Research* 28, no. 9 (2018): 1395–1405; Elizabeth Boskey and Oren Ganor, "Sexual Health and Gender-Affirming Care," *Harvard Health Blog*, 7 January 2021, https:// www.health.harvard.edu/blog/sexual-health-and-gender-affirming-care -2021010721688.

14. Irina D. Burd, Nicole Nevadunsky, and Gloria Bachmann, "Impact of Physician Gender on Sexual History Taking in a Multispecialty Practice," *Journal of Sexual Medicine* 3, no. 2 (2006): 194–200.

15. Jordan Rosenfeld, "Rooting out Gender Bias in Sexual Health Treatment," *Medical Economics*, 14 November 2019, https://www.medicaleconomics .com/sexual-health/rooting-out-gender-bias-sexual-health-treatment.

16. Janelle N. Sobecki, Farr A. Curlin, and Kenneth A. Rasinski, "What We Don't Talk about When We Don't Talk about Sex: Results of a National Survey of U.S. Obstetrician/Gynecologists," *Journal of Sexual Medicine* 9, no. 5 (2012): 1285–94.

17. Jack Ende, Susan Rockwell, and Marian Glasgow, "The Sexual History in General Medical Practice," *Archives of Internal Medicine* 144 (1983): 558–61.

18. "Patient Sexual Health History: What You Need to Know to Help" (video) (American Medical Association, 2008). This video was previously accessible online; I watched it on 23 March 2017.

19. Only in 1993, after seven previous failed attempts, did the AMA amend its nondiscrimination clause to include reference to sexual orientation. Jason Schneider and Saul Levin, "Uneasy Partners: The Lesbian and Gay Health Care Community and the AMA," *msJAMA* 282 (1999): 1287–88. A few years later, the association repealed a previous policy

recommendation that endorsed attempts to "reverse" sexual orientation in selected cases. American Medical Association Council on Scientific Affairs, "Health Care Needs of Gay Men and Lesbians in the United States," *JAMA* 275, no. 17 (1996): 1354–59.

20. For a sense of the prevalence of medical mnemonics, see "List of Medical Mnemonics," Wikipedia, accessed 20 February 2021, https://en.wikipedia .org/wiki/List_of_medical_mnemonics.

21. Althof et al., "Standard Operating Procedures."

22. The Five Ps are rendered slightly differently in different iterations, perhaps to some degree belying the standardization they suggest. For example, the final "P" sometimes stands for "Pregnancy Plans."

23. Centers for Disease Control and Prevention, *A Guide to Taking a Sexual History*, report 99-8445 (Atlanta: US Department of Health and Human Services, 2005), https://stacks.cdc.gov/view/cdc/12303.

24. See, for example, Richard A. Pessagno, "Don't Be Embarrassed: Taking a Sexual Health History," *Nursing* 43, no. 9 (2013): 60–64. Of course, some publications resist the pressure to simplify and standardize. The book *Sexual Health across the Lifecycle: A Practical Guide for Clinicians* is lengthy enough to cover a wide range of topics, including alternative therapies, the sexuality of disabled people, and domestic violence. Margaret Nusbaum and Jo Ann Rosenfeld, *Sexual Health across the Lifecycle: A Practical Guide for Clinicians* (Cambridge: Cambridge University Press, 2004).

25. National LGBT Health Education Center, *Taking Routine Histories of Sexual Health: A System-Wide Approach for Health Centers* (Boston: Fenway Institute, November 2015), 8.

26. Ibid., 30–33. On the history of the medical record as a form of medical standardization, see Marc Berg and Paul Harterink, "Embodying the Patient: Records and Bodies in Early 20th-Century US Medical Practice," *Body and Society* 10, nos. 2–3 (2004): 13–41.

27. Faculty of Sexual and Reproductive Healthcare Clinical Standards Committee, *Service Standards for Sexual and Reproductive Healthcare* (London: Royal College of Obstetricians and Gynaecologists, 2013), https://www .fsrh.org/standards-and-guidance/documents/fsrh-service-standards -for-sexual-and-reproductive-healthcare/.

28. Steffie Goodman, "Venturing beyond the Binary Sexual Health Interview," *American Journal of Public Health* 108, no. 8 (2018): 965.

29. Arlene Stein, *Unbound: Transgender Men and the Remaking of Identity* (New York: Pantheon Books, 2018), 266.

30. This is an adaptation of Bowker and Star's definition; they also note that standards span more than one "community of practice" or activity site; that they make things work together over distance or heterogeneous metrics; and that they are backed up by bodies such as professional organizations,

manufacturers' associations, or the state. See Geoffrey C. Bowker and Susan Leigh Star, *Sorting Things Out: Classification and Its Consequences* (Cambridge, MA: MIT Press, 1999), 13–14.

31.   For an overview of the sociological implications of standardization, see Stefan Timmermans and Steven Epstein, "A World of Standards but Not a Standard World: Toward a Sociology of Standards and Standardization," *Annual Review of Sociology* 36 (2010): 69–89. See also Nils Brunsson and Bengt Jacobsson, *A World of Standards* (Oxford: Oxford University Press, 2000); Martha Lampland and Susan Leigh Star, eds., *Standards and Their Stories: How Quantifying, Classifying, and Formalizing Practices Shape Everyday Life* (Ithaca, NY: Cornell University Press, 2009); Laurent Thévenot, "Governing Life by Standards: A View from Engagements," *Social Studies of Science* 39 (2009): 793–813; Lawrence Busch, *Standards: Recipes for Reality* (Cambridge, MA: MIT Press, 2011).

32.   Stefan Timmermans and Marc Berg, *The Gold Standard: The Challenge of Evidence-Based Medicine and Standardization in Health Care* (Philadelphia: Temple University Press, 2003), 24–25.

33.   Steven Epstein, "Beyond the Standard Human?," in *Standards and Their Stories: How Quantifying, Classifying, and Formalizing Practices Shape Everyday Life*, ed. Martha Lampland and Susan Leigh Star (Ithaca, NY: Cornell University Press, 2009), 35–53; Susan Leigh Star, "Power, Technologies and the Phenomenology of Conventions: On Being Allergic to Onions," in *A Sociology of Monsters: Essays on Power, Technology and Domination*, ed. John Law, Sociological Review Monograph (London: Routledge, 1991), 26–56.

34.   Stefan Timmermans and Alison Angell, "Evidence-Based Medicine, Clinical Uncertainty, and Learning to Doctor," *Journal of Health and Social Behavior* 42, no. 4 (2001): 342–59; Timmermans and Berg, *Gold Standard*; Eric Mykhalovskiy and Lorna Weir, "The Problem of Evidence-Based Medicine: Directions for Social Science," *Social Science & Medicine* 59, no. 5 (2004): 1059–69; Tiago Moreira, "Diversity in Clinical Guidelines: The Role of Repertoires of Evaluation," *Social Science & Medicine* 60 (2005): 1975–85; Epstein, "Beyond the Standard Human?"; Teun Zuiderent-Jerak, *Situated Intervention: Sociological Experiment in Health Care* (Cambridge, MA: MIT Press, 2015).

35.   Timmermans and Epstein, "World of Standards," 81.

36.   Ibid., 82.

37.   G. Corona, E.A. Jannini, and M. Maggi, "Inventories for Male and Female Sexual Dysfunctions," *International Journal of Impotence Research* 18 (2006): 236–50, esp. 237.

38.   See, for example, Raymond C. Rosen et al., "The International Index of Erectile Function (IIEF): A Multidimensional Scale for Assesment of Erectile Dysfunction," *Urology* 49, no. 6 (1997): 822–30; Raymond C. Rosen et al., "Male Sexual Health Questionnaire (MSHQ): Scale Development and Psy-

chometric Validation," *Urology* 64, no. 4 (2004): 777–82; Markus Wiegel, Cindy Meston, and Raymond Rosen, "The Female Sexual Function Index (FSFI): Cross-Validation and Development of Clinical Cutoff Scores," *Journal of Sex & Marital Therapy* 31 (2005): 1–20; Patrick Jern, Juhana Piha, and Pekka Santtila, "Validation of Three Early Ejaculation Diagnostic Tools: A Composite Measure Is Accurate and More Adequate for Diagnosis by Updated Diagnostic Criteria," *PLOS One* 8, no. 10 (2013): e77676.

39.   See, for example, Raymond Rosen et al., "The Female Sexual Function Index (FSFI): A Multidimensional Self-Report Instrument for the Assessment of Female Sexual Function," *Journal of Sex & Marital Therapy* 26 (2000): 191–208, esp. 194.

40.   Rosen et al., "Male Sexual Health," 778.

41.   "Male Sexual Health Questionnaire (MSHQ)," eProvide, last modified February 2021, https://eprovide.mapi-trust.org/instruments/male-sexual -health-questionnaire.

42.   R. C. Rosen, J. C. Cappeleri, and N. Gendrano, "The International Index of Erectile Function (IIEF): A State-of-the-Science Review," *International Journal of Impotence Research* 14 (2002): 226–44.

43.   "Sexual Health Inventory for Men," Pfizer, https://s3.amazonaws.com /pfizerpro.com/fixtures/viagra/docs/SHIM.pdf.

44.   I accessed this page on 23 October 2015 at https://www.seekwellness.com /mens_sexuality/shim_questionnaire.htm, but it is no longer accessible.

45.   These might be examples of what Tom Waidzunas and I (building on earlier work by Lisa Jean Moore) called "technosexual scripts"—a hybrid concept drawing together the STS literature on technological scripts and the sexuality studies literature on sexual scripts. See Tom Waidzunas and Steven Epstein, "'For Men Arousal Is Orientation': Bodily Truthing, Technosexual Scripts, and the Materialization of Sexualities through the Phallometric Test," *Social Studies of Science* 45, no. 2 (2015): 1–27; Lisa Jean Moore, "'It's Like You Use Pots and Pans to Cook. It's the Tool': The Technologies of Safer Sex," *Science, Technology & Human Values* 22, no. 4 (1997): 434–71, esp. 459.

46.   Demetrios Psihopaidas, "Intimate Standards: Medical Knowledge and Self-Making in Digital Transgender Groups," *Sexualities* 20, no. 4 (2016): 412–27.

47.   Ayo Wahlberg and Nikolas Rose, "The Governmentalization of Living: Calculating Global Health," *Economy and Society* 44, no. 1 (2015): 60–90, esp. 74, 85.

CHAPTER FIVE

1.   "WHO Releases New International Classification of Diseases (ICD 11)," World Health Organization, last modified 18 June 2018, http://www.who

.int/news-room/detail/18-06-2018-who-releases-new-international-clas
sification-of-diseases-(icd-11); "World Health Assembly Update, 25 May
2019," World Health Organization, https://www.who.int/news/item/25
-05-2019-world-health-assembly-update. My discussion here and in what
follows is based on interviews with participants; published commentary
about the ICD revision process; and the following online sources for ICD-10
and ICD-11 codes, respectively: "ICD-10 Version:2019," World Health Organization, https://icd.who.int/browse10/2019/en; "ICD-11 for Mortality
and Morbidity Statistics," World Health Organization, https://icd.who
.int/browse11/l-m/en.

2. "Classification of Diseases: ICD," World Health Organization, http://www
.who.int/classifications/icd/en/.

3. WHO, "WHO Releases." The ICD therefore plays an important role in
shoring up what scholars have described more generally as the regulated
and "legalized" character of present-day biomedicine at the global level.
See Carol A. Heimer, JuLeigh C. Petty, and Rebecca J. Culyba, "Risk and
Rules: The 'Legalization' of Medicine," in *Organizational Encounters with
Risk*, ed. Bridget Hutter and Michael Power (Cambridge: Cambridge University Press, 2005), 92–131; Alberto Cambrosio, Peter Keating, Thomas
Schlich, and George Weisz, "Regulatory Objectivity and the Generation
and Management of Evidence in Medicine," *Social Science & Medicine* 63
(2006): 189–99.

4. These are ICD-10 codes.

5. Geoffrey M. Reed, "Diagnostic Classifications in Psychiatry: Why Do We
Have Two Systems and Is That a Bad Thing?" (video), Columbia University Department of Psychiatry Grand Rounds, 4 October 2017, https://
www.youtube.com/watch?v=d_9sE3fXmUs&list=PLVeamqkJbnWir3bsyu
_w6G4HeAOv46HyP&index=21.

6. Annemarie Jutel, "Sociology of Diagnosis: A Preliminary Review," *Sociology
of Health & Illness* 31, no. 2 (2009): 278–99, esp. 278.

7. Geoffrey C. Bowker and Susan Leigh Star, *Sorting Things Out: Classification
and Its Consequences* (Cambridge, MA: MIT Press, 1999), 110, 135.

8. I checked by using the search function at "ICD-10 Version:2019," WHO.

9. Author's field notes, National Sexual Health Conference, Chicago, 10 July
2019.

10. Michel Foucault, *The Order of Things: An Archaeology of the Human Sciences*
(New York: Vintage Books, 1973); Mary Douglas, *Purity and Danger* (New
York: Routledge & Kegan Paul, 1979); Pierre Bourdieu, "The Social Space
and the Genesis of Groups," *Theory and Society* 14, no. 6 (1985): 723–44; Evi-
atar Zerubavel, "Lumping and Splitting: Notes on Social Classification,"
Sociological Forum 11, no. 3 (1996): 421–33; Bowker and Star, *Sorting Things Out*.

11. Bowker and Star, *Sorting Things Out*, 53–161.

12. Ibid., 111.

13. Ibid., 66. For the analysis in this chapter, I am indebted to the substantial literature on changes to the DSM, of which I cite many examples. In contrast, there has been less work done on the ICD, but see David Armstrong, "Diagnosis and Nosology in Primary Care," *Social Science & Medicine* 73 (2011): 801–7; Alain Giami, "Between DSM and ICD: Paraphilias and the Transformation of Sexual Norms," *Archives of Sexual Behavior* 44 (2015): 1127–38.

14. However, while Bowker and Star may be right to describe an existing version of the ICD as a classification system where the politics have been carefully scrubbed away, the debates over changing the ICD may bring political and ethical considerations into the foreground in ways that, especially nowadays, no one seeks to hide. I develop this point in detail in Steven Epstein, "Cultivated Co-Production: Sexual Health, Human Rights, and the Revision of the ICD," *Social Studies of Science*, advance online publication, 30 April 2021, https://journals.sagepub.com/doi/10.1177/030631 27211014283.

15. On normality and pathology in the case of the DSM, see Paige L. Sweet and Claire Laurier Decoteau, "Contesting Normal: The DSM-5 and Psychiatric Subjectivation," *BioSocieties* 13, no. 1 (2017): 103–22; Damien W. Riggs et al., "Transnormativity in the Psy Disciplines: Constructing Pathology in the Diagnostic and Statistical Manual of Mental Disorders and Standards of Care," *American Psychologist* 74, no. 8 (2019): 912–24.

16. The first edition was called the International List of Causes of Death, and it was adopted by the International Statistical Institute. "Classification of Diseases: ICD," WHO. On the prehistory of the ICD, see Armstrong, "Diagnosis and Nosology."

17. WHO, "WHO Releases." In saying that ICD-11 was temporarily finalized, I mean that it was "frozen" in 2018 in preparation for the ratification vote. After implementation it will continue to be updated, and it is conceived of as a "living document."

18. Joanne J. Meyerowitz, *How Sex Changed: A History of Transsexuality in the United States* (Cambridge, MA: Harvard University Press, 2002), 14–50, 120–24.

19. Mary C. Burke, "Resisting Pathology: GID and the Contested Terrain of Diagnosis in the Transgender Rights Movement," *Advances in Medical Sociology* 12 (2011): 183–210. In 2012, Argentina became a leader in bypassing this dilemma: its passage of a gender identity law removed the requirement of a diagnosis in order to fulfill legal and medical aspects of gender transitioning. By 2016, three European countries—Denmark, Malta, and Ireland—had followed Argentina's lead. Sam Winter et al., "Transgender People: Health at the Margins of Society," *Lancet* 388 (2016): 390–400, esp. 395.

20. Sandy Stone, "The *Empire* Strikes Back: A Posttranssexual Manifesto," in *Body Guards: The Cultural Politics of Gender Ambiguity*, ed. Julia Epstein and

Kristina Straub (New York: Routledge, 1991), 280–304; Dean Spade, "Mutilating Gender," in *The Transgender Studies Reader*, ed. Susan Stryker and Stephen Whittle (New York: Routledge, 2006), 315–32; Susan Stryker, *Transgender History* (Berkeley: Seal Press, 2008).

21.   Dr. Jack Drescher, paraphrased in Camille Beredjick, "DSM-V to Rename Gender Identity Disorder 'Gender Dysphoria,'" *Advocate*, 23 July 2012, http://www.advocate.com/politics/transgender/2012/07/23/dsm -replaces-gender-identity-disorder-gender-dysphoria.

22.   Furthermore, transgender people have been subject to "a particular and narrow set of tropes to which all transgender people are expected to adhere." Riggs et al., "Transnormativity," 913. On the dilemmas of diagnosis, the movement to depathologize trans experiences, and the complex history of collaboration and conflict in trans healthcare and politics, see also David Valentine, *Imagining Transgender: An Ethnography of a Category* (Durham, NC: Duke University Press, 2007); Demetrios Psihopaidas, "Intimate Standards: Medical Knowledge and Self-Making in Digital Transgender Groups," *Sexualities* 20, no. 4 (2016): 412–27; stef m. shuster, "Uncertain Expertise and the Limitations of Clinical Guidelines in Transgender Healthcare," *Journal of Health and Social Behavior* 57, no. 3 (2016): 319–32; Teun Zuiderent-Jerak and Sonja Jerak-Zuiderent, "'Trans* Health Guides as Doing Human Rights: Activism, Evidence, and Standardizing from the Zero Point" (paper presented to the Science and Technology Studies Department, Cornell University, 3 October 2016); Christoph Hanssmann, "Care in Transit: The Political and Clinical Emergence of Trans Health" (PhD diss., University of California, San Francisco, 2017); Florence Ashley, "Gatekeeping Hormone Replacement Therapy for Transgender Patients Is Dehumanising," *Journal of Medical Ethics* 45 (2019): 480–82; Florence Ashley, "The Misuse of Gender Dysphoria: Toward Greater Conceptual Clarity in Transgender Health," *Perspectives on Psychological Science*, advance online publication, 20 November 2019, https://doi.org/10.1177/1745691619872987; Austin H. Johnson, "Rejecting, Reframing, and Reintroducing: Trans People's Strategic Engagement with the Medicalisation of Gender Dysphoria," *Sociology of Health & Illness* 41, no. 3 (2019): 517–32; Cal Lee Garrett, "Finding Natural Variation: Assembling Underdetermined Evidence of Gender Dysphoria, Doing Trans Therapeutics," *BioSocieties*, advance online publication, 28 July 2020, https://doi.org/10.1057/s41292-020-00201-9; Tara Gonsalves, "Gender Identity, the Sexed Body, and the Medical Making of Transgender," *Gender & Society* 34, no. 6 (2020): 1005–33.

23.   Arlene Stein, *Unbound: Transgender Men and the Remaking of Identity* (New York: Pantheon Books, 2018), 73. Florence Ashley refers to this situation as "an unjustified double standard in contrast to other forms of clinical care." Ashley, "Gatekeeping," 480.

24. "F64: Gender Identity Disorders [in ICD-10]," World Health Organization, https://icd.who.int/browse10/2019/en#/F64.0.

25. Mauro Cabral Grinspan, "Right Answers," *Archives of Sexual Behavior* 46 (2017): 2505–6; Zowie Davy, Anniken Sørlie, and Amets Suess Schwend, "Democratising Diagnoses? The Role of the Depathologisation Perspective in Constructing Corporeal Trans Citizenship," *Critical Social Policy* 38, no. 1 (2018): 13–34; Riggs et al., "Transnormativity"; Ashley, "Misuse of Gender Dysphoria."

26. Beredjick, "DSM-V to Rename." See also Riggs et al., "Transnormativity."

27. Garrett, "Finding Natural Variation."

28. Ashley, "Misuse of Gender Dysphoria."

29. Garrett, "Finding Natural Variation."

30. Eli Coleman, interviewed by author, 11 July 2019.

31. Doris Chou et al., "Sexual Health in the International Classification of Diseases (ICD): Implications for Measurement and Beyond," *Reproductive Health Matters* 23, no. 46 (2015): 185–92, esp. 187.

32. Doris Chou, interviewed by author, 29 August 2019. The views expressed by Dr. Chou (here and elsewhere in this chapter) are her own and do not represent the official policies or positions of the WHO.

33. Peter Galison, "Trading Zone: Coordinating Action and Belief," in *The Science Studies Reader*, ed. Mario Biagioli (New York: Routledge, 1999), 137–60.

34. Chou, interview. See also "Sexual Health in the Revised 11th Version of the International Classification of Diseases (ICD)," World Health Organization, http://www.who.int/reproductivehealth/topics/sexual_health/icd_revision/en/.

35. Geoffrey M. Reed et al., "Disorders Related to Sexuality and Gender Identity in the ICD-11: Revising the ICD-10 Classifications Based on Current Scientific Evidence, Best Clinical Practices, and Human Rights Considerations," *World Psychiatry* 15 (2016): 205–21; Richard B. Krueger et al., "Proposals for Paraphilic Disorders in the International Classification of Diseases and Related Health Problems, Eleventh Revision (ICD-11)," *Archives of Sexual Behavior* 46 (2017): 1529–45; Reed, "Diagnostic Classifications." For an analysis of the management of sexuality in previous editions of the DSM and the ICD, see Giami, "Between DSM and ICD."

36. In a survey conducted in 2010–2011 by the World Psychiatric Association and the WHO, 70.1 percent of 4,887 participating psychiatrists in forty-four countries reported that ICD-10 was the classification system they used most in their day-to-day clinical work, versus 23.0 percent who cited DSM-4. Geoffrey M. Reed et al., "The WPA-WHO Global Survey of Psychiatrists' Attitudes towards Mental Disorders Classification," *World Psychiatry* 10, no. 2 (2011): 118–31, esp. 124. Doris Chou similarly noted

the significance of DSM categories in working group discussions while underscoring the point that the DSM is understood to originate with the American Psychiatric Association and is not necessarily endorsed by all psychiatric societies globally. Chou, interview.

37. I am grateful to Doris Chou (interview) for helpful discussion of what might be called the ontology of the ICD: what sorts of entities are included within it?

38. Mauro Cabral Grinspan, interviewed by author, 15 November 2019. On "spoiled identity," see Erving Goffman, *Stigma: Notes on the Management of Spoiled Identity* (Englewood Cliffs, NJ: Prentice-Hall, 1963).

39. Johannes Fuss et al., "Public Stakeholders' Comments on ICD-11 Chapters Related to Mental and Sexual Health," *World Psychiatry* 18, no. 2 (2019): 233–35, esp. 233.

40. Krueger et al., "Proposals for Paraphilic," 1530.

41. Cabral Grinspan, interview.

42. On patient groups and health advocacy, see Steven Epstein, *Impure Science: AIDS, Activism, and the Politics of Knowledge* (Berkeley: University of California Press, 1996); Steven Epstein, "Patient Groups and Health Movements," in *The Handbook of Science and Technology Studies*, ed. Edward J. Hackett et al. (Cambridge, MA: MIT Press, 2008), 499–539; Vololona Rabeharisoa and Michel Callon, "The Involvement of Patients' Associations in Research," *International Social Science Journal* 54, no. 171 (2002): 57–63; Phil Brown et al., "Embodied Health Movements: New Approaches to Social Movements in Health," *Sociology of Health & Illness* 26, no. 1 (2004): 50–80; Vololona Rabeharisoa, Tiago Moreira, and Madeleine Akrich, "Evidence-Based Activism: Patients', Users' and Activists' Groups in Knowledge Society," *BioSocieties* 9, no. 2 (2014): 111–28.

43. Véronique Mottier and Robbie Duschinsky, "Introduction to the Special Section on DSM-5: Classifying Sex," *Archives of Sexual Behavior* 44 (2015): 1087–90, esp. 1087. See also Kristin Barker and Tasha R. Galardi, "Diagnostic Domain Defense: Autism Spectrum Disorder and the *DSM-5*," *Social Problems* 62 (2015): 120–40.

44. Davy et al., "Democratising Diagnoses," 15.

45. Cabral Grinspan, interview.

46. Ibid.

47. Ibid.

48. Ibid. See *supra* note 19.

49. Krueger et al., "Proposals for Paraphilic," 1530.

50. Coleman, interview.

51. Reed et al., "Disorders," 216.

52. "The Yogyakarta Principles: Principles on the Application of International Human Rights Law in Relation to Sexual Orientation and Gender Iden-

tity" (Yogyakarta, Indonesia, March 2007), 6, http://yogyakartaprinciples
.org/principles-en/official-versions-pdf/.

53. See chapter 3, note 59.
54. Yogyakarta Principles, 23.
55. Reed et al., "Disorders." The quote is from the article title.
56. Eli Coleman et al., "Commentary: Revising the International Classification of Diseases (ICD-11) and Improving Global Sexual Health: Time for an Integrated Approach That Moves beyond the Mind-Body Divide," *International Journal of Sexual Health* 29, no. 2 (2017): 113–14, esp. 114.
57. However, the subcategory of sexual dysfunction associated with pelvic organ prolapse retains a primary home in the chapter on diseases of the genitourinary system.
58. Reed et al., "Disorders," 207.
59. Coleman et al., "Commentary."
60. Coleman, interview.
61. As noted above, DSM-5 defined gender dysphoria in terms of incongruence ("a marked incongruence between one's experienced/expressed gender and assigned gender"). Therefore the break between DSM-5 and ICD-11 is less sharp than might be supposed.
62. Reed et al., "Disorders," 209–10. See also Jack Drescher, Peggy Cohen-Kettenis, and Sam Winter, "Minding the Body: Situating Gender Identity Diagnoses in the ICD-11," *International Review of Psychiatry* 24, no. 6 (2012): 568–77, esp. 573.
63. Fuss et al., "Public Stakeholders."
64. "Reflections from STP Regarding the ICD Revision Process and Publication of the DSM-5," STP (International Campaign Stop Trans Pathologization), last modified August 2013, https://www.stp2012.info/STP_Commu nique_August2013.pdf.
65. Valentine, *Imagining Transgender*; Alyssa Lynne, "Paired Double Consciousness: A Du Boisian Approach to Gender and Transnational Double Consciousness in Thai *Kathoey* Self-Formation," *Social Problems* 68, no. 2 (2021): 250–66. See also the special issue on "Decolonizing the Transgender Imaginary" in *TSQ: Transgender Studies Quarterly* 1, no. 3 (2014).
66. Chou, interview.
67. Reed et al., "Disorders," 211.
68. Ibid.
69. Cabral Grinspan, interview.
70. Chou, interview.
71. Coleman, interview.
72. Griet De Cuypere and Gail Knudson, *WPATH Consensus Process Regarding Transgender and Transsexual-Related Diagnoses in ICD-11* (World Professional Association for Transgender Health, 31 May 2013), 8–9.

73. Cabral Grinspan, interview.
74. Drescher et al., "Minding the Body," 574.
75. Caroline Simon, "Being Transgender No Longer Classified as Mental Illness," *USA Today*, 20 June 2018, https://www.usatoday.com/story/news/2018/06/20/transgender-not-mental-illness-world-health-organization/717758002/.
76. Jessica Ravitz, Ben Pickman, and Brandon Griggs, "Transgender People Are Not Mentally Ill, the WHO Decrees," *CNN*, 28 May 2019, https://www.cnn.com/2019/05/28/health/who-transgender-reclassified-not-mental-disorder/index.html.
77. The working group proposed criteria for diagnosing "gender incongruence of childhood" that were stricter than those for the previous category of "gender identity disorder of childhood" so as to avoid capturing within the diagnosis children who are "merely gender variant." Reed et al., "Disorders," 211. However, many transgender activists continued to oppose the childhood category altogether. See Sam Winter, "Gender Trouble: The World Health Organization, the International Statistical Classification of Diseases and Related Health Problems (ICD)-11and the Trans Kids," *Sexual Health* 14 (2017): 422–30.
78. "New Developments in the ICD Revision Process," CLAM (Latin American Center on Sexuality and Human Rights), last modified 20 August 2014, http://www.clam.org.br/en/news/conteudo.asp?cod=11752.
79. "'WHO Still Calls Trans Identity a Disorder': Mexican Activists," *TeleSur*, 20 June 2018, https://www.telesurenglish.net/news/WHO-Still-Calls-Trans-Identity-A-Disorder-Mexican-Activists-20180620-0024.html; Aryn Plax, "Trans Identity Not Mental Illness, Says World Health Organization," *Advocate*, 19 June 2018, https://www.advocate.com/transgender/2018/6/19/transgender-identity-not-mental-illness-says-world-health-organization.
80. Cabral Grinspan, "Right Answers," 2505.
81. "Joint Statement on ICD-11 Process for Trans & Gender Diverse People," Global Action for Trans* Equality (GATE), 24 May 2019, https://transactivists.org/icd-11-trans-process/ (emphasis in the original).
82. See *supra* note 65.
83. Stone, "*Empire* Strikes Back"; Eric D. Plemons, "Description of Sex Difference as Prescription for Sex Change: On the Origins of Facial Feminization Surgery," *Social Studies of Science* 44, no. 5 (2014): 657–79; J. R. Latham, "Axiomatic: Constituting 'Transexuality' and Trans Sexualities in Medicine," *Sexualities* 22, nos. 1–2 (2019): 13–30. This phenomenon has been termed "transnormativity" (on the analogy with heteronormativity and homonormativity). See Riggs et al., "Transnormativity."
84. Reed et al., "Disorders," 212–16. See also Krueger et al., "Proposals for Paraphilic." On the history of the concept of paraphilia and its medical classification, see Giami, "Between DSM and ICD," 1131–32.

85. Ronald Bayer, *Homosexuality and American Psychiatry: The Politics of Diagnosis* (New York: Basic Books, 1981).

86. Tom Waidzunas, *The Straight Line: How the Fringe Science of Ex-Gay Therapy Reoriented Sexuality* (Minneapolis: University of Minnesota Press, 2015), 70–86.

87. Susan D. Cochran et al., "Proposed Declassification of Disease Categories Related to Sexual Orientation in the *International Statistical Classification of Diseases and Related Health Problems* (ICD-11)," *Bulletin of the World Health Organization* 92 (2014): 672–79, esp. 674–75.

88. Ibid., 675.

89. Ibid., 676. On the efficacy and ethics of "reorientation" or "conversion" therapy for gay people, see Waidzunas, *Straight Line*.

90. Cochran et al., "Proposed Declassification," 676.

91. Chou, interview.

92. Giami, "Between DSM and ICD," 1136.

93. See Chapter 10. I am grateful to Cathy Gere for suggesting I think more about the place of discourses of consent in the ICD.

94. Winter, "Gender Trouble," 424.

95. "6D36: Paraphilic Disorder Involving Solitary Behaviour or Consenting Individuals [in ICD-11]," World Health Organization, https://icd.who.int /browse11/1-m/en#/http%3a%2f%2fid.who.int%2ficd%2fentity%2f2055 403635. See also Reed et al., "Disorders," 214–15; Krueger et al., "Proposals for Paraphilic," 1534–41.

96. Winter, "Gender Trouble," 424.

97. Janice M. Irvine, "Reinventing Perversion: Sex Addiction and Cultural Anxieties," *Journal of the History of Sexuality* 5, no. 3 (1995): 429–50, esp. 431.

98. Janna A. Dickenson, Neal Gleason, Eli Coleman, and Michael H. Miner, "Prevalence of Distress Associated with Difficulty Controlling Sexual Urges, Feelings, and Behaviors in the United States," *JAMA Network Open* 1, no. 7 (2018): e184468, https://jamanetwork.com/journals/jamanetworkopen /fullarticle/2713037. The research involved the application of survey results to the Compulsive Sexual Behavior Inventory—thereby combining two distinct modes of "operationalization" of sexual health discussed in part 2: scales and surveys.

99. Jon E. Grant et al., "Impulse Control Disorders and 'Behavioural Addictions' in the ICD-11," *World Psychiatry* 13, no. 2 (2014): 125–27, esp. 126.

100. "AASECT: From a Scientific Perspective, Sex Addiction Is Not Real," *Business Wire*, 13 December 2016, https://www.businesswire.com/news/home /20161213005309/en/AASECT-From-a-Scientific-Perspective-Sex-Addic tion-is-Not-Real.

101. This category is also distinct from the disorders related to addictive behaviors—that is, the ICD has avoided the controversial nomenclature of "sex addiction."

102. See Cochran et al., "Proposed Declassification"; Reed et al., "Disorders."

103. Grant et al., "Impulse Control Disorders," 126.

104. See Liana Schreiber, Brian L. Odlaug, and Jon E. Grant, "Impulse Control Disorders: Updated Review of Clinical Characteristics and Pharmacological Management," *Frontiers in Psychiatry* 2 (21 February 2011), https://doi.org/10.3389/fpsyt.2011.00001. I am grateful to Aaron Norton for suggesting this implication.

105. Fuss et al., "Public Stakeholders," 233.

106. "6C72: Compulsive Sexual Behaviour Disorder [in ICD-11]," World Health Organization, https://icd.who.int/browse11/l-m/en#/http://id.who.int/icd/entity/1630268048.

107. "WAS Statement about the WHO/ICD 11," World Association for Sexual Health, last modified 6 July 2018, https://worldsexualhealth.net/2018/07/.

108. On obligatory passage points in science, see Michel Callon, "Some Elements of a Sociology of Translation: Domestication of the Scallops and the Fishermen of St Brieuc Bay," in *Power, Action, and Belief*, ed. John Law (London: Routledge & Kegan Paul, 1986), 196–233; Bruno Latour, *Science in Action: How to Follow Scientists and Engineers through Society* (Cambridge, MA: Harvard University Press, 1987), 145–76.

109. For a similar point about the DSM, see Andrew Lakoff, "Diagnostic Liquidity: Mental Illness and the Global Trade in DNA," *Theory and Society* 34, no. 1 (2005): 63–92, esp. 86.

110. Ibid., esp. 67.

111. Armstrong, "Diagnosis and Nosology"; Amber D. Nelson, "Diagnostic Dissonance and Negotiations of Biomedicalisation: Mental Health Practitioners' Resistance to the DSM Technology and Diagnostic Standardisation," *Sociology of Health & Illness* 41, no. 5 (2019): 933–49.

112. Chou, interview.

113. Peter Cryle and Elizabeth Stephens, *Normality: A Critical Genealogy* (Chicago: University of Chicago Press, 2017), esp. 164.

114. Gayle S. Rubin, "Thinking Sex: Notes for a Radical Theory of the Politics of Sexuality," in *Pleasure and Danger: Exploring Female Sexuality*, ed. Carole S. Vance (New York: Routledge, 1984), 267–318, esp. 283.

115. On the limits of the depathologization strategy for achieving social change in the domain of sexuality, see Waidzunas, *Straight Line*, 231–53; Geeti Das, "Mostly Normal: American Psychiatric Taxonomy, Sexuality, and Neoliberal Mechanisms of Exclusion," *Sexuality Research & Social Policy* 13, no. 4 (2016): 390–401.

116. See Burke, "Resisting Pathology." I am grateful to Daniel Navon for suggesting I think more about this implication of the ICD-11 changes.

117. Cryle and Stephens, *Normality*, esp. 359.

118. "Millennium Development Goals (MDGs)," World Health Organization, last modified 19 February 2018, https://www.who.int/news-room/fact-sheets/detail/millennium-development-goals-(mdgs).

119. "Indicators and a Monitoring Framework," Sustainable Development Solutions Network, http://indicators.report/targets/3-7/. I also discuss the SDGs in chapter 3.

120. World Health Organization, *Measuring Sexual Health: Conceptual and Practical Considerations and Related Indicators*, report WHO/RHR/10.12 (Geneva: World Health Organization, 2010), 2.

121. Ibid., 1–2, 11–12.

122. The matrix focused on measures of determinants of sexual health, access, use of services, and outcomes. Ibid., 13–15.

123. Chou et al., "Sexual Health," 186.

124. Ibid., 187.

125. Wendy Nelson Espeland and Mitchell L. Stevens, "A Sociology of Quantification," *European Journal of Sociology* 49, no. 3 (2008): 401–36.

126. Mary Morgan, "Observing Poverty, Measuring the Good Life" (paper presented to the Science in Human Culture Program, Northwestern University, 17 April 2017).

127. Sally Engle Merry, *The Seductions of Quantification: Measuring Human Rights, Gender Violence, and Sex Trafficking* (Chicago: University of Chicago Press, 2016).

128. Bowker and Star, *Sorting Things Out*, 86–87.

129. Reed et al., "Disorders," 205.

130. In these respects, the development of the sexual health chapter is a textbook illustration of what Sheila Jasanoff has termed "co-production"—or of the canonical claim in STS scholarship, by Steven Shapin and Simon Schaffer, that in the history of scientific controversies, problems of knowledge and problems of order are often solved together. At the same time, the self-conscious way in which these health experts went about such negotiations suggests a kind of co-production that, more unusually, is both transparent and orchestrated. Using the example of the ICD, I have characterized this as "cultivated co-production." Epstein, "Cultivated Co-Production." See also Sheila Jasanoff, "The Idiom of Co-Production," in *States of Knowledge: The Co-Production of Science and Social Order*, ed. Sheila Jasanoff (London: Sage, 2004), 1–12; Steven Shapin and Simon Schaffer, *Leviathan and the Air-Pump: Hobbes, Boyle and the Experimental Life* (Princeton, NJ: Princeton University Press, 1985).

131. I made a similar argument about the biomedicalizing of governance (within the United States) in Steven Epstein, *Inclusion: The Politics of Difference in Medical Research* (Chicago: University of Chicago Press, 2007), esp. 17–18.

132. Steven Epstein, "The Construction of Lay Expertise: AIDS Activism and the Forging of Credibility in the Reform of Clinical Trials," *Science, Technology & Human Values* 20, no. 4 (1995): 408–37; Steven Epstein, "The Meaning and Significance of Lay Expertise," in *The Oxford Handbook of Expertise*, ed. Gil Eyal and Thomas Medvetz (Oxford: Oxford University Press, forthcoming).

133. Riggs et al., "Transnormativity," 913.
134. I am grateful to Helen Tilley for discussion of this point.
135. Alyssa Lynne, personal communication, based on attendance of the 26th Scientific Symposium of the World Professional Association for Transgender Health (WPATH), 6–10 November 2020. On the sexual and reproductive health needs of trans and nonbinary people, see Nik M. Lampe and Alexandra C. H. Nowakowski, "New Horizons in Trans and Non-Binary Health Care: Bridging Identity Affirmation with Chronicity Management in Sexual and Reproductive Services," *International Journal of Transgender Health* 22, nos. 1–2 (2021): 141–53.
136. Chou, interview.
137. Bowker and Star, *Sorting Things Out*, 139.
138. To be sure, disease taxonomists are not unaware of the problems that cultural variability and language translation pose for stable diagnostic criteria. See Neil Krishan Aggarwal, "Culture, Communication, and DSM-5 Diagnostic Reliability," *Journal of the National Medical Association* 109, no. 3 (2017): 150–52.
139. Didier Fassin, "That Obscure Object of Global Health," in *Medical Anthropology at the Intersections: Histories, Activisms, and Futures*, ed. Marcia C. Inhorn and Emily A. Wentzell (Durham, NC: Duke University Press, 2012), 95–115, esp. 106.
140. Krueger et al., "Proposals for Paraphilic," 1542.
141. Bowker and Star, *Sorting Things Out*, 131. See also Owen Whooley, "Nosological Reflections: The Failure of *DSM-5*, the Emergence of RDoC, and the Decontextualization of Mental Distress," *Society and Mental Health* 4, no. 2 (2014): 92–110, esp. 93.
142. "Eleventh Revision of the International Classification of Diseases: Report by the Director-General" (Seventy-Second World Health Assembly, provisional agenda item 12.7, 4 April 2019), World Health Organization, http://apps.who.int/gb/ebwha/pdf_files/WHA72/A72_29-en.pdf.
143. Jeffrey Weeks, "Beyond the Categories," *Archives of Sexual Behavior* 44 (2015): 1091–97, esp. 1095.
144. Ian Hacking, "Kinds of People: Moving Targets," *Journal of the British Academy* 151 (2007): 285–318.

CHAPTER SIX

1. Enumeration is a prime example of social uses of quantification. Wendy Nelson Espeland and Mitchell L. Stevens, "A Sociology of Quantification," *European Journal of Sociology* 49, no. 3 (2008): 401–36. On the politics of enumeration, see Melissa Nobles, *Shades of Citizenship: Race and the Census in Modern Politics* (Stanford, CA: Stanford University Press, 2000); Steven Epstein, *Inclusion: The Politics of Difference in Medical Research* (Chicago: Uni-

versity of Chicago Press, 2007); Sarah Elizabeth Igo, *The Averaged American: Surveys, Citizens, and the Making of a Mass Public* (Cambridge, MA: Harvard University Press, 2007); Rebecca Jean Emigh, Dylan Riley, and Patricia Ahmed, *Antecedents of Censuses from Medieval to Nation States: How Societies and States Count* (Houndmills, UK: Palgrave Macmillan, 2016); Michael Rodríguez-Muñiz, *Figures of the Future: Latino Civil Rights and the Politics of Demographic Change* (Princeton, NJ: Princeton University Press, 2021).

2. Robert N. Proctor, *Cancer Wars: How Politics Shapes What We Know and Don't Know about Cancer* (New York: Basic Books, 1995), 8. See also Robert Proctor and Londa L. Schiebinger, *Agnotology: The Making and Unmaking of Ignorance* (Stanford, CA: Stanford University Press, 2008); Scott Frickel et al., "Undone Science: Charting Social Movement and Civil Society Challenges to Research Agenda Setting." *Science, Technology & Human Values* 35 (2010): 444–73. On agnotology in relation to sexuality, see Steven Epstein, "The Great Undiscussable: Anal Cancer, HPV, and Gay Men's Health," in *Three Shots at Prevention: The HPV Vaccine and the Politics of Medicine's Simple Solutions*, ed. Keith Wailoo et al. (Baltimore: Johns Hopkins University Press, 2010), 61–90.

3. Janice M. Irvine, "The Other Sex Work: Stigma in Sexuality Research," *Social Currents* 2, no. 2 (2015): 116–25.

4. Michel Foucault, *The History of Sexuality, Volume 1: An Introduction*, trans. Robert Hurley (New York: Vintage Books, 1980).

5. Igo, *Averaged American*, 236–38, 256.

6. Robert T. Michael, John H. Gagnon, Edward O. Laumann, and Gina Kolata, *Sex in America: A Definitive Survey* (Boston: Little, Brown, 1994), 20–21; Julia A. Ericksen, *Kiss and Tell: Surveying Sex in the Twentieth Century* (Cambridge, MA: Harvard University Press, 1999), 59; Janice M. Irvine, "'The Sociologist as Voyeur': Social Theory and Sexuality Research, 1910–1978," *Qualitative Sociology* 26, no. 4 (2003): 429–56, esp. 451; Igo, *Averaged American*, 236–58.

7. Igo, *Averaged American*, 297.

8. Ibid., 278.

9. Edward O. Laumann, Robert T. Michael, and John H. Gagnon, "A Political History of the National Sex Survey of Adults," *Family Planning Perspectives* 26, no. 1 (1994): 34–38, esp. 34–35.

10. Ibid., 35.

11. Morton Hunt, *The New Know-Nothings: The Political Foes of the Scientific Study of Human Nature* (New Brunswick, NJ: Transaction, 1999), 187; Ericksen, *Kiss and Tell*, 205.

12. Diane di Mauro, *Sexuality Research in the United States: An Assessment of the Social and Behavioral Sciences* (New York: Sexuality Research Assessment Project, 1995), 8–12; Ericksen, *Kiss and Tell*, 80–89; Hunt, *New Know-Nothings*, 185–91.

13. Ericksen, *Kiss and Tell*, 188. On the politics of estimating the size of the gay population, see Wendy Espeland and Stuart Michaels, "The Biography of 10%: Measures of Sexual Behavior and the Gay Rights Movement in the U.S., 1948–1994" (unpublished manuscript, Evanston, IL, n.d.). On the widespread fear that producing knowledge about sexuality inevitably functions as advocacy, see Mary Poovey, "Sex in America," *Critical Inquiry* 24, no. 2 (2009): 366–92, esp. 385.

14. Edward O. Laumann, John H. Gagnon, Robert T. Michael, and Stuart Michaels, *The Social Organization of Sexuality: Sexual Practices in the United States* (Chicago: University of Chicago Press, 1994); Michael et al., *Sex in America*.

15. Of course, sex surveys with probability samples have also been performed in other countries. For example, the British National Survey of Sexual Attitudes and Lifestyles (Natsal) has been conducted in three separate waves: 1990–91, 1999–2001, and 2010–12. See Kaye Wellings and Anne M. Johnson, "Framing Sexual Health Research: Adopting a Broader Perspective," *Lancet* 382 (2013): 1759–62.

16. "National Survey of Sexual Health and Behavior," Indiana University School of Public Health, http://www.nationalsexstudy.indiana.edu/.

17. Debby Herbenick et al., "Sexual Behavior in the United States: Results from a National Probability Sample of Men and Women Ages 14–94," *Journal of Sexual Medicine* 7, suppl. 5 (2010): 255–65.

18. Indiana University, "National Survey."

19. Michael Reece et al., "Background and Considerations on the National Survey of Sexual Health and Behavior (NSSHB) from the Investigators," *Journal of Sexual Medicine* 7, suppl. 5 (2010): 243–45, esp. 245.

20. Debby Herbenick, "America Undercovers" (plenary presentation at the National Sexual Health Conference, Chicago, 11 July 2019) (author's field notes). The characterization of the study as providing a "snapshot" was offered by the team in Herbenick et al., "Sexual Behavior," 256.

21. Ibid., 256–57; Reece et al., "Background and Considerations."

22. Herbenick, "America Undercovers."

23. See the discussion of this issue in chapters 2 and 9.

24. Brian Dodge et al., "Sexual Health among U.S Black and Hispanic Men and Women: A Nationally Representative Study," *Journal of Sexual Medicine* 7, suppl. 5 (2010): 330–45; Michael Reece et al., "Condom Use Rates in a National Probability Sample of Males and Females Ages 14 to 94 in the United States," *Journal of Sexual Medicine* 7, suppl. 5 (2010): 266–76.

25. Herbenick, "America Undercovers."

26. Indiana University, "National Survey."

27. Herbenick et al., "Sexual Behavior," 260.

28. Laurel Westbrook, Jamie Budnick, and Aliya Saperstein, "Dangerous Data: Seeing Social Surveys through the Sexuality Prism," *Sexualities*, advance

online publication, 10 February 2021, https://doi.org/10.1177/13634607
20986927. For a thorough review of how attitudes about sexuality and
identity inform surveys on sexual orientation and gender minorities, see
also Jamie Louise Budnick, "The New Gay Science: Sexuality Knowledge,
Demography, and the Politics of Population Measurement" (PhD diss.,
University of Michigan, 2020), 60–122. To be sure, surveys in general tend
to focus on problems much more than pleasures, so it may not seem surprising that they would do so in relation to sexuality. However, Westbrook
(personal communication) found that the set of surveys they studied did,
in fact, sometimes address issues related to pleasure—for example, by
asking questions about happiness and satisfaction—but generally did not
do so in relation to sexuality.

29.   Megan B. Ivankovich, Jami S. Leichliter, and John M. Douglas, "Measurement of Sexual Health in the U.S.: An Inventory of Nationally Representative Surveys and Surveillance Systems," *Public Health Reports* 128, suppl. 1
(2013): 62–72, esp. 70.

30.   Angela Jones, "Sex Is Not a Problem: The Erasure of Pleasure in Sexual
Science Research," *Sexualities* 22, no. 4 (2019): 643–68, esp. 661–62. Jones
also found that the body of research tended to presume and reinforce
heteronormativity while insufficiently incorporating diversity of various
kinds.

31.   Wellings and Johnson, "Framing Sexual Health," 1759.

32.   Ibid., 1759–61.

33.   Indiana University, "National Survey." See also the articles devoted to the
study in the *Journal of Sexual Medicine*, volume 7, supplement 5.

34.   Herbenick, "America Undercovers."

35.   Ericksen, *Kiss and Tell*, 223.

36.   This is the phenomenon that Espeland and Stevens refer to as the "reactiv-
ity" of numbers: "Measurement intervenes in the social world it depicts."
Wendy Nelson Espeland and Mitchell L. Stevens, "A Sociology of Quantification," *European Journal of Sociology* 49, no. 3 (2008): 401–36, esp. 412.
On the cultural impact of surveys and their effects on those who absorb
lessons from them, see Igo, *Averaged American*; John Law, "Seeing Like a
Survey," *Cultural Sociology* 3, no. 2 (2009): 239–56. More specifically on the
effects of sex surveys, see the discussion of Kinsey in Igo, *Averaged American*, 191–228, as well as Ericksen, *Kiss and Tell*, 27; Poovey, "Sex in America";
Budnick, "New Gay Science"; Westbrook et al., "Dangerous Data"; and
Aaron Norton's analysis of the survey as "a discursive technology . . . that
communicates particular information to its readers" and as "a device that
creates particular subject positions for respondents": Aaron T. Norton,
"Surveying Risk Subjects: Public Health Surveys as Instruments of Biomedicalization," *BioSocieties* 8 (2013): 265–88, esp. 270–71.

37.   Igo, *Averaged American*, 6.

38. Leonore Tiefer, "Unpacking the Popularity of a Paper on Feigning Sexual Pleasure: Consider Both Sexual Politics and 21st-Century Profits," *Sexualities* 21, no. 4 (2018): 706–9, esp. 707.

39. Igo, *Averaged American*, 281–82.

40. Charles Briggs and Daniel Hallin have coined the term "biocommunicability" to describe the ways in which health communication in the media not only reflects assumptions about how medical knowledge is made but also shapes a wide array of social beliefs. In discussions of sexual health surveys in the public sphere, we see the dynamics of what might be called "biosexual communicability." Charles L. Briggs and Daniel C. Hallin, "Health Reporting as Political Reporting: Biocommunicability and the Public Sphere," *Journalism* 11, no. 2 (2010): 149–65.

41. Mary Robertson, "Sex in America," cable television episode in *Curiosity* series (Discovery Channel, 11 November 2012).

42. Curt Wagner, "Sex in America: Discovery's 'Curiosity' Reveals Sexual Habits," *Chicago Tribune*, 8 November 2012, http://www.chicagotribune.com /redeye/redeye-sex-in-america-discoverys-curiosity-reveals-sexual-habits -tv-20121108-story.html.

43. Logan Levkoff, "Sex: 5 Things You May Be Missing Out on in Bed," *Huffington Post*, 25 September 2012, https://www.huffpost.com/entry/sex _b_1697938.

44. "A Tale of Two Studies," Family Research Institute, last modified November 2010, http://www.familyresearchinst.org/2010/12/frr-nov-2010-%E2 %80%94-a-tale-of-two-studies/. Interestingly, the Family Research Institute author introduced the NSSHB by claiming (incorrectly), "The *Kinsey Institute* is at it again"—although "of course they've changed their name"— thereby proposing a connection between the agendas of the two Indiana University–based studies that were conducted at different research centers, more than half a century apart.

45. These issues were addressed in several articles in the special issue of the *Journal of Sexual Medicine*, including Reece et al., "Condom Use"; Vanessa Schick et al., "Sexual Behaviors, Condom Use, and Sexual Health of Americans over 50: Implications for Sexual Health Promotion for Older Adults," *Journal of Sexual Medicine* 7, suppl. 5 (2010): 315–29.

46. Belinda Luscombe, "Study of American Sex Habits Suggests Boomers Need Sex Ed," *Time*, 4 October 2010, http://healthland.time.com/2010/10/04 /study-suggests-boomers-need-sex-ed/.

47. Roni Caryn Rabin, "Condom Use Is Highest for Young, Study Finds," *New York Times*, 4 October 2010, A13; Roni Caryn Rabin, "Grown-up, but Still Irresponsible," *New York Times*, 9 October 2010, https://www.nytimes.com /2010/10/10/weekinreview/10rabin.html.

48. As compared to gender, race has been less of a focus of public and mass media discussion of the NSSHB—perhaps because, as noted earlier, the

most distinctive findings positioned racial and ethnic minorities as be-having more responsibly, with African Americans and Hispanics reporting more frequent condom use than did Whites.

49. Katherine Speller, "Losing Your Chill Would Be Great for Your Sex Life," *MTV News*, 6 November 2015, http://www.mtv.com/news/2369922/the -orgasm-gap-has-no-chill/.

50. Mona Chalabi, "The Gender Orgasm Gap," *FiveThirtyEight*, 20 August 2015, https://fivethirtyeight.com/datalab/the-gender-orgasm-gap/; Samantha Allen, "Can Virtual Vaginas Help Close the Orgasm Gap?" (2015), *Daily Beast*, 26 June 2017, http://www.thedailybeast.com/articles/2015/12/30 /can-kinsey-approved-virtual-vaginas-help-close-the-orgasm-gap.html; Linda Blair, "Mind the Orgasm Gap," *The Guardian*, 5 October 2010, https:// www.theguardian.com/lifeandstyle/2010/oct/05/orgasm-gap-sex.

51. Research based on in-depth interviews has suggested greater complexity to the heterosexual orgasm gap, which may vary in size depending on the context of the sexual interaction (for example, hookups versus relation-ships). See Elizabeth A. Armstrong, Paula England, and Alison C. K. Fog-arty, "Accounting for Women's Orgasm and Sexual Enjoyment in College Hookups and Relationships," *American Sociological Review* 77, no. 3 (2012): 435–62.

52. David Rosen, "America's Changing Sexual Appetites," *Counterpunch*, 25 February 2011, http://www.counterpunch.org/2011/02/25/america-s -changing-sexual-appetites/. The Discovery Channel episode mentioned earlier sounded similar notes. Of course, the comparability of these differ-ent sex studies, conducted according to different methodologies, is itself a matter of debate.

53. Lea Rose Emery, "7 Reasons to Integrate Anal Stimulation into Your Sex Life," 18 January 2016, https://www.bustle.com/articles/136225-7-reasons -to-integrate-anal-stimulation-into-your-sex-life.

54. Igo, *Averaged American*, 279. See also Peter Cryle and Elizabeth Stephens, *Normality: A Critical Genealogy* (Chicago: University of Chicago Press, 2017), 336–37.

55. Thomas Walter Laqueur, *Solitary Sex: A Cultural History of Masturbation* (New York: Zone Books, 2003); Helen Lefkowitz Horowitz, *Rereading Sex: Battles over Sexual Knowledge and Suppression in Nineteenth-Century America* (New York: Knopf, 2002), 86–122.

56. Rachel Grumman Bender, "How Much Masturbation Is Too Much?," *Grea-tist*, 20 November 2015, http://greatist.com/grow/masturbate-too-much. Accessed 6 April 2017 but no longer available in this form.

57. Mona Chalabi, "Dear Mona, I Masturbate More Than Once a Day. Am I Normal?," *FiveThirtyEight*, 30 May 2014, https://fivethirtyeight.com/data lab/dear-mona-i-masturbate-more-than-once-a-day-am-i-normal/.

58. Herbenick, "America Undercovers."

59.   Joshua R. Goldstein and Ann J. Morning, "Back in the Box: The Dilemma of Using Multiple-Race Data for Single Race Laws," in *The New Race Question: How the Census Counts Multiracial Individuals*, ed. Joel Perlmann and Mary C. Waters (New York: Russell Sage, 2002), 119–36; Alexandra C. H. Nowakowski, J. E. Sumerau, and Lain A. B. Mathers, "None of the Above: Strategies for Inclusive Teaching with 'Representative' Data," *Teaching Sociology* 44, no. 2 (2016): 96–105; Patrick Grzanka, "Queer Survey Research and the Ontological Dimensions of Heterosexism," in *Imagining Queer Methods*, ed. Amin Ghaziani and Matt Brim (New York: NYU Press, 2019), 84–102.

CHAPTER SEVEN

1.   For a concise summary of the contemporary tensions around expertise, see Gil Eyal, *The Crisis of Expertise* (Cambridge, UK: Polity, 2019). My approach to expertise is shaped by a significant body of work in STS and other fields, including Stephen Hilgartner, *Science on Stage: Expert Advice as Public Drama* (Stanford, CA: Stanford University Press, 2000); H. M. Collins and Robert Evans, *Rethinking Expertise* (Chicago: University of Chicago Press, 2007); Michel Callon, Pierre Lascoumes, and Yannick Barthe, *Acting in an Uncertain World: An Essay on Technical Democracy* (Cambridge, MA: MIT Press, 2009); Frank Fischer, *Democracy and Expertise: Reorienting Policy Inquiry* (Oxford: Oxford University Press, 2009); E. Summerson Carr, "Enactments of Expertise," *Annual Review of Anthropology* 39 (2010): 17–32; Gil Eyal, "For a Sociology of Expertise: The Social Origins of the Autism Epidemic," *American Journal of Sociology* 118, no. 4 (2013): 863–907; Reiner Grundmann, "The Problem of Expertise in Knowledge Societies," *Minerva* 55, no. 1 (2017): 25–48; Sheila Jasanoff, "Science and Democracy," in *The Handbook of Science and Technology Studies*, ed. Ulrike Felt et al. (Cambridge, MA: MIT Press, 2017), 259–87.
2.   Michèle Lamont, "Toward a Comparative Sociology of Valuation and Evaluation," *Annual Review of Sociology* 38 (2012): 201–21.
3.   Grundmann, "Problem of Expertise," 27.
4.   Holger Strassheim, "Politics and Policy Expertise: Towards a Political Epistemology," in *Handbook of Critical Policy Studies*, ed. Frank Fischer et al. (Cheltenham, UK: Edward Elgar, 2015), 319–40, esp. 326.
5.   Eyal, *Crisis of Expertise*.
6.   Steven Epstein, "The Construction of Lay Expertise: AIDS Activism and the Forging of Credibility in the Reform of Clinical Trials," *Science, Technology & Human Values* 20, no. 4 (1995): 408–37; Steven Epstein, "The Meaning and Significance of Lay Expertise," in *The Oxford Handbook of Expertise*, ed. Gil Eyal and Thomas Medvetz (Oxford: Oxford University Press, forthcoming).

7. On the understanding of expertise as a network of people, tools, and techniques, see Eyal, "For a Sociology of Expertise."

8. Author's field notes, National Sexual Health Conference, 10–12 July 2019, Chicago.

9. "About ISSM," International Society for Sexual Medicine, https://www .issm.info/who-we-are/; "Journals," International Society for Sexual Medicine, https://professionals.issm.info/journals/; "Events," International Society for Sexual Medicine, https://professionals.issm.info/meetings/.

10. Kristen Thometz, "Northwestern Opens Center for Sexual Medicine and Menopause," *WTTV Chicago Tonight*, 18 October 2017, https://chicago tonight.wttw.com/2017/10/18/northwestern-opens-center-sexual-medi cine-and-menopause.

11. "World Association for Sexual Health Definitions of Professional Specialties," World Association for Sexual Health, last modified 17 April 2007, http://176.32.230.27/worldsexology.org/wp-content/uploads/2013/08 /definitions-of-professional-specialties.pdf.

12. This text is no longer available, but it was posted previously at http:// www.aasect.org (accessed 14 September 2013).

13. I am grateful to Kellie Owens for performing this analysis (with advice from Loet Leydesdorff) using a technique called science overlay mapping. See Ismael Rafols, Alan L. Porter, and Loet Leydesdorff, "Science Overlay Maps: A New Tool for Research Policy and Library Management," *Journal of the American Society for Information Science and Technology* 61, no. 9 (2010): 1871–87.

14. I. Simms, M. Gibin, and J. Petersen, "Location, Location, Location: What Can Geographic Information Science (GIS) Offer Sexual Health Research?," *Sexually Transmitted Infections* 90, no. 6 (2014): 442–43.

15. Ross Shegog et al., "Serious Games for Sexual Health," *Games for Health Journal* 4, no. 2 (2015): 69–77, esp. 74.

16. "Sexual Health Certificate Program," University of Michigan School of Social Work, https://ssw.umich.edu/offices/continuing-education/certi ficate-courses/sexual-health.

17. "Sexual Health Educator Certification (SHEC)," Options for Sexual Health, https://www.optionsforsexualhealth.org/sex-ed/shec/; "SHEC FAQ," Options for Sexual Health, https://www.optionsforsexualhealth.org/sex-ed /shec/shec-faq/.

18. "Hypnotic Relaxation Therapy Improves Sexual Health for Postmenopausal Women with Hot Flashes," *Medical News Today*, 19 August 2013, http://www.medicalnewstoday.com/releases/264942.

19. "Hypnotherapy for Sex and Intimacy Issues," A Time for Change Hypnotherapy, https://www.atfchypnotherapy.com/services/sex-intimacy-issues/.

20. "Hypnosis Denver: Lynda Pulford C.Ht.," A Time for Change Hypnotherapy, https://www.atfchypnotherapy.com/about/.

21.   This argument is developed in Steven Epstein and Stefan Timmermans, "From Medicine to Health: The Proliferation and Diversification of Cultural Authority," *Journal of Health and Social Behavior* 62, no. 3 (2021): 240–54.

22.   Kristin K. Barker, "Mindfulness Meditation: Do-It-Yourself Medicalization of Every Moment," *Social Science & Medicine* 106 (2014): 168–76.

23.   Gemma Mangione, "The Art and Nature of Health: A Study of Therapeutic Practice in Museums," *Sociology of Health & Illness* 40, no. 2 (2018): 283–96, esp. 283.

24.   Leonore Tiefer, "Medicalizations and Demedicalizations of Sexuality Therapies," *Journal of Sex Research* 49, no. 4 (2012): 311–18, esp. 311, 313.

25.   Ibid., 313.

26.   M. E. Melody and Linda M. Peterson, *Teaching America about Sex: Marriage Guides and Sex Manuals from the Late Victorians to Dr. Ruth* (New York: NYU Press, 1999); Rodney A. Buxton, "Dr. Ruth Westheimer: Upsetting the Normalcy of the Late-Night Talk Show," *Journal of Homosexuality* 21, nos. 1–2 (1991): 139–54; Victoria Davion, "Not Really a 'New Attitude': Dr. Laura on Gender and Morality," in *Fundamental Differences: Feminists Talk Back to Social Conservatives*, ed. Cynthia Burack and Jyl J. Josephson (Lanham, MD: Rowman & Littlefield, 2004), 143–55.

27.   I return to the topic of Christian conservative sex advice, and its political functions, in chapter 10.

28.   "Who Is Dan Savage?," *Savage Lovecast* (podcast), https://www.savagelove cast.com/about#about.

29.   Miranda Nelson, "Dan Savage named 2013's Sexual Health Champion by Options for Sexual Health," *Georgia Straight*, 12 December 2012, https:// www.straight.com/blogra/dan-savage-named-2013s-sexual-health-cham pion-options-sexual-health.

30.   "Dan Savage," Wikipedia, accessed 21 February 2021, https://en.wikipedia .org/wiki/Dan_Savage.

31.   Neve Fear-Smith, "The Influencers Normalising Conversations around Sexual Health and Wellbeing," *Talking Influence*, 9 February 2021, https:// talkinginfluence.com/2021/02/09/the-influencers-normalising-conver sations-around-sexual-health-and-wellbeing/.

32.   Amanda Hess, "The Sex-Ed Queens of Youtube Don't Need a PhD," *New York Times*, 30 September 2016, http://www.nytimes.com/2016/10/01 /arts/the-sex-ed-queens-of-youtube-dont-need-a-phd.html.

33.   Ibid.

34.   Savas Abadsidis, "How Did a Boy from Rural Georgia Become the King of Kink?," *Towelroad*, 18 January 2019, https://www.towleroad.com/2019/01 /how-did-a-boy-from-rural-georgia-become-the-king-of-kink/; Alexander Cheves, *Love, Beastly* (blog), https://thebeastlyexboyfriend.com. Emphasis in the original.

35.   Alisha Haridasani Gupta, "The Sex Adviser Will See You Now. On Insta-
      gram," *New York Times*, 13 February 2021, https://www.nytimes.com/2021
      /02/13/style/emily-morse-masterclass-instagram-podcast.html.

36.   "Welcome to the Pornhub Sexual Wellness Center," Pornhub, https://www
      .pornhub.com/sex/; "Contributors," Pornhub, https://www.pornhub.com
      /sex/contributors/.

37.   "Pornhub Launches Sexual Wellness Center for Advice and Information
      on Sexuality, Sexual Health and Relationships," Pornhub, last modified
      1 February 2017, https://www.pornhub.com/press/show?id=1162.

38.   "Contact Us," Pornhub, https://www.pornhub.com/sex/contact-us/.

39.   Kimberly Truong, "Pornhub Might Be Your New Source for Sex Ed,"
      Refinery29, 1 February 2017, https://www.refinery29.com/2017/01/138743
      /pornhub-sex-ed-site.

40.   Pornhub, "Contributors."

41.   "jessica drake," Guide to Wicked Sex, http://www.guidetowickedsex.com.

42.   "Jessica Drake Addresses UCLA Class of Licensed Therapists," *AVN*, 15 May
      2012, https://avn.com/business/articles/video/jessica-drake-addresses
      -ucla-class-of-licensed-therapists-475744.html. For a parallel example, see
      the discussion of Nina Hartley in Tiefer, "Medicalizations and Demedical-
      izations," 313.

43.   Nick Wilson, E. Jane MacDonald, Osman David Mansoor, and Jane Morgan,
      "In Bed with Siri and Google Assistant: A Comparison of Sexual Health
      Advice," *BMJ* 359 (13 December 2017), https://doi.org/10.1136/bmj.j5635.

44.   "Introducing Roo," Planned Parenthood, https://www.plannedparenthood
      .org/learn/roo-sexual-health-chatbot. On expertise as a heterogeneous
      network, see Eyal, "For a Sociology of Expertise."

45.   Eyal, *Crisis of Expertise*. Because of his close focus on the state and the poli-
      tics of regulatory science, Eyal misses the chance to paint the crisis of
      expertise as a broadly cultural phenomenon, one that might involve such
      matters as sexuality. Steven Epstein, "Comments on Gil Eyal's *The Crisis of
      Expertise*," *Perspectives* (newsletter of the Theory Section of the American
      Sociological Association) 41, no. 2 (Winter 2019): 20–23.

46.   Emma McGowan, "How to Tell If a Sexual Health Resource Is Legit, Ac-
      cording to a Sex Educator," *Bustle*, 31 July 2019, https://www.bustle.com
      /p/how-to-tell-if-a-sexual-health-resource-is-legit-according-to-a-sex
      -educator-18367105.

47.   McGowan doesn't explain, but the acronym appears to refer to a group
      called San Francisco Sex Information.

48.   Joshua Gamson, *Freaks Talk Back: Television Talk and Sexual Nonconformity*
      (Chicago: University of Chicago Press, 1998), 15–16, 100. On the "evidence
      of experience," see Joan Scott, "The Evidence of Experience," *Critical In-
      quiry* 17, no. 4 (1991): 773–97.

49.   Rob Cover, "Populist Contestations: Cultural Change and the Competing Languages of Sexual and Gender Identity," *Sexualities*, advance online publication, 23 December 2020, https://doi.org/10.1177/1363460720982924.

50.   Epstein, "Construction of Lay Expertise"; Epstein, "Meaning and Significance of Lay Expertise."

51.   See chapter 5, note 42.

52.   The many examples of new forms of expertise that are emerging at the junctures of diverse social worlds bear out Eyal's suggestion that we look for expertise not only within established fields of social practice but also in the hybrid and interstitial "spaces between fields." Gil Eyal, "Spaces between Fields," in *Pierre Bourdieu and Historical Analysis*, ed. Philip S. Gorski (Durham, NC: Duke University Press, 2013), 158–82.

53.   Jeffrey Escoffier, "The Invention of Safer Sex: Vernacular Knowledge, Gay Politics, and HIV Prevention," *Berkeley Journal of Sociology* 43 (1999): 1–30, esp. 2.

54.   Ibid., 19–23; Epstein, *Impure Science*, 63–64, 97.

55.   Dennis Altman, *AIDS in the Mind of America* (Garden City, NJ: Anchor Press, 1986), 153.

56.   See chapter 3, note 25.

57.   Penelope Green, "Betty Dodson, 91, Guru of Self-Pleasure for Generations of Women, Dies," *New York Times*, 4 November 2020, B10.

58.   Ibid.

59.   Stephanie Theobald, "How Is Betty Dobson, the Queen of Female Masturbation, Dying? Not Quietly . . . ," *Daily Beast*, 27 August 2020, https://www.thedailybeast.com/how-is-betty-dodson-the-queen-of-female-masturbation-dying-not-quietly.

60.   Betty Dodson, *Sex by Design: The Betty Dodson Story* (New York: Betty A. Dodson Foundation, 2015), esp. locs. 2427 and 2342, Kindle.

61.   Green, "Betty Dodson."

62.   "Dr. Carol Queen," Good Vibrations, https://www.goodvibes.com/s/content/c/carol_queen.

63.   Robert Morgan Lawrence and Carol Queen, "Bisexuals Help Create the Standards for Safer Sex: San Francisco, 1981–1987," *Journal of Bisexuality* 1, no. 1 (2000): 145–62, esp. 156.

64.   "Susie Bright," Wikipedia, accessed 21 February 2021, https://en.wikipedia.org/wiki/Susie_Bright; "C.V.," Annie Sprinkle, http://anniesprinkle.org/cv/.

65.   On such communities, see Tiefer, "Medicalizations and Demedicalizations," 313.

66.   Salma Haidrani, "'Black Fly' Is the Foremost Sex Zine for People of Colour," *Vice*, 27 March 2017, https://www.vice.com/en/article/vvj878/black-fly-is-the-foremost-sex-zin.

67.   Oliver Taylor, "Skin Deep Meets: Black Fly Zine," *Skin Deep*, 4 November 2020, https://skindeepmag.com/articles/skin-deep-meets-black-fly-zine

-sexual-health-sex-positive-community-poc/; "Black Fly Zine: The Community for Sexual Wellbeing," The Sassy Show, last modified 14 October 2020, https://www.thesassyshow.com/post/black-fly-zine-the-community-for-sexual-wellbeing.

68. Ibid.
69. Ibid.
70. Taylor, "Skin Deep."
71. "Swallow It Whole: A Zine about PrEP for Women," Black Fly and Prepster, last modified 2019, https://prepster.info/wp-content/uploads/2019/11/swallowitwhole.pdf.
72. Michel Foucault, *The History of Sexuality, Volume 1: An Introduction*, trans. Robert Hurley (New York: Vintage Books, 1980), 41–49, 144.
73. Gayle S. Rubin, "Thinking Sex: Notes for a Radical Theory of the Politics of Sexuality," in *Pleasure and Danger: Exploring Female Sexuality*, ed. Carole S. Vance (New York: Routledge, 1984), 267–318, esp. 281–83.
74. On the various critiques of Rubin's "charmed circle," see Rebecca L. Jones, "Later Life Sex and Rubin's 'Charmed Circle,'" *Sexuality & Culture* 24 (2020): 1480–98, esp. 1481. See also Ken Plummer, *Cosmopolitan Sexualities: Hope and the Humanist Imagination* (Cambridge, UK: Polity, 2015), 146. On the enduring impact of Rubin's essay, see Steven Epstein, "Thinking Sex Ethnographically," *GLQ* 17, no. 1 (2010): 85–88.
75. As Michèle Lamont has observed, heterarchies (or plurarchies) of worth may be preferable in processes of evaluation, precisely because of their more pluralistic character. Lamont, "Valuation and Evaluation." On the multiplicity of orders of worth, see Luc Boltanski and Laurent Thévenot, *On Justification: Economies of Worth* (Princeton, NJ: Princeton University Press, 2006).
76. Science studies scholars have emphasized that the production of trustworthy knowledge (especially in laboratory settings, but elsewhere, too) depends on the creation of what Lorraine Daston and Peter Galison have called "working objects." See Lorraine Daston and Peter Galison, "The Image of Objectivity," *Representations* 40 (1992): 81–128. See also Adele E. Clarke and Joan H. Fujimura, eds., *The Right Tools for the Job: At Work in Twentieth-Century Life Sciences* (Princeton, NJ: Princeton University Press, 1992).
77. Fernando Domínguez Rubio, "Preserving the Unpreservable: Docile and Unruly Objects at MoMA," *Theory and Society* 43 (2014): 617–45, esp. 633. Domínguez Rubio clarifies (p. 622) that "docility" and "unruliness" are not inherent characteristics of an object but rather ways in which the materiality of the object is expressed in particular organizational and institutional contexts. Extrapolating to sexuality, we might say that there is nothing necessarily or essentially "unruly" about sexuality but that some of its features may quite often lend themselves to being rendered "problematic."

78. On the "materialization" of sexuality, see Tom Waidzunas and Steven Epstein, "'For Men Arousal Is Orientation': Bodily Truthing, Technosexual Scripts, and the Materialization of Sexualities through the Phallometric Test," *Social Studies of Science* 45, no. 2 (2015): 1–27.

79. Standardization, classification, enumeration, and evaluation are examples of what Charles Tilly called "robust" social processes that are marked by their presence "across a variety of settings and circumstances." Charles Tilly, *Explaining Social Processes* (Boulder, CO: Paradigm Publishers, 2008), 139. My approach here is influenced not only by much work on these topics in science and technology studies but also by Michèle Lamont's theorization of the deep significance and impact of these fundamental cultural processes. See Lamont, "Valuation and Evaluation"; Michèle Lamont, Stefan Beljean, and Matthew Clair, "What Is Missing? Cultural Processes and Causal Pathways to Inequality," *Socio-Economic Review* 12, no. 3 (2014): 573–608.

80. When I began work on this book, I thought, perhaps naively, that the terminology of "operationalizing" sexual health was my own gloss on a set of activities that its practitioners would be more inclined to describe using other words. However (as I discussed in chapter 3), as the WHO has become more invested in sexual health, it has also demonstrated an increasing commitment to what it calls "operationalizing." See Lianne Gonsalves, *Sexual Health and Its Linkages to Reproductive Health: An Operational Approach* (Geneva: World Health Organization, 2017), https://www.who.int/reproductivehealth/publications/sexual_health/sh-linkages-rh/en/.

81. Stefan Vogler, *Sorting Sexualities: Expertise and the Politics of Legal Classification* (Chicago: University of Chicago Press, 2021), 10.

82. See Nelly Oudshoorn and Trevor Pinch, eds., *How Users Matter: The Co-Construction of Users and Technology* (Cambridge, MA: MIT Press, 2003).

CHAPTER EIGHT

1. "Tantus Participates in Spring Sexual Health Expo," *Tantus* (blog), https://www.tantusinc.com/blogs/news/18043168-tantus-participates-in-spring-sexual-health-expo; "Our Story," Tantus, https://www.tantusinc.com/pages/about-us.

2. "Global $108 Billion Sexual Wellness Industry Outlook 2020–2027: Rise in Millennial Population, Surge in Disposable Income," *Cision PR Newswire*, 2 September 2020, https://www.prnewswire.com/news-releases/global-108-billion-sexual-wellness-industry-outlook-2020-2027-rise-in-millennial-population-surge-in-disposable-income-301123244.html.

3. Nora Caley, "Cashing in on Sexual Wellness as a Self-Care Category," *Drug Store News*, 16 September 2019, https://drugstorenews.com/otc/cashing-in-on-sexual-wellness-as-a-self-care-category.

4. On sexuopharmaceuticals, see chapter 2, note 17.

5. On direct-to-consumer advertising, see Julie Donohue, "A History of Drug Advertising: The Evolving Roles of Consumers and Consumer Protection," *Milbank Quarterly* 84, no. 4 (2006): 659–99.

6. Meika Loe, *The Rise of Viagra: How the Little Blue Pill Changed Sex in America* (New York: NYU Press, 2004), 79.

7. Ibid., 83.

8. Maria Gurevich et al., "Propping up Pharma's (Natural) Neoliberal Phallic Man: Pharmaceutical Representations of the Ideal Sexuopharmaceutical User," *Culture, Health & Sexuality* 19, no. 4 (2017): 422–37, esp. 426.

9. David Tuller, "Gentlemen, Start Your Engines?," *New York Times*, 21 June 2004, http://www.nytimes.com/2004/06/21/health/sex-medicine-gen tlemen-start-your-engines.html.

10. Matthew Schneier, "Marketing Viagra without Walks on the Beach," *New York Times*, 30 November 2017, D11.

11. For some examples of Viagra counternarratives, see Annie Potts, "Deleuze on Viagra (or, What Can a 'Viagra-Body' Do?)," *Body & Society* 10, no. 1 (2004): 17–36.

12. The hope, of course, is that this indefinite extension into the future of one's sexual potency does not manifest as that dreaded and well-advertised side effect: the erection lasting more than four hours.

13. On the relation between treatment and enhancement, see Sheila M. Roth-man and David J. Rothman, *The Pursuit of Perfection: The Promise and Perils of Medical Enhancement* (New York: Pantheon Books, 2003).

14. Carl Elliott, *Better Than Well: American Medicine Meets the American Dream* (New York: W. W. Norton, 2003).

15. Kristina Gupta, "'Screw Health': Representations of Sex as a Health-Promoting Activity in Medical and Popular Literature," *Journal of Medical Humanities* 32 (2011): 127–40, esp. 130.

16. Carl Cederström and André Spicer, *The Wellness Syndrome* (Cambridge, UK: Polity, 2015), 3.

17. Anna Kirkland, "What Is Wellness Now?," *Journal of Health Politics, Policy & Law* 39, no. 5 (2014): 957–70, esp. 957.

18. Anna Kirkland, "Critical Perspectives on Wellness," *Journal of Health Politics, Policy and Law* 39, no. 5 (2014): 971–88, esp. 973; Gordon Hull and Frank Pasquale, "Toward a Critical Theory of Corporate Wellness," *BioSocieties* 13 (2018): 190–212.

19. Justin Lee, "Investigating the Hybridity of 'Wellness' Practices," e-Scholarship, UCLA Department of Sociology, Theory and Research in Comparative Social Analysis, 2005, https://escholarship.org/uc/item/88c4t567, 2.

20. Steven Epstein and Stefan Timmermans, "From Medicine to Health: The Proliferation and Diversification of Cultural Authority," *Journal of Health and Social Behavior* 62, no. 3 (2021): 240–54.

21. Kelly Moore, "Neoliberal Wellness and the Routinization of Harm" (paper presented at the annual meeting of the American Sociological Association, Chicago, 22–25 August 2015), emphasis in the original. My analysis in this chapter is in conversation with much work on the "neoliberal subject" (in general, and in the domains of health and sexuality), although I use the term "neoliberal" with reservations because of its disparate uses. See Peter A. Hall and Michèle Lamont, "Introduction: Social Resilience in the Neoliberal Era," in *Social Resilience in the Neoliberal Era*, ed. Peter A. Hall and Michèle Lamont (Cambridge: Cambridge University Press, 2013), 1–31; Kirsten Bell and Judith Green, "On the Perils of Invoking Neoliberalism in Public Health Critique," *Critical Public Health* 26, no. 3 (2016): 239–43; Patrick Grzanka, Emily S. Mann, and Sinikka Elliott, "The Neoliberalism Wars, or Notes on the Persistence of Neoliberalism," *Sexuality Research & Social Policy* 13, no. 4 (2016): 297–307.

22. Vincanne Adams, Michelle Murphy, and Adele E. Clarke, "Anticipation: Technoscience, Life, Affect, Temporality," *Subjectivity* 28 (2009): 246–65.

23. Nikolas Rose, "The Politics of Life Itself," *Theory, Culture & Society* 18, no. 6 (2001): 1–30, esp. 17–18.

24. See chapter 2, note 83.

25. Laura Mamo, Amber Nelson, and Aleia Clark, "Producing and Protecting Risky Girlhoods," in *Three Shots at Prevention: The HPV Vaccine and the Politics of Medicine's Simple Solutions*, ed. Keith Wailoo et al. (Baltimore: Johns Hopkins University Press, 2010), 121–45; Nicole Charles, "Mobilizing the Self-Governance of Pre-Damaged Bodies: Neoliberal Biological Citizenship and HPV Vaccination Promotion in Canada," *Citizenship Studies* 17, no. 6–7 (2013): 770–84.

26. See the introduction, note 37.

27. For an analysis of one instructive case, see Abigail Cope Saguy, *What's Wrong with Fat?* (New York: Oxford University Press, 2013).

28. Robert Crawford, "Healthism and the Medicalization of Everyday Life," *International Journal of Health Services* 10, no. 3 (1980): 365–88, esp. 365, 368. Subsequently, Crawford connected the "new health consciousness" to a "neoliberal restructuring of American society" and described health as "the language of a [middle] class that, even as it disintegrates, continues to believe in its self-making salvation." Robert Crawford, "Health as a Meaningful Social Practice," *Health* 10, no. 4 (2006): 401–20, esp. 419.

29. Jonathan M. Metzl, "Introduction: Why Against Health?," in *Against Health: How Health Became the New Morality*, ed. Jonathan M. Metzl and Anna Kirkland (New York: NYU Press, 2010), 1–11, esp. 1–2.

30. "Manila Luzon Owns It" (YouTube video), OraQuick, last modified 16 October 2017, https://www.youtube.com/watch?v=9x5VM-wSVGO.

31. On risk assessment in recent genetic science and changing boundaries of normality and pathology, see Daniel Navon, *Mobilizing Mutations: Human Genetics in the Age of Patient Advocacy* (Chicago: University of Chicago Press, 2019).

32. Natasha Dow Schüll, "Our Metrics, Ourselves," *Public Books*, 26 January 2017, https://www.publicbooks.org/our-metrics-ourselves/.

33. Deborah Lupton, "Quantified Sex: A Critical Analysis of Sexual and Reproductive Self-Tracking Using Apps," *Culture, Health & Sexuality* 17, no. 4 (2015): 440–53.

34. See the Ngram Viewer at https://books.google.com/ngrams (accessed 29 January 2021).

35. "Sexual Wellness," Walgreens, accessed 21 February 2021, https://www.walgreens.com/store/c/sexual-wellness/ID=359445-tier1.

36. Search conducted on 10 May 2017 at https://www.amazon.com/Best-Sellers-Health-Personal-Care-Sexual-Wellness-Products/zgbs/hpc/3777371. According to the web page, this list of "most popular products based on sales" is updated hourly.

37. Such sanitizing can be distinguished from a more thoroughgoing "camouflaging" of sexual accessories in early twentieth-century catalog advertising. See Rachel P. Maines, *The Technology of Orgasm: "Hysteria," the Vibrator, and Women's Sexual Satisfaction* (Baltimore: Johns Hopkins University Press, 1999), 19–20, 100–110.

38. Gary W. Dowsett, "'And Next, Just for Your Enjoyment!': Sex, Technology and the Constitution of Desire," *Culture, Health & Sexuality* 17, no. 4 (2015): 527–39, esp. 536.

39. Home Page, *Sexual Health*, https://www.sexualhealthmagazine.com.

40. These are all examples from the January 2020 issue of *Sexual Health*.

41. I accessed this page, https://bewell.usc.edu/sexual-health/, on 11 May 2017, but it is no longer available.

42. Charles Shepherd, representing Durex, 23 September 2013, at the 21st Congress of the World Association for Sexual Health, Porto Alegre, Brazil (author's field notes).

43. Caitlin Gibson, "The Future of Sex Includes Robots and Holograms. What Does That Mean for Us?," *Washington Post*, 14 January 2016, https://www.washingtonpost.com/news/soloish/wp/2016/01/14/the-future-of-sex-includes-robots-and-holograms-what-does-that-mean-for-us/?utm_term=.8a47198e1117.

44. Kirkland, "Critical Perspectives on Wellness," 976.

45. Alanna Vagianos, "You Can Send a Vibrator to Your Congressperson to Protest the Health Care Bill," *Huffington Post*, 28 June 2017, https://www.huffpost.com/entry/you-can-send-a-vibrator-to-your-congressperson-to-protest-the-health-care-bill_n_595283b0e4b0da2c731ed86e.

46. Sarah Parvini, "This California University Has a Vending Machine That Sells the Morning-after Pill," *Los Angeles Times*, 25 April 2017, http://www.latimes.com/local/lanow/la-me-ln-morning-after-pill-machine-201704 25-story.html.

47. Ibid.

48. "Not Just for Snacks! University Offers Abortifacient Plan B Vending Machine," Texas Right to Life, https://www.texasrighttolife.com/not-just -for-snacks-university-offers-abortifacient-plan-b-vending-machine/; Alayna Lee and Larissa Jimenez, "Sexual Wellness Vending Machine Opens," *Yale Daily News*, 5 September 2019, https://yaledailynews.com/blog/2019 /09/05/sexual-wellness-vending-machine-opens/.

49. "Sex Expo," SHE Media, http://www.sexexpo.com/; "Frequently Asked Questions," SHE Media, http://www.sexualhealthexpo.com/faq.php.

50. Lynn Comella, *Vibrator Nation: How Feminist Sex-Toy Stores Changed the Business of Pleasure* (Durham, NC: Duke University Press, 2017), 2.

51. Ibid., 7, 13, 140. See also April Huff, "Liberation and Pleasure: Feminist Sex Shops and the Politics of Consumption," *Women's Studies* 47, no. 4 (2018): 427–46, esp. 434–36.

52. "About Good Vibrations," Good Vibrations, https://www.goodvibes.com /s/content/c/about-good-vibrations.

53. Huff, "Liberation and Pleasure," 428–29.

54. Shelly Ronen, "Gendered Morality in the Sex Toy Market: Entitlements, Reversals, and the Irony of Heterosexuality," *Sexualities*, advance online publication, 27 July 2020, https://doi.org/10.1177/1363460720914601, esp. 3, 18.

55. "Sexual Health Brand Nuelle™ Unveils Its Latest Innovation to Aid Couples Intimacy during Showstoppers at CES 2017," *Cision PR Newswire*, 5 January 2017, https://www.prnewswire.com/news-releases/sexual-health -brand-nuelle-unveils-its-latest-innovation-to-aid-couples-intimacy -during-showstoppers-at-ces-2017-300383662.html.

56. "Legalize V," Twitter, https://twitter.com/legalizev?lang=en.

57. Alyson K. Spurgas, "Interest, Arousal, and Shifting Diagnoses of Female Sexual Dysfunction, Or: How Women Learn about Desire," *Studies in Gender and Sexuality* 14, no. 3 (2013): 187–205, esp. 199. Of course, the concern about those who express "too little" sexual desire mirrors and inverts the concern about those whose sexual desires are deemed "excessive," as discussed in chapter 5. On attempts to conceptualize and treat female sexual dysfunction, see also Jennifer R. Fishman, "Manufacturing Desire: The Commodification of Female Sexual Dysfunction," *Social Studies of Science* 34, no. 2 (2004): 187–218; Loe, *Rise of Viagra*, 125–65; Thea Cacchioni, *Big Pharma, Women, and the Labour of Love* (Toronto: University of Toronto Press, 2015); Alyson K. Spurgas, *Diagnosing Desire: Biopolitics and Femininity into the Twenty-First Century* (Columbus: Ohio State University Press,

2020). I thank Jennifer Fishman for first bringing many of the issues concerning flibanserin to my attention via her presentation in a panel on "The Medicalization and Demedicalization of Sexuality" at the annual meeting of the American Sociological Association, Chicago, 22 August 2015.

58. Rob Stein, "Female Libido Pill Fires up Debate about Women and Sex," *NPR*, 16 February 2015, https://www.npr.org/sections/health-shots/2015/02/16/384043661/female-libido-pill-fires-up-debate-about-women-and-sex; Daniel Bergner, "Unexcited? There May Be a Pill for That," *New York Times Magazine*, 22 May 2013, http://www.nytimes.com/2013/05/26/magazine/unexcited-there-may-be-a-pill-for-that.html?pagewanted=all&_r=0&pagewanted=print.

59. Hylton V. Joffe et al., "FDA Approval of Flibanserin—Treating Hypoactive Sexual Desire Disorder," *New England Journal of Medicine* 374 (2015): 101–4.

60. The Sprout Pharmaceutical website is no longer retrievable. I accessed it on 10 September 2018.

61. Andrew Pollack, "'Viagra for Women' Gets Push for F.D.A. Approval," *New York Times*, 31 May 2015, B1; Jennifer Block and Liz Canner, "The 'Grassroots Campaign' for 'Female Viagra' Was Actually Funded by Its Manufacturer," *New York Magazine*, 8 September 2016, https://www.thecut.com/2016/09/how-addyi-the-female-viagra-won-fda-approval.html; Judy Z. Segal, "Sex, Drugs, and Rhetoric: The Case of Flibanserin for 'Female Sexual Dysfunction,'" *Social Studies of Science* 48, no. 4 (2018): 459–82.

62. Pollack, "Viagra for Women."

63. From http://eventhescore.org/take-action/ (accessed 11 October 2015 and no longer available).

64. "#WomenDeserve," Even the Score (YouTube video), last modified 16 October 2014, https://www.youtube.com/watch?v=KVdJ5AdmhSQ.

65. "Even The Score Marks 17th Viagra Anniversary with Release of New Letter from Members of Congress to FDA Calling for Equity in Sexual Health," *Cision PR Newswire*, 26 March 2015, http://www.prnewswire.com/news-releases/even-the-score-marks-17th-viagra-anniversary-with-release-of-new-letter-from-members-of-congress-to-fda-calling-for-equity-in-sexual-health-300056528.html.

66. Home page, New View Campaign, http://www.newviewcampaign.org.

67. Sharon Kirkey, "On the Eve of Its Release, Question Remains: Is 'Pink Viagra' Solving a Problem That Doesn't Exist?," *National Post*, 18 September 2015, https://nationalpost.com/health/on-the-eve-of-its-release-the-question-remains-if-pink-viagra-is-solving-a-problem-that-doesnt-exist; Stein, "Female Libido Pill."

68. "End Deceptive PR about Women's Sexual Health," ipetitions, https://www.ipetitions.com/petition/end-deceptive-pr-about-womens-sexual-health.

69. For a critique of the FDA approval process for flibanserin, see Segal, "Sex, Drugs."

70. Walid F. Gellad, Kathryn E. Flynn, and G. Caleb Alexander, "Evaluation of Flibanserin: Science and Advocacy at the FDA," *Journal of the American Medical Association* 314, no. 9 (2015): 869–70. In 2019 the FDA changed the boxed warning to indicate that women need not abstain altogether from alcohol but should discontinue alcohol two hours before taking the medication and not resume until the following day.

71. Andrew Pollack and Chad Bray, "Maker of Addyi, 'Female Viagra' Drug, Being Sold to Valeant for $1 Billion," *New York Times*, 21 August 2015, B1.

72. Joffe et al., "FDA Approval," 103.

73. Loes Jaspers, Frederik Feys, and Wichor Bramer, "Efficacy and Safety of Flibanserin for the Treatment of Hypoactive Sexual Desire Disorder in Women," *JAMA Internal Medicine* 176, no. 4 (2016): 453–62.

74. Sonia Sadha, "Feminists, Stop Lecturing Women about 'Female Viagra,'" *The Guardian*, 22 August 2015, https://www.theguardian.com/commentis free/2015/aug/23/female-viagra-fliibanserin-feminists-womens-sexuality.

75. Lynn Barclay, interviewed by author, 22 July 2019.

76. Laura Lorenzetti, "CEO Behind 'Female Viagra' Leaves Company after Valeant Purchase," *Fortune*, 10 December 2015, http://fortune.com/2015 /12/10/valeant-sprout-ceo-departure/; Katie Thomas and Gretchen Morgenson, "The Female Viagra, Undone by a Drug Maker's Dysfunction," *New York Times*, 9 April 2016, http://www.nytimes.com/2016/04/10/business /female-viagra-addyi-valeant-dysfunction.html. In 2019 the FDA approved another drug to treat hypoactive sexual desire disorder in women—Vyleesi, which requires auto-injection into the thigh or abdomen.

77. Steven Epstein, "Activism, Drug Regulation, and the Politics of Therapeutic Evaluation in the AIDS Era: A Case Study of ddC and the 'Surrogate Markers' Debate," *Social Studies of Science* 27, no. 5 (1997): 691–726.

78. Spurgas, *Diagnosing Desire*, 66. Spurgas adds that "it is more useful to critique the gendered foundation upon which these sexual dysfunction drugs operate than the marketing of the drugs or corporate 'profiteering'" (94).

79. The discussion that follows is based on documents that appeared at http:// healthysexual.tumblr.com (accessed 21 March 2017 but no longer available). I am grateful to Kristen Schilt for pointing me to this website.

80. Héctor Carrillo and Amanda Hoffman, "'Straight with a Pinch of Bi': The Construction of Heterosexuality as an Elastic Category among Adult US Men," *Sexualities* 21 (2017): 90–108; J. E. Sumerau, Lain A. B. Mathers, and Dawne Moon, "Foreclosing Fluidity at the Intersection of Gender and Sexual Normativities," *Symbolic Interaction* 43, no. 2 (2019): 205–34.

81. On "looping effects" and "making up people," see Ian Hacking, "Kinds of People: Moving Targets," *Journal of the British Academy* 151 (2007): 285–318.

82. See chapter 3, note 25.

83. @pupbones, "I am a Truvada Whore," My PrEP Experience, 28 March 2014, http://myprepexperience.blogspot.com/2014/03/i-am-truvada-whore

.html; Christopher Glazek, "Why I Am a Truvada Whore," *OUT Magazine*, 20 May 2014, http://www.out.com/entertainment/popnography/2014 /05/20/why-i-am-truvada-whore; Tim Dean, "Mediated Intimacies: Raw Sex, Truvada, and the Biopolitics of Chemoprophylaxis," *Sexualities* 18, nos. 1–2 (2015): 224–46; Kane Race, "Reluctant Objects: Sexual Pleasure as a Problem for HIV Biomedical Prevention," *GLQ* 22, no. 1 (2016): 1–31.

84. Ronald O. Valdiserri and David R. Holtgrave, "Pre-Exposure Prophylaxis for HIV Infection: Preventing Disease or Promoting Sexual Health?," *Journal of Community Health* 44 (2019): 423–27, esp. 423, 426. See also Walter Gómez, Ian W. Holloway, David W. Pantalone, and Christian Grov, "PrEP Uptake as a Social Movement among Gay and Bisexual Men," *Culture, Health & Sexuality*, advance online publication, 29 October 2020, https:// doi.org/10.1080/13691058.2020.1831075.

85. On cost and insurance barriers and disparities of access, see Valdiserri and Holtgrave, "Pre-Exposure Prophylaxis."

86. Renato Barucco, "Beyond "Poz" and "Neg": Five HIV Statuses, Plus a New One," *Huffington Post*, 27 March 2014, http://www.huffingtonpost.com /renato-barucco/beyond-poz-and-neg-five-h_b_5039729.html.

87. Cary Courtenay-Quirk et al., "Is HIV/AIDS Stigma Dividing the Gay Community? Perceptions of HIV-Positive Men Who Have Sex with Men," *AIDS Education and Prevention* 18, no. 1 (2006): 56–67; Dean, "Mediated Intimacies," 241.

88. Asha Persson, "'The World Has Changed': Pharmaceutical Citizenship and the Reimagining of Serodiscordant Sexuality among Couples with Mixed HIV Status in Australia," *Sociology of Health & Illness* 38, no. 3 (2016): 380–95.

89. Jason Orne and James Gall, "Converting, Monitoring, and Policing PrEP Citizenship: Biosexual Citizenship and the PrEP Surveillance Machine," *Surveillance & Society* 17, no. 5 (2019): 641–61, esp. 642. On biosexual citizenship, see chapter 9.

90. Lauren Suchman, "HIV Pre-Exposure Prophylaxis (PrEP) for Women: Claiming Risk and Recognizing Responsibility to End the AIDS Epidemic in New York," *Journal of Health and Social Sciences* 5, no. 3 (2020): 501–12.

91. Juan Michael Porter, II, "'PrEP for Women Too' Campaign Aims to Bring This Empowering HIV Prevention Tool to More Black and Latinx Women," *The BodyPro*, 5 November 2020, https://www.thebodypro.com/article /prep-for-women-too-campaign-hiv-prevention-black-latinx-women.

92. Linda Goler Blount and Oni J. Blackstock, "'Let's Talk about PrEP' Targets Black Women for HIV Prevention," *NBC News*, 17 February 2016, https:// www.nbcnews.com/news/nbcblk/let-s-talk-about-prep-targets-black -women-hiv-prevention-n504731; Porter, "PrEP for Women."

93. "Ready, Set, PrEP," US Department of Health and Human Services, https:// www.hiv.gov/federal-response/ending-the-hiv-epidemic/prep-program.

94. Clay Davis, "*Homo Adhaerens*: Risk and Adherence in Biomedical HIV Pre-
     vention Research," *Social Studies of Science* 50, no. 6 (2020): 860–80, esp. 863.
     Potential marketing of long-acting injectable forms of PrEP may shift the
     dynamics of adherence.

CHAPTER NINE

1.   Nahal Toosi and Dan Diamond, "Trump's State Department Eyes Ban on
     Terms Like 'Sexual Health,'" *Politico*, 31 October 2018, https://www.poli
     tico.com/story/2018/10/31/state-department-ban-terms-sexual-health
     -907134.
2.   Robbie Gramer and Colum Lynch, "Inside Trump's Plans to Scale Back U.N.
     Resolutions on Sexual Health, Violence against Women," *Foreign Policy*,
     30 October 2018, https://foreignpolicy.com/2018/10/30/inside-trump
     -state-department-plan-to-scale-back-united-nations-resolutions-on-sex
     ual-reproductive-health-violence-against-women-abortion-global-gag
     -rule-gender-equality/.
3.   Ibid.
4.   Erica L. Green, Katie Benner, and Robert Pear, "Trump May Limit How
     Government Defines One's Sex," *New York Times*, 21 October 2018, A1.
5.   This policy was first established in 1984 by Ronald Reagan, rescinded by
     Bill Clinton in 1993, put back in place by George W. Bush in 2001, rescinded
     again by Barack Obama in 2009, and then reinstated and expanded by
     Donald Trump in 2017. "Sexual Health and Reproductive Rights at a Cross-
     road," *Lancet* 390 (2017): 1. The policy was then rescinded by Joe Biden in
     2021.
6.   The Trump administration also faced pushback from other nations. See
     Edith M. Lederer, "US Fails to Weaken UN References to Sexual Health,"
     Associated Press, 16 November 2018, https://www.apnews.com/7be9101de1
     77451ca33dfc61983d8ff5.
7.   Office of the Surgeon General, *The Surgeon General's Call to Action to Promote
     Responsible Sexual Health and Responsible Sexual Behavior* (Washington, DC:
     US Department of Health and Human Services, 9 July 2001), http://www
     .ncbi.nlm.nih.gov/pubmed/20669514.
8.   National Prevention Council, *National Prevention Strategy* (Washington,
     DC: Office of the Surgeon General, US Department of Health and Human
     Services, 2011).
9.   While I emphasize the role of the federal government, it is worth noting
     that city and state governments have also pursued the goal of strategic
     planning around sexual health and have issued policy documents.
10. Kimberly J. Morgan and Ann Shola Orloff, eds., *The Many Hands of the State:
     Theorizing Political Authority and Social Control* (New York: Cambridge Uni-
     versity Press, 2017).

11. Kimberly J. Morgan and Ann Shola Orloff, "Introduction: The Many Hands of the State," in Morgan and Orloff, *Many Hands*, 1–32, esp. 3.

12. Elisabeth S. Clemens and James M. Cook, "Politics and Institutionalism: Explaining Durability and Change," *Annual Review of Sociology* 25, no. 1 (1999): 441–66, esp. 443. See also Philip Abrams, "Notes on the Difficulty of Studying the State (1977)," *Journal of Historical Sociology* 1, no. 1 (1988): 58–89; Timothy Mitchell, "Society, Economy, and the State Effect," in *Culture: State-Formation after the Cultural Turn*, ed. George Steinmetz (Ithaca, NY: Cornell University Press, 1999), 76–97; Patrick Joyce and Chandra Mukerji, "The State of Things: State History and Theory Reconfigured," *Theory and Society* 46 (2017): 1–19.

13. Morgan and Orloff, "Introduction," 17.

14. Steven Shapin and Simon Schaffer, *Leviathan and the Air-Pump: Hobbes, Boyle and the Experimental Life* (Princeton, NJ: Princeton University Press, 1985); Sheila Jasanoff, *Designs on Nature: Science and Democracy in Europe and the United States* (Princeton, NJ: Princeton University Press, 2005); Patrick Carroll, *Science, Culture, and Modern State Formation* (Berkeley: University of California Press, 2006).

15. On governmentality and the "conduct of conduct," see Michel Foucault, *Security, Territory, Population: Lectures at the Collège de France, 1977–78* (Houndmills, UK: Palgrave Macmillan, 2007); Thomas Lemke, "Foucault, Governmentality, and Critique," *Rethinking Marxism* 14, no. 3 (2002): 49–64.

16. Mark Wolfson, *The Fight against Big Tobacco: The Movement, the State, and the Public's Health* (New York: Aldine de Gruyter, 2001); John David Skrentny, *The Minority Rights Revolution* (Cambridge, MA: Harvard University Press, 2002), 5.

17. Margot Canaday, *The Straight State: Sexuality and Citizenship in Twentieth-Century America* (Princeton, NJ: Princeton University Press, 2009). See also Lisa Duggan, "Queering the State," *Social Text*, no. 39 (1994): 1–14; Kristin Luker, "Sex, Social Hygiene, and the State: The Double-Edged Sword of Social Reform," *Theory and Society* 27, no. 5 (1998): 601–34.

18. Stefan Vogler, *Sorting Sexualities: Expertise and the Politics of Legal Classification* (Chicago: University of Chicago Press, 2021). On the role of state surveillance practices in the production of gender and sexual identities, see also Toby Beauchamp, *Going Stealth: Transgender Politics and U.S. Surveillance Practices* (Durham, NC: Duke University Press, 2019).

19. Jyoti Puri, *Sexual States: Governance and the Struggle over the Antisodomy Law in India* (Durham, NC: Duke University Press, 2016), 10, 13.

20. In general terms, citizenship refers to differentiated modes of incorporation of individuals or groups fully or partially into a polity through the articulation of notions of rights and responsibilities. See Stuart Hall and David Held, "Citizens and Citizenship," in *New Times: The Changing Face of Politics in the 1990s*, ed. Stuart Hall and Martin Jacques (London: Verso,

1990), 173–88; Gershon Shafir, ed., *The Citizenship Debates: A Reader* (Minneapolis: University of Minnesota Press, 1998).

21.   Claire Rasmussen and Michael Brown, "Radical Democratic Citizenship: Amidst Political Theory and Geography," in *Handbook of Citizenship Studies*, ed. Engin F. Isin and Bryan S. Turner (London: Sage, 2002), 175–88, esp. 179.

22.   Carole Pateman, "Equality, Difference, Subordination: The Politics of Motherhood and Women's Citizenship," in *Beyond Equality and Difference: Citizenship, Feminist Politics, and Female Subjectivity*, ed. Gisela Bock and Susan James (New York: Routledge, 1992), 17–31; Melissa Nobles, *Shades of Citizenship: Race and the Census in Modern Politics* (Stanford, CA: Stanford University Press, 2000); Steven Epstein and Héctor Carrillo, "Immigrant Sexual Citizenship: Intersectional Templates among Mexican Gay Immigrants to the United States," *Citizenship Studies* 18, nos. 3–4 (2014): 259–76.

23.   Aaron T. Norton, "Cutting the Risk: The Emergence of Male Circumcision Status as an HIV-Risk Reduction Strategy" (PhD diss., University of California, Davis, 2014), 193–237, esp. 196. I draw here on my approach to citizenship, biocitizenship, sexual citizenship, and biosexual citizenship as presented in Steven Epstein, "Governing Sexual Health: Bridging Biocitizenship and Sexual Citizenship," in *Biocitizenship: The Politics of Bodies, Governance, and Power*, ed. Kelly Happe, Jenell Johnson, and Marina Levina (New York: NYU Press, 2018), 21–50.

24.   As Diane Richardson has described, sexual citizenship and sexual rights are concepts that overlap but do not coincide; moreover, the two have different "historical configuration[s] and disciplinary origin[s]." Diane Richardson, *Sexuality and Citizenship* (Cambridge, England: Polity Press, 2018), 33. On sexual rights, see the discussion in chapter 3 as well as chapter 2, note 22.

25.   Epstein and Carrillo, "Immigrant Sexual Citizenship." On sexual citizenship, see also Jeffrey Weeks, "The Sexual Citizen," *Theory, Culture & Society* 15, nos. 3–4 (1998): 35–52; David Bell and Jon Binnie, *The Sexual Citizen: Queer Politics and Beyond* (Cambridge, England: Polity, 2000); Diane Richardson, *Rethinking Sexuality* (London: Sage, 2000), 86–115; Carl F. Stychin, "Sexual Citizenship in the European Union," *Citizenship Studies* 5, no. 3 (2001): 285–301; Ken Plummer, *Intimate Citizenship* (Seattle: University of Washington Press, 2003); Richardson, *Sexuality and Citizenship*. On "recentering" sexual citizenship beyond the global North, see Sharyn Graham Davies, "Sexual Citizenship Re-Centred: Gender and Sexuality Diversity in Indonesia," in *The Sage Handbook of Global Sexualities*, ed. Zowie Davy et al. (London: Sage, 2020).

26.   Barbara Cruikshank, *The Will to Empower: Democratic Citizens and Other Subjects* (Ithaca, NY: Cornell University Press, 1999), 2.

27.   For a useful overview, see Torsten Heinemann, "Biological Citizenship," in *Encyclopedia of Global Bioethics*, ed. Henk Ten Have (New York: Springer,

2015), http://link.springer.com/referenceworkentry/10.1007/978-3-319
-05544-2_453-1. See also Adriana Petryna, *Life Exposed: Biological Citizens
after Chernobyl* (Princeton, NJ: Princeton University Press, 2002), 5; Deborah Heath, Rayna Rapp, and Karen-Sue Taussig, "Genetic Citizenship," in
A Companion to the Anthropology of Politics, ed. David Nugent and Joan Vincent (London: Blackwell, 2004), 152–67; Nikolas Rose and Carlos Novas,
"Biological Citizenship," in *Global Assemblages: Technology, Politics, and Ethics
as Anthropological Problems*, ed. Aihwa Ong and Stephen J. Collier (Malden,
MA: Blackwell, 2005), 439–63, esp. 445–46; Steven Epstein, *Inclusion: The
Politics of Difference in Medical Research* (Chicago: University of Chicago
Press, 2007), esp. 21.

28. Jonathan M. Metzl, "Introduction: Why against Health?," in *Against Health:
How Health Became the New Morality*, ed. Jonathan M. Metzl and Anna Kirkland (New York: NYU Press, 2010), 1–11, esp. 6–7.

29. Office of the Surgeon General, *Surgeon General's Call*, 24–25. See also John
Bancroft, "Promoting Responsible Sexual Behavior," *Sexual and Relationship
Therapy* 17, no. 1 (2002): 9–12; Alain Giami, "Sexual Health: The Emergence,
Development, and Diversity of a Concept," *Annual Review of Sex Research* 13
(2002): 1–35, esp. 21.

30. In a public statement, Elders had proposed teaching children that masturbation could be a way of avoiding HIV infection. Critics portrayed her as
having proposed that children be taught how to masturbate in sex education classes. Douglas Jehl, "Surgeon General Forced to Resign by White
House," *New York Times*, 10 December 1994, A1.

31. Eli Coleman, interviewed by author, 11 July 2019. I was not able to verify
this account with Dr. Satcher, who declined to be interviewed for this book.

32. Bancroft, "Promoting Responsible," 10.

33. Office of the Surgeon General, *Surgeon General's Call*, ii, 10, 15.

34. Giami, "Sexual Health," 23. For more positive takes on the report's focus
on responsibility, see Weston M. Edwards and Eli Coleman, "Defining Sexual Health: A Descriptive Overview," *Archives of Sexual Behavior* 33, no. 3
(2004): 189–95, esp. 193; Bancroft, "Promoting Responsible," 12.

35. World Health Organization, *Defining Sexual Health: Report of a Technical
Consultation on Sexual Health, 28–31 January 2002, Geneva* (Geneva: World
Health Organization, 2006), 1.

36. Jessie V. Ford et al., "The Need to Promote Sexual Health in America: A
New Vision for Public Health Action," *Sexually Transmitted Diseases* 44,
no. 10 (2017): 579–85, esp. 579–80.

37. Office of the Surgeon General, *Surgeon General's Call*, ii.

38. Ibid., 1.

39. On neoliberalism, see chapter 8, note 21.

40. Dorothy Roberts, *Killing the Black Body: Race, Reproduction, and the Meaning
of Liberty*, 2nd ed. (New York: Vintage, 2017).

41.   Teresa Kominos, "What Do Marriage and Welfare Reform Really Have in Common? A Look into TANF Marriage Promotion Programs," *Journal of Civil Rights and Economic Development* 21, no. 3 (2007): 915–45, esp. 916–17.

42.   David Satcher, "Addressing Sexual Health: Looking Back, Looking Forward," *Public Health Reports* 128, suppl. 1 (2013): 111–14.

43.   Andrea Swartzendruber and Jonathan M. Zenilman, "A National Strategy to Improve Sexual Health," *Journal of the American Medical Association* 304, no. 9 (2010): 1005–6.

44.   "Leading Health Indicators," Healthy People 2010, http://www.healthy people.gov/2010/Document/html/uih/uih_bw/uih_4.htm. The previous version, "Healthy People 2000," had no equivalent category, although "HIV infection" and "sexually transmitted diseases" were included in the list of twenty-two priority areas. "Healthy People 2000 Priority Areas," Centers for Disease Control and Prevention, http://www.cdc.gov/nchs /healthy_people/hp2000/hp2000_priority_areas.htm.

45.   "Reproductive and Sexual Health," Healthy People 2020, https://www .healthypeople.gov/2020/leading-health-indicators/2020-lhi-topics /Reproductive-and-Sexual-Health.

46.   Office of National AIDS Policy, National HIV/AIDS Strategy for the United States (Washington, DC: White House, 2010). See also Kevin A. Fenton, "Time for Change: Rethinking and Reframing Sexual Health in the United States," *Journal of Sexual Medicine* 7, suppl. 5 (2010): 250–52, esp. 250.

47.   National Prevention Council, *National Prevention Strategy*. The other six health priorities were tobacco-free living, preventing drug abuse and excessive alcohol use, healthy eating, active living, injury- and violence-free living, and mental and emotional well-being.

48.   Ibid., 44.

49.   Ibid., 46–47.

50.   Kevin Fenton, interviewed by author, 12 July 2019; "Kevin Fenton," Wikipedia, accessed 21 February 2021, https://en.wikipedia.org/wiki/Kevin _Fenton.

51.   Fenton, interview.

52.   Centers for Disease Control and Prevention, *A Public Health Approach for Advancing Sexual Health in the United States: Rationale and Options for Implementation* (Atlanta: US Department of Health and Human Services, December 2010), 10, 33.

53.   Fenton, interview.

54.   John M. Douglas and Kevin A. Fenton, "Understanding Sexual Health and Its Role in More Effective Prevention Programs," *Public Health Reports* 128, suppl. 1 (2013): 1–4, esp. 1.

55.   CDC/HRSA Advisory Committee on HIV, *Viral Hepatitis and STD Prevention and Treatment: Record of the Proceedings* (Atlanta: US Department of Health and Human Services, 8–9 May 2012).

56. Fenton, interview.

57. State-level statutes from recent decades that criminalize sexual contact by HIV-positive individuals in the name of public health hark back to the regulation of sex workers and the policing and condemnation of male same-sex activity in the social hygiene era. However, as I suggested in chapter 3, criminalization is not so much an example of sexual health governance as it is an alternative paradigm. See Trevor Hoppe, "Controlling Sex in the Name of 'Public Health': Social Control and Michigan HIV Law," *Social Problems* 60, no. 1 (2013): 27–49.

58. Julian B. Carter, *The Heart of Whiteness: Normal Sexuality and Race in America, 1880–1940* (Durham, NC: Duke University Press, 2007), 152.

59. Fenton, interview.

60. See also Emily Mann, "Regulating Latina Youth Sexualities through Community Health Centers: Discourses and Practices of Sexual Citizenship," *Gender & Society* 27, no. 5 (2013): 681–703.

61. Juan Battle and Sandra L. Barnes, eds., *Black Sexualities: Probing Powers, Practices, Passions, and Policies* (New Brunswick, NJ: Rutgers University Press, 2010).

62. Jenny Dyck Brian, Patrick R. Grzanka, and Emily S. Mann, "The Age of LARC: Making Sexual Citizens on the Frontiers of Technoscientific Healthism," *Health Sociology Review* 29, no. 3 (2020), 312–28, esp. 316, 322–23. I also discuss this example in chapter 3.

63. Chris A. Barcelos, *Distributing Condoms and Hope: The Racialized Politics of Youth Sexual Health* (Berkeley: University of California Press, 2020), esp. 197.

64. On the rise of a concept of sexual rights, see chapter 3, as well as chapter 2, note 22.

65. On the "interpenetration" of social movements and the state, see Wolfson, *Fight against Big Tobacco*, 7, 144–45.

66. John D'Emilio and Estelle B. Freedman, *Intimate Matters: A History of Sexuality in America* (New York: Harper & Row, 1988), 205.

67. CDC, *Public Health Approach*, 33.

68. Michael R. (Bob) MacDonald, "Sexual Health and Responsibility Program (SHARP): Preventing HIV, STIs, and Unplanned Pregnancies in the Navy and Marine Corps," *Public Health Reports* 128, suppl. 1 (2013): 81–88, esp. 82.

69. Ibid., 87.

70. On the rise and consequences of these efforts, see Epstein, *Inclusion*.

71. "National CLAS Standards," US Department of Health and Human Services, https://www.thinkculturalhealth.hhs.gov/clas.

72. Steven Epstein, "Sexualizing Governance and Medicalizing Identities: The Emergence of 'State-Centered' LGBT Health Politics in the United States," *Sexualities* 6, no. 2 (2003): 131–71; Kenneth H. Mayer et al., "Sexual and Gender Minority Health: What We Know and What Needs to Be Done," *American Journal of Public Health* 98, no. 6 (2008): 989–95. On the

outsider-citizen distinction in LGBTQ politics, see Seidman, "From Outsider to Citizen."

73.   Institute of Medicine Committee on Lesbian, Gay, Bisexual, and Trans-
       gender Health Issues and Research Gaps and Opportunities, *The Health of
       Lesbian, Gay, Bisexual, and Transgender People: Building a Foundation for Better
       Understanding* (Washington, DC: National Academies Press, 2011); Wil-
       liam Byne, "A New Era for LGBT Health," *LGBT Health* 1, no. 1 (2013): 1–3;
       Rashada Alexander, Karen Parker, and Tara Schwetz, "Sexual and Gender
       Minority Health Research at the National Institutes of Health," *LGBT
       Health* 3, no. 1 (2016): 7–10.

74.   National Institutes of Health Sexual and Gender Minority Research Coor-
       dinating Committee, *NIH FY 2016–20 Strategic Plan to Advance Research on
       the Health and Well-Being of Sexual and Gender Minorities* (Bethesda, MD: US
       Department of Health and Human Services, n.d. [ca. 2013]); Alexander
       et al., "Sexual and Gender"; "Appointment of Dr. Karen L. Parker as Direc-
       tor of the Sexual & Gender Minority Research Office, NIH," National Insti-
       tutes of Health, last modified 30 June 2017, https://dpcpsi.nih.gov/sgmro
       /directorsannouncement.

75.   Eliseo J. Pérez-Stable, "Sexual and Gender Minorities Formally Designated
       as a Health Disparity Population for Research Purposes," National Insti-
       tute on Minority Health and Health Disparities, National Institutes of
       Health, 6 October 2016, https://www.nimhd.nih.gov/about/directors
       -corner/messages/message_10-06-16.html. On the consolidation of sexual
       orientation and gender identity into health data infrastructures during
       the Obama years, see Stephen Molldrem, "Remaking Biomedical Sexu-
       alities: Health Technologies and the Governance of HIV in the United
       States" (PhD diss., University of Michigan, 2019), 208–86.

76.   "National Institutes of Health Pride 2016 Observance," National Institutes
       of Health Office of Equity, Diversity, and Inclusion, https://www.edi.nih
       .gov/people/sep/lgbti/pride-2016.

77.   These include organizations such as the Gay and Lesbian Medical Asso-
       ciation and advocacy and research projects organized by the Fenway In-
       stitute in Boston. The increasing attention to SGM health and health
       disparities has also been accompanied and furthered by the founding of
       a new medical journal, *LGBT Health*, and it has been taken up by health
       insurers as a demonstration of their commitment to equity, diversity, and
       inclusion.

78.   Epstein, "Sexualizing Governance."

79.   Here I leave to one side the complex question of how sexual health agen-
       das may differ for specific sexual and gender minority groups—and
       whether the concerns of some, such as bisexuals, genderqueer, and trans-
       gender people, become obscured when subsumed within larger concat-
       enations such as "LGBTQ" or "SGM."

80. Institute of Medicine, *Health of LGBT People*, chs. 5–6.
81. This framework may be both enabling and constraining for LGBTQ individuals and social movement organizations. Although inclusion may be preferable to its opposite, a particular risk here is that of reifying gender and sexual identity categories—solidifying a sense of the biopsychological "naturalness" of these categories while eliding the many potential slippages between identity, desire, and behavior. Epstein, "Sexualizing Governance."
82. "GLMA Statement on HHS Secretary Selection," GLMA, http://glma.org /index.cfm?fuseaction=Feature.showFeature&CategoryID=1&FeatureID =798. Price served as secretary of Health and Human Services only from February to September 2017 and left office following widespread criticism of his use of chartered and military planes for travel.
83. Jamie O'Quinn and Jessica Fields, "The Future of Evidence: Queerness in Progressive Visions of Sexuality Education," *Sexuality Research & Social Policy* 17 (2020): 175–87.
84. Scott Schoettes, "Trump Doesn't Care about HIV. We're Outta Here," *Newsweek*, 16 June 2017, http://www.newsweek.com/trump-doesnt-care-about -hiv-were-outta-here-626285; Callum Paton, "Trump Fires HIV/AIDS Council in Its Entirety by Fedex Letter, Report Claims," *Newsweek*, 29 December 2017, https://www.newsweek.com/trump-fires-hivaids-council -its-entirety-fedex-letter-report-claims-763737.
85. Alex M. Azar II, "Remarks on Universal Health Coverage," in *U.N. General Assembly Press, New York City, NY* (Washington, DC: US Department of Health and Human Services, 2019).
86. Divya Mallampati, "Evolving State-Based Contraceptive and Abortion Policies," *JAMA* 317, no. 24 (2017): 2481–82.
87. "HHS Denial of Care Rule FAQ," Lambda Legal, https://www.lambdalegal .org/faq_hhs-denial-of-care. See also Gilbert Gonzales and Tara McKay, "What an Emerging Trump Administration Means for Lesbian, Gay, Bisexual, and Transgender Health," *Health Equity* 1, no. 1 (2017): 83–86; William Byne, "Sustaining Progress toward LGBT Health Equity: A Time for Vigilance, Advocacy, and Scientific Inquiry," *LGBT Health* 4, no. 1 (2017): 1–3.
88. Allegra Kirkland, "The CDC Abruptly Cancelled an LGBT Youth Health Summit after Trump Got Elected," *Talking Points Memo*, 26 January 2017, http://www.businessinsider.com/cdc-trump-lgbt-2017-1.
89. Alfredo Morabia, "Notes from the Editor-in-Chief: Who Wants to Exclude Older LGBT Persons from Public Health Surveillance?," *American Journal of Public Health* 107, no. 6 (2017): 844–45.
90. Sean R. Cahill and Harvey J. Makadon, "If They Don't Count Us, We Don't Count: Trump Administration Rolls Back Sexual Orientation and Gender Identity Data Collection," *LGBT Health* 4, no. 3 (2017): 171–73; "Sexual Orientation Questions Added Back into National Survey of LGBT Older Adults,"

Rainbow Times, 23 June 2017, http://www.therainbowtimesmass.com/sex
ual-orientation-questions-added-back-national-survey-lgbt-older-adults/.

91.   Christopher Ingraham, "The Military Spends Five Times as Much on
Viagra as It Would on Transgender Troops' Medical Care," *Washington Post*,
26 July 2017, https://www.washingtonpost.com/news/wonk/wp/2017/07
/26/the-military-spends-five-times-as-much-on-viagra-as-it-would-on
-transgender-troops-medical-care/. (While the article headline notes that
the military spends five time as much on Viagra, the article text clarifies
that the amount spent is actually ten times as much when all erectile
dysfunction medications are considered.)

92.   Lena H. Sun and Juliet Eilperin, "CDC Gets List of Forbidden Words: Fetus,
Transgender, Diversity," *Washington Post*, 15 December 2017, https://www
.washingtonpost.com/national/health-science/cdc-gets-list-of-forbidden
-words-fetus-transgender-diversity/2017/12/15/f503837a-e1cf-11e7-89e8
-edec16379010_story.html?utm_term=.acd319bd2f76.

93.   Elizabeth Cohen, "The Truth about Those 7 Words 'Banned' at the CDC,"
CNN, 31 January 2018, https://edition.cnn.com/2018/01/11/health/cdc
-word-ban-hhs-document/index.html.

94.   "Leading Health Indicators," Healthy People 2030, https://health.gov
/healthypeople/objectives-and-data/leading-health-indicators; "LGBT,"
Healthy People 2030, https://health.gov/healthypeople/objectives-and
-data/browse-objectives/lgbt; "Sexually Transmitted Infections," Healthy
People 2030, https://health.gov/healthypeople/objectives-and-data
/browse-objectives/sexually-transmitted-infections.

95.   "Strategic Plan FY 2018–2022," US Department of Health and Human
Services, last modified 28 February 2018, https://www.hhs.gov/about
/strategic-plan/index.html. Previous strategic plans are available at "Divi-
sion of Strategic Planning," US Department of Health and Human Services, https://aspe.hhs.gov/strategic-planning.

96.   See also Jordan Dashow, "HHS Strategic Plan Removes All Mentions of
LGBTQ People and Health Disparities," 3 October 2017, https://www.hrc
.org/blog/hhs-strategic-plan-removes-all-mentions-of-lgbtq-people-and
-health-disparit.

97.   On symbolic boundaries, see Michèle Lamont and Virág Molnár, "The
Study of Boundaries in the Social Sciences," *Annual Review of Sociology* 28,
no. 1 (2002): 167–95. On the maintenance, as well as the shifting over
time, of moral boundaries between accepted and forbidden sexualities,
see Gayle S. Rubin, "Thinking Sex: Notes for a Radical Theory of the Politics of Sexuality," in *Pleasure and Danger: Exploring Female Sexuality*, ed. Carole S. Vance (New York: Routledge, 1984), 267–318.

98.   Epstein, "Governing Sexual Health," 35.

99.   Michelle Yee Hee Lee, "Donald Trump's False Comments Connecting Mexican Immigrants and Crime," *Washington Post*, 8 July 2015, https://www

.washingtonpost.com/news/fact-checker/wp/2015/07/08/donald-trumps
-false-comments-connecting-mexican-immigrants-and-crime/?utm
_term=.87573c5cfc2a.

100. Michel Foucault, *The History of Sexuality, Volume 1: An Introduction*, trans. Robert Hurley (New York: Vintage Books, 1980), 12.

101. See Gil Eyal, *The Crisis of Expertise* (Cambridge, England: Polity, 2019).

102. More generally, on the historical shift toward the use of quantification and formal methods as a solution to the problem of distrust of experts in the United States, see Theodore M. Porter, *Trust in Numbers: The Pursuit of Objectivity in Science and Public Life* (Princeton, NJ: Princeton University Press, 1995).

103. CDC, *Public Health Approach*, 6, 10; MacDonald, "Sexual Health and Responsibility," 84; Megan B. Ivankovich, Kevin A. Fenton, and John M. Douglas, "Considerations for National Public Health Leadership in Advancing Sexual Health," *Public Health Reports* 128, suppl. 1 (2013): 102–10, esp. 105.

104. Megan B. Ivankovich, Jami S. Leichliter, and John M. Douglas, "Measurement of Sexual Health in the U.S.: An Inventory of Nationally Representative Surveys and Surveillance Systems," *Public Health Reports* 128, suppl. 1 (2013): 62–72.

105. Fenton, "Time for Change," 251.

106. See, for example, Jeffrey S. Becasen, Jessie Ford, and Matthew Hogben, "Sexual Health Interventions: A Meta-Analysis," *Journal of Sex Research* 52, no. 4 (2015): 433–43.

107. Fenton, interview.

108. Sun and Eilperin, "CDC Gets List."

109. Lawrence O. Gostin, "Language, Science, and Politics: The Politicization of Public Health," *JAMA* 319, no. 6 (2018): 541–42.

110. For critical discussion, see Susan Kippax, "Sexual Health Interventions Are Unsuitable for Experimental Evaluation," in *Effective Sexual Health Interventions: Issues in Experimental Evaluation*, ed. Judith M. Stephenson, John Imrie, and Chris Bonell (Oxford: Oxford University Press, 2003), 17–34; Judith D. Auerbach, Juston O. Parkhurst, and Carlos F. Cáceres, "Addressing Social Drivers of HIV/AIDS for the Longterm Response: Conceptual and Methodological Considerations," *Global Public Health* 6, suppl. 3 (2011): S293–S309; Adam Isaiah Green, "Keeping Gay and Bisexual Men Safe: The Arena of HIV Prevention Science and Praxis," *Social Studies of Science* 46, no. 2 (2016): 210–35. For critical reflections on evidence and the authority of science in sexual health education, see O'Quinn and Fields, "Future of Evidence."

111. Barbara Klugman, "Complexity versus the Technical Fix or How to Put Sexuality Back into Sexual Health," *Global Public Health* 9, no. 6 (2014): 653–60.

112.   Steven Epstein, "The New Attack on Sexuality Research: Morality and the Politics of Knowledge Production," *Sexuality Research and Social Policy* 3, no. 1 (2006): 1–12.

113.   Sexual and Gender Minority Research Office, *Sexual and Gender Minority Populations in NIH-Supported Research*, Notice Number NOT-OD-19-139 (Bethesda, MD: National Institutes of Health, 28 August 2019).

114.   Sexual and Gender Minority Research Office, *Strategic Plan to Advance Research on the Health and Well-Being of Sexual and Gender Minorities: Fiscal Years 2021–2025* (Bethesda, MD: National Institutes of Health, 2020).

115.   "NIH Pride 2020," National Institutes of Health, https://www.edi.nih.gov /people/sep/lgbti/pride-2020.

116.   For example, the draft referred only once to "sexual and gender minorities," while the final version does so six times. The draft also failed to reference contraception, while the final version does so once. *Sexually Transmitted Infections National Strategic Plan for the United States: 2021–2025* (Washington, DC: US Department of Health and Human Services, 2020), https:// www.hhs.gov/programs/topic-sites/sexually-transmitted-infections/plan -overview/index.html.

117.   "LGBT," Healthy People 2030.

118.   David T. Huang et al., "Seven Prevention Priorities of USPHS Scientist Officers," *American Journal of Public Health* 107, no. 1 (2017): 39–40.

119.   Katie Keith, "Court Vacates New 1557 Rule That Would Roll Back Antidiscrimination Protections for LGBT Individuals," *Health Affairs Blog*, 18 August 2020, https://www.healthaffairs.org/do/10.1377/hblog20200818 .468025/full/.

120.   Ford et al., "Need to Promote," 580.

121.   Giami, "Sexual Health," 25–30.

122.   From the 1994 Canadian Guidelines for Sexual Health Education, quoted in Ilsa Lottes, "New Perspectives on Sexual Health," in *New Views on Sexual Health: The Case of Finland*, ed. Ilsa Lottes and Osmo Kontula (Helsinki: Population Research Institute, Family Federation of Finland, 2000), 7–28, esp. 20.

123.   A volume by Tony Sandset and coauthors, published just as I was completing this one, analyzes the representations of sexual health in the recent policy documents of six European countries: Norway, England, Denmark, France, Sweden, and Ireland. Tony Sandset, Eivind Engebretsen, and Kristin Heggen, *Sustainable Sexual Health: Analyzing the Implementation of the SDGs* (Oxford, UK: Routledge, 2020), ch. 5. The authors locate these national plans in a global context by linking them to the United Nations' Sustainable Development Goals. Consistent with my analysis of sexual health governance in the United States, they find in these documents "the near-absolute absence of pleasure as part of sexual health" (84). Their

analysis also aligns with mine in their critical discussion of the use of metrics (117).

124. Giami, "Sexual Health," 26–27.

125. Inuit Five-Year Strategic Plan on Sexual Health (Ottawa: Pauktuuit Inuit Women of Canada, 2010), https://www.pauktuutit.ca/project/inuit-five -year-strategic-plan-sexual-health/.

126. Jennifer M. Piscopo, "Female Leadership and Sexual Health Policy in Argentina," *Latin American Research Review* 49, no. 1 (2014): 104–27.

127. "National Document on Sexual Health Training Being Prepared," *Tehran Times*, 15 January 2019, https://www.tehrantimes.com/news/431887 /National-document-on-sexual-health-training-being-prepared.

128. Tracy Morison and Sarah Herbert, "Rethinking 'Risk' in Sexual and Reproductive Health Policy: The Value of the Reproductive Justice Framework," *Sexuality Research & Social Policy* 16 (2019): 434–45.

129. Kevin Fenton made this observation at the National Sexual Health Conference (author's field notes, 10 July 2019, Chicago). See "A Framework for Sexual Health Improvement in England," Gov.UK, https://www.gov.uk /government/publications/a-framework-for-sexual-health-improvement -in-england.

130. For a model of such comparative analysis in a different context, see Sheila Jasanoff's discussion of nation-specific "civic epistemologies." Jasanoff, *Designs on Nature*, ch. 10. In contrast with these national projects are moves toward what we might call *transnational* sexual health governance—the outgrowth of the definitional, classificatory, and policy-making work of the WHO that I have described in previous chapters.

131. In 2016, California became the third state, after Vermont and Mississippi, to provide condoms to prisoners. Joe Watson, "Condoms Now Available to Prisoners in Three States," *Prison Legal News*, September 2016, https:// www.prisonlegalnews.org/news/2016/sep/2/condoms-now-available -prisoners-three-states/. On sexual health in prisons, see also James Horley, "Sexuality and Sexual Health in Prisons," *Sexuality & Culture* 23 (2019): 1372–86.

132. Sheila Jasanoff and Sang-Hyun Kim, "Containing the Atom: Sociotechnical Imaginaries and Nuclear Power in the United States and South Korea," *Minerva* 27, no. 2 (2009): 119–46, esp. 120.

CHAPTER TEN

1. Sexual Health Program of National Center for Primary Care, Interim Report of the National Consensus Process on Sexual Health and Responsible Sexual Behavior (Atlanta: Morehouse School of Medicine, 18 May 2006), 2, 4.

2. Ibid., 2, 5, 7–10.

3.   Todd Melby, "Consensus Is Never Easy," *Contemporary Sexuality* 40, no. 11 (2006): 1, 4–7, esp. 6.

4.   Ibid., 5; Sexual Health Program, *Interim Report*, 8, 17–25.

5.   Sexual Health Program, *Interim Report*, 7.

6.   Ibid., 9–10.

7.   Ibid., 3.

8.   Melby, "Consensus Is Never Easy," 4.

9.   See, for example, Arlene Stein, *The Stranger Next Door: The Story of a Small Community's Battle over Sex, Faith, and Civil Rights* (Boston: Beacon Press, 2001); Elizabeth Bernstein and Laurie Schaffner, *Regulating Sex: The Politics of Intimacy and Identity* (New York: Routledge, 2005); Diane Di Mauro and Carole Joffe, "The Religious Right and the Reshaping of Sexual Policy: An Examination of Reproductive Rights and Sexuality Education," *Sexuality Research and Social Policy* 4, no. 1 (2007): 67–92; Laurel Westbrook and Kristen Schilt, "Doing Gender, Determining Gender: Transgender People, Gender Panics, and the Maintenance of the Sex/Gender/Sexuality System," *Gender & Society* 28, no. 1 (2014): 32–57.

10.   On sex education, see chapter 2, note 28.

11.   Inderpal Grewal and Caren Kaplan, "Global Identities: Theorizing Transnational Studies of Sexuality," *GLQ* 7, no. 4 (2001): 663–79; Dennis Altman, *Global Sex* (Chicago: University of Chicago Press, 2001); Sonia Corrêa and Cymene Howe, "Global Perspectives on Sexual Rights," in *21st Century Sexualities: Contemporary Issues in Health, Education, and Rights*, ed. Gilbert Herdt and Cymene Howe (London: Routledge, 2007), 170–73; Ken Plummer, *Cosmopolitan Sexualities: Hope and the Humanist Imagination* (Cambridge, UK: Polity, 2015).

12.   By "politics," I refer to both the "capital P" politics of formal organizations and movements and the various kinds of "lowercase p" politics enacted in everyday encounters and life experiences. See Claudio E. Benzecry and Gianpaolo Baiocchi, "What Is Political about Political Ethnography? On the Context of Discovery and the Normalization of an Emergent Subfield," *Theory and Society* 46 (2017): 229–47, esp. 231–32.

13.   Laura Briggs has argued that, in the United States in recent years, "all politics became reproductive politics," insofar as concerns about reproductive rights became intertwined with a remarkably broad set of political concerns. Somewhat similarly, I am suggesting the tight interplay between sexual and reproductive health issues and a wide range of political matters. Laura Briggs, *How All Politics Became Reproductive Politics: From Welfare Reform to Foreclosure to Trump* (Oakland: University of California Press, 2017).

14.   Ernesto Laclau and Chantal Mouffe, *Hegemony and Socialist Strategy: Towards a Radical Democratic Politics* (London: Verso, 1985), 112–13.

15. My conception here of education as a broad-ranging political project is loosely Gramscian. Antonio Gramsci, *Selections from the Prison Notebooks* (New York: International Publishers, 1971).

16. As Iddo Tavory and Nina Eliasoph have observed, "ghosts of many potential futures haunt any interaction." Iddo Tavory and Nina Eliasoph, "Coordinating Futures: Toward a Theory of Anticipation," *American Journal of Sociology* 118, no. 4 (2013): 908–42, esp. 910. On the political and cultural potency of imagined futures, see Ann Mische, "Measuring Futures in Action: Projective Grammars in the Rio+20 Debate," *Theory and Society* 43 (2014): 437–64; Michael Rodríguez-Muñiz, *Figures of the Future: Latino Civil Rights and the Politics of Demographic Change* (Princeton, NJ: Princeton University Press, 2021).

17. Sarah Kliff and Shane Goldmacher, "Planned Parenthood's Struggle: Is It a Service or an Advocate?," *New York Times*, 17 July 2019, A1.

18. David A. Snow and Robert D. Benford, "Ideology, Frame Resonance, and Participant Mobilization," *International Social Movement Research* 1 (1988): 197–217.

19. On the multivocality of discourse often employed by political advocates, see Marc W. Steinberg, "Tilting the Frame: Considerations on Collective Action Framing from a Discursive Turn," *Theory and Society* 27 (1998): 845–72; Ann Mische, "Cross-Talk in Movements: Reconceiving the Culture-Network Link," in *Social Movements and Networks: Relational Approaches to Collective Action*, ed. Mario Diani and Doug McAdam (Oxford: Oxford University Press, 2003), 258–80; Francesca Polletta, *It Was Like a Fever: Storytelling in Protest and Politics* (Chicago: University of Chicago Press, 2006), esp. 10, 172.

20. David A. Snow, E. Burke Rochford, Jr., Steven K. Worden, and Robert D. Benford, "Frame Alignment Processes, Micromobilization, and Movement Participation," *American Sociological Review* 51, no. 4 (1986): 464–81, esp. 467–69.

21. The idea behind this movement is that the legalization of cannabis will facilitate its employment as a treatment for various sexual ailments and a means to increase blood flow to the genitals. Allison Tierney, "Meet the Woman Taking Charge of the Cannabis Sexual Health Movement in Canada," *The Fresh Toast*, 15 October 2018, https://thefreshtoast.com/can nabis/meet-one-of-the-women-taking-charge-of-the-cannabis-sexual -health-movement/.

22. "Sexual and Reproductive Health and Climate Change," *Lancet* 374 (2009): 949.

23. "#BlackSexualHealthMatters: Understanding The Role of PrEP In HIV Prevention," National Coalition for Sexual Health, last modified 1 September 2015, http://nationalcoalitionforsexualhealth.org/media-center

/ncsh-in-the-news/blacksexualhealthmatters-understanding-the-role
-of-prep-in-hiv-prevention. Arguably, though, the article promoting the
#BlackSexualHealthMatters campaign missed the opportunity for more
meaningful frame bridging from sexual health to the concerns of the
Black Lives Matter movement: it did not indicate how systemic racism
might contribute to Black Americans' greater epidemiological risk for
HIV. In contrast, when the Black Women's Health Imperative used the
work of Black feminist, activist, and poet Audre Lorde to inform its PrEP
campaign, its frame bridging tied matters of sexuality and health more
compellingly to histories of oppression and resistance among Black
women. See Barbara Lee Jackson, "The Role of PrEP in HIV Prevention for
Black Women: Power in Service," HIV.gov, last modified 4 August 2016,
https://www.hiv.gov/blog/power-in-service-the-role-of-prep-in-hiv-pre
vention-for-black-women.

24.   More generally, on the history of the Christian Right's entry into political
advocacy (on matters related to sexuality, among others) beginning in the
1980s in the United States, see Rebecca E. Klatch, *Women of the New Right*
(Philadelphia: Temple University Press, 1987).

25.   Dagmar Herzog, *Sex in Crisis: The New Sexual Revolution and the Future of
American Politics* (New York: Basic Books, 2008), 31.

26.   Amy DeRogatis, *Saving Sex: Sexuality and Salvation in American Evangelical-
ism* (Oxford: Oxford University Press, 2015), 1–2.

27.   Ibid. See also Emma Green, "The Warrior Wives of Evangelical Christian-
ity," *The Atlantic*, 9 November 2014, https://www.theatlantic.com/national
/archive/2014/11/the-warrior-wives-of-evangelical-christianity/382365/.
On evangelical sex advice books, see also Herzog, *Sex in Crisis*, 32–41.

28.   DeRogatis, *Saving Sex*, 129–49, esp. 130–31. In describing the writing and
preaching by African American evangelicals, DeRogatis notes that "the expectation of living up to strict biblical sexual ideals and the shaming that
has repercussions for a lifetime (and eternity), are often softened" (149).

29.   Kelsy Burke, *Christians under Covers: Evangelicals and Sexual Pleasure on the
Internet* (Berkeley: University of California Press, 2016), 3.

30.   Ibid., 17.

31.   Ibid.

32.   Ibid., 144, 148. See also Kelsy Burke, "What Makes a Man: Gender and
Sexual Boundaries on Evangelical Christian Sexuality Websites," *Sexualities* 17, nos. 1–2 (2014): 3–22.

33.   Home page, Christian Sexual Health, http://www.christiansexualhealth
.com/.

34.   "The 'Sex Is Dirty' Mindset," Christian Sexual Health, http://www.christian
sexualhealth.com/before-marriage/correcting-the-sex-is-dirty-mindset/.

35.   "Masturbation," Christian Sexual Health, http://www.christiansexual
health.com/issues/masturbation/.

36. "Physical Preparation," Christian Sexual Health, http://www.christian sexualhealth.com/before-marriage/physical-preparation/.

37. Herzog, *Sex in Crisis*, xi–xii.

38. This is a common feature of conservative Christian discourse in recent decades, manifested, for example, in discussions of creation science. See Dorothy Nelkin, *The Creation Controversy: Science or Scripture in the Schools* (New York: W. W. Norton, 1982); Kathleen C. Oberlin, *Creating the Creation Museum: How Fundamentalist Beliefs Come to Life* (New York: New York University Press, 2020).

39. "6 Marks of Healthy Sexuality." GaryThomas.com, last modified 17 October 2015, http://www.garythomas.com/6-marks-of-healthy-sexuality/.

40. Ibid.

41. Ibid.

42. Home page, Christian Association of Sexual Educators, https://case.sex ualwholeness.com.

43. This wording no longer appears on the website but was available at http://sexualwholeness.com/casehome/vision.html.

44. On the New Right's critique of narcissism going back to the 1980s, see Klatch, *Women of the New Right*, 127–31.

45. "6 Marks," GaryThomas.com.

46. Rob Jackson, "Teaching Children Healthy Sexuality," Focus on the Family, 1 January 2004, https://www.focusonthefamily.com/parenting/teaching -children-healthy-sexuality/.

47. "Focus on the Family," Wikipedia, accessed 22 February 2021, https://en .wikipedia.org/wiki/Focus_on_the_Family.

48. "Consolidated Financial Statement with Independent Auditors Report," Focus on the Family, http://media.focusonthefamily.com/fotf/pdf/about -us/financial-reports/fotf-2018-financial-statements.pdf.

49. Brian Eason, "Pence Heralds Plan to Thwart Planned Parenthood, Neil Gorsuch's Supreme Court Seat at Focus on the Family," *Denver Post*, 23 June 2017, https://www.denverpost.com/2017/06/23/mike-pence-focus-family -colorado-springs/.

50. "Counseling Consultation & Referrals," Focus on the Family, https://www .focusonthefamily.com/get-help/counseling-services-and-referrals/.

51. Rob Jackson, "Healthy Childhood Sexual Development," Focus on the Family, 1 January 2004, https://www.focusonthefamily.com/parenting /healthy-childhood-sexual-development/; Rob Jackson, "Sex Education: How to Start Early," Focus on the Family, 24 January 2020, https://www .focusonthefamily.com/parenting/sex-education-how-to-start-early/.

52. Jackson, "Teaching Children."

53. Jackson, "Healthy Childhood."

54. Ibid.

55. Jackson, "Sex Education."

56. "Sexuality," Focus on the Family, https://www.focusonthefamily.com/topic/get-help/sexuality/.

57. Ibid. Of course, not all of Focus on the Family's political stances involve matters directly related to gender and sexuality (although the proportion that does is substantial).

58. Chad Hills, "National Survey: Parents Support Sexual-Risk Avoidance," Focus on the Family, 2010 (accessed 2 August 2017 and no longer available), http://www.focusonthefamily.com/socialissues/education/sex-education/national-survey-parents-support-sexual-risk-avoidance.

59. Andy Birkey, "Focus on the Family Distorts Work," originally published circa 2008 on the Minnesota Monitor website (no longer accessible), re-posted on Respect My Research, last modified 2 May 2008, http://respectmyresearch.org/articles/minnesota-monitor-focus-on-the-family-distorts-work/.

60. Crystal Kupper, "Changing the Conversation" (2016), *Daily Citizen*, 2 December 2019, http://www.focusonthefamily.com/socialissues/citizen-magazine/changing-the-conversation.

61. See Steven Epstein and April N. Huff, "Sex, Science, and the Politics of Biomedicine: Gardasil in Comparative Perspective," in *Three Shots at Prevention: The HPV Vaccine and the Politics of Medicine's Simple Solutions,* ed. Keith Wailoo et al. (Baltimore: Johns Hopkins University Press, 2010), 213–28.

62. Interview with Linda Klepacki, conducted by April N. Huff, 27 September 2007. For analysis of the role of conservative advocacy groups in debates about the HPV vaccine, see Epstein and Huff, "Sex, Science."

63. The quotes that follow are from my interview with Chad Hills, Jeff Johnston, and Glenn Stanton, conducted on February 27, 2013, in Colorado Springs, Colorado.

64. Jeff Johnston, "Just a Good Christian Boy," *Daily Citizen*, 17 May 2012, https://dailycitizen.focusonthefamily.com/just-a-good-christian-boy/.

65. Lynne Gerber, *Seeking the Straight and Narrow: Weight Loss and Sexual Reorientation in Evangelical America* (Chicago: University of Chicago Press, 2011), 54.

66. Quoted in Green, "Warrior Wives."

67. "SIECUS Announces Major Rebrand, Changing Conversations around Sex Ed after 55 Years," SIECUS, last modified 12 November 2019, https://siecus.org/siecus-rebrand-announcement/.

68. Jennifer Driver, "It's Time to Rethink Sex Ed," SIECUS, https://siecus.org/time-to-rethink-sex-ed/.

69. Kate Kollars, "The Kids Could Be Alright: A Call for Comprehensive Sexual Education," *Harvard Public Health Review* 22 (Fall 2019): 1–3.

70. Sara Gentzler, "Washington Voters Approved Comprehensive Sex Ed. Now What?," *The Olympian*, 1 December 2020, https://www.theolympian.com/news/local/education/article247463565.html.

71. Jaimie Morse, "Legal Mobilization in Medicine: Nurses, Rape Kits, and the Emergence of Forensic Nursing in the United States since the 1970s," *Social Science & Medicine* 222 (2019): 323–34.

72. Adrienne D. Davis, "Slavery and the Roots of Sexual Harassment," in *Directions in Sexual Harassment Law*, ed. Catherine A. MacKinnon and Reva B. Siegel (New Haven, CT: Yale University Press, 2004), 437–78; Elizabeth Armstrong, Laura Hamilton, and Brian Sweeney, "Sexual Assault on Campus: A Multilevel, Integrative Approach to Party Rape," *Social Problems* 53, no. 4 (2006): 483–99; Elizabeth Armstrong, Miriam Gleckman-Krut, and Lanora Johnson, "Silence, Power, and Inequality: An Intersectional Approach to Sexual Violence," *Annual Review of Sociology* 44 (2018): 99–122; Jennifer S. Hirsch and Shamus Khan, *Sexual Citizens: A Landmark Study of Sex, Power, and Assault on Campus* (New York: W. W. Norton, 2020), xi–xii, xxi, 255; Abigail C. Saguy and Mallory E. Rees, "Gender, Power, and Harassment: Sociology in the #MeToo Era," *Annual Review of Sociology* 47 (2021): 13.1–13.19.

73. Elizabeth A. Armstrong et al., *Defining Sexual Consent on Campus: What's in Media vs. What's in the Policies* (Austin, TX: Council on Contemporary Families, 21 October 2019), https://contemporaryfamilies.org/defining-consent -symposium-2019-armstrong-et-al-defining-sexual-consent-on-campus/. For critical discussion of affirmative consent, see Janet Halley, "The Move to Affirmative Consent," *Signs* 42, no. 1 (2016): 257–79. On the complexities of sexual consent, see also Joseph J. Fischel, *Sex and Harm in the Age of Consent* (Minneapolis: University of Minnesota Press, 2016).

74. Laura Kipnis, *Unwanted Advances: Sexual Paranoia Comes to Campus* (New York: HarperCollins, 2017).

75. Elizabeth A. Armstrong, Paula England, and Allsun C.K. Fogarty, "Accounting for Women's Orgasm and Sexual Enjoyment in College Hookups and Relationships," *American Sociological Review* 77, no. 3 (2012): 435–62; Lisa Wade, *American Hookup: The New Culture of Sex on Campus* (New York: W. W. Norton, 2017).

76. "Sexual Health and Assault Peer Educators (SHAPE)", Northwestern University, https://www.northwestern.edu/care/get-involved/student-involvement/shape/.

77. Beth Howard, "How Colleges Handle Sexual Assault in the #MeToo Era," *US News & World Report*, 1 October 2018, https://www.usnews.com/edu cation/best-colleges/articles/2018-10-01/how-colleges-handle-sexual -assault-in-the-metoo-era.

78. Emma Pettit, "The Next Wave of #MeToo," *Chronicle of Higher Education*, 16 February 2020.

79. Hirsch and Khan, *Sexual Citizens*, xvi. On sexual citizenship, see the discussion in chapter 9.

80. Ibid., xii, 255–56.

81.   See also Jennifer S. Hirsch, "The Next Step for #MeToo Is Better Sex Edu-cation," *The Hill*, 6 December 2018, https://thehill.com/opinion/civil-rights/420039-the-next-step-for-metoo-is-better-sex-education.

82.   Hirsch and Khan, *Sexual Citizens*, xvi.

83.   Ibid., xi–xii.

84.   Melissa Chan, "Utah Governor Declares Pornography a Public Health Crisis," *Time*, 19 April 2016, http://time.com/4299919/utah-porn-public-health-crisis/; Camila Domonoske, "Utah Declares Porn a Public Health Hazard," *NPR*, 20 April 2016, http://www.npr.org/sections/thetwo-way/2016/04/20/474943913/utah-declares-porn-a-public-health-hazard.

85.   Jacqueline Howard, "Republicans Are Calling Porn a 'Public Health Crisis,' but Is It Really?," *CNN*, 2 September 2016, http://www.cnn.com/2016/07/15/health/porn-public-health-crisis/.

86.   Kimberly M. Nelson and Emily F. Rothman, "Should Public Health Profes-sionals Consider Pornography a Public Health Crisis?," *American Journal of Public Health* 110, no. 2 (2020): 151–53, esp. 152.

87.   Paul J. Wright, "U.S. Males and Pornography, 1973–2010: Consumption, Predictors, Correlates," *Journal of Sex Research* 50, no. 1 (2013): 60–71; Mi-chael Castleman, "Dueling Statistics: How Much of the Internet Is Porn?," *Psychology Today*, 3 November 2016, https://www.psychologytoday.com/intl/blog/all-about-sex/201611/dueling-statistics-how-much-the-inter net-is-porn.

88.   Kelsy Burke and Alice MillerMacPhee, "Constructing Pornography Addic-tion's Harms in Science, News Media, and Politics," *Social Forces* 99, no. 3 (2020): 1334–62.

89.   Chira Brambilla, "How Porn Addiction Is Harming Our Sexual Health," *Newsweek*, 4 December 2018, https://www.newsweek.com/porn-addiction-harming-sexual-health-1242994.

90.   For a critique by public health scholars, see Nelson and Rothman, "Should Public Health."

91.   James Hamblin, "Inside the Movement to Declare Pornography a 'Health Crisis,'" *The Atlantic*, 14 April 2016, https://www.theatlantic.com/health/archive/2016/04/a-crisis-of-education/478206/.

92.   Samantha Allen, "'Porn Kills Love': Mormons' Anti-Smut Crusade," *Daily Beast*, 20 October 2015, http://www.thedailybeast.com/porn-kills-love-mormons-anti-smut-crusade; Hamblin, "Inside the Movement." The group Fight the New Drug denies any formal connection to the Church of Jesus Christ of Latter-day Saints.

93.   Gail Dines, "Is Porn Immoral? That Doesn't Matter: It's a Public Health Crisis," *Washington Post*, 8 April 2016, https://www.washingtonpost.com/posteverything/wp/2016/04/08/is-porn-immoral-that-doesnt-matter-its-a-public-health-crisis/?utm_term=.28c6f7ba8444. Dines's influence on Weiler is described in Hamblin, "Inside the Movement." Dines's self-

characterization appeared on her academic website, http://www.wheelock
.edu/academics/faculty-and-administration/dines-gail, but is no longer
available following her retirement from Wheelock.

94. Although Dines called the science in support of her conclusions "beyond
dispute," research in this area has been quite controversial. Critics of hy-
perbole have noted that reported "associations" between porn consumption and unhealthy attitudes and behaviors do not prove causation and
that experimental studies involve highly artificial conditions that may
not be generalizable to everyday life. Megan S. C. Lim, Elise R. Carrotte,
and Margaret E. Hellard, "The Impact of Pornography on Gender-Based
Violence, Sexual Health and Well-Being: What Do We Know?," *Journal of
Epidemiology and Community Health* 70, no. 1 (2016): 3–5.

95. Home page, "Culture Reframed," http://www.culturereframed.org.

96. Lisa Duggan and Nan D. Hunter, *Sex Wars: Sexual Dissent and Political Culture* (New York: Routledge, 1995), 16–73.

97. Elizabeth Bernstein, *Brokered Subjects: Sex, Trafficking, and the Politics of
Freedom* (Chicago: University of Chicago Press, 2018), esp. 11, 21, 70, 77, 155.

CONCLUSION

1. Andrew Lakoff, *Unprepared: Global Health in a Time of Emergency* (Oakland:
University of California Press, 2017), 8.

2. Ibid., 5, 76. See also Richard Parker et al., "Global Transformations and Intimate Relations in the 21st Century: Social Science Research on Sexuality
and the Emergence of *Sexual Health* and *Sexual Rights* Frameworks," *Annual
Review of Sex Research* 15 (2004): 362–98; Allan M. Brandt, "How AIDS Invented Global Health," *New England Journal of Medicine* 368 (2013): 2149–52.

3. Philip Dawkins, "Phone Sex Is Safe Sex," *New York Times*, 20 March 2020,
https://www.nytimes.com/2020/03/20/opinion/coronavirus-sex.html.

4. Elizabeth Anne Bernstein, "Sex in the Time of Coronavirus," *Wall Street
Journal*, 19 April 2020, https://www.wsj.com/articles/sex-in-the-time-of
-coronavirus-11587301200?mod=searchresults&page=1&pos=3.

5. Jera Brown, "Making Safer Sexual Health Choices During the Pandemic,"
Rebellious, 2020, https://rebelliousmagazine.com/making-safer-sexual
-health-choices-during-the-pandemic/.

6. A. Sansone et al., "Addressing Male Sexual and Reproductive Health in the
Wake of COVID-19 Outbreak," *Journal of Endocrinological Investigation* 44
(2021): 223–31.

7. See chapter 3, note 25.

8. "Sex & Covid-19," Howard Brown Health Center, last modified 24 March
2020, https://howardbrown.org/sex-covid-19-get-the-facts/. Not only have
the lessons of the AIDS epidemic been mobilized to confront COVID-19,
but also COVID-19 has been invoked, sometimes problematically, as a way

to revisit strategies to address HIV/AIDS. Chase Ledin and Benjamin Weil, "'Test Now, Stop HIV': COVID-19 and the Idealisation of Quarantine as the 'End of HIV,'" *Culture, Health & Sexuality*, advance online publication, 1 April 2021, https://doi.org/10.1080/13691058.2021.1906953.

9.   Stephen Petrow, "Stop Handshakes, Hugs or Kisses—Jazz Hands Now to Combat Coronavirus," *USA Today*, 12 March 2020, https://www.usatoday .com/story/opinion/2020/03/12/jazz-hands-now-and-stop-handshakes -fight-coronavirus-column/5005368002/.

10.   Megan Nolan, "The Joys of Frivolous Sex," *New York Times*, 22 December 2020, https://www.nytimes.com/2020/12/22/opinion/sex-relationships -covid.html.

11.   "Unintended Pregnancy in the United States," Guttmacher Institute, https://www.guttmacher.org/fact-sheet/unintended-pregnancy-united -states; Rebecca J. Kreitzer, Candis Watts Smith, Kellen A. Kane, and Tracee M. Saunders, "Affordable but Inaccessible? Contraception Deserts in the US States," *Journal of Health Politics, Policy & Law* 46, no. 2 (2021): 277–304.

12.   David C. Harvey, "Our Nation's Deadly Disregard for Sexual Health," *The Hill*, 21 October 2019, https://thehill.com/opinion/healthcare/466771-our -nations-deadly-disregard-for-sexual-health. STI rates dropped in 2020, but perhaps mostly because many people avoided screening and testing out of fear of contracting COVID-19 in medical facilities. Jan Hoffman, "People Are Still Having Sex. So Why Are STD Rates Dropping?," *New York Times*, 28 October 2020, https://www.nytimes.com/2020/10/28/health /covid-std-testing.html.

13.   David M. Halperin and Trevor Hoppe, eds., *The War on Sex* (Durham, NC: Duke University Press, 2017).

14.   "Statement on President Trump's State of the Union Remarks on Ending the U.S. HIV Epidemic by 2030 from the Act Now: End AIDS Coalition," Treatment Action Group, last modified 5 February 2019, http://www .treatmentactiongroup.org/content/statement-president-trump's-sotu -remarks-ending-us-hiv-epidemic-2030-act-now-end-aids-coalition; Steven W. Thrasher, "HIV Is Coming to Rural America," *New York Times*, 2 December 2019, A27.

15.   For one articulation of a new agenda for sexual and reproductive health and rights, in light of the disruptions caused by the COVID-19 pandemic and the opportunities presented by the inauguration of the Biden ad-ministration, see Sophia Sadinsky and Zara Ahmed, "A Time for Change: Advancing Sexual and Reproductive Health and Rights in a New Global Era," *Guttmacher Policy Review* 24 (2021): 14–21.

16.   Chris A. Barcelos, *Distributing Condoms and Hope: The Racialized Politics of Youth Sexual Health* (Berkeley: University of California Press, 2020).

17. This paragraph adapts text from Steven Epstein and Laura Mamo, "The Proliferation of Sexual Health: Diverse Social Problems and the Legitimation of Sexuality," *Social Science & Medicine* 188 (2017): 176–90, esp. 188.

18. Laura Mamo and I also developed this point in ibid., 187–88.

19. Didier Fassin, "That Obscure Object of Global Health," in *Medical Anthropology at the Intersections: Histories, Activisms, and Futures,* ed. Marcia C. Inhorn and Emily A. Wentzell (Durham, NC: Duke University Press, 2012), 95–115, esp. 96. See also George Weisz, Alberto Cambrosio, and Jean-Philippe Cointet, "Mapping Global Health: A Network Analysis of a Heterogeneous Publication Domain," *BioSocieties* 12, no. 4 (2017): 520–42.

20. Sara Shostak, *Exposed Science: Genes, the Environment, and the Politics of Population Health* (Berkeley: University of California Press, 2013).

21. Author's field notes, National Sexual Health Conference, Chicago, 10 July 2019.

22. As I see it, this vision of sexual health is agnostic on the complicated question of whether individual sexual desires and societal requirements can ever be made fully compatible or whether (as the Freudian and Freudo-Marxist traditions would have it) there always remains a fundamental tension between the two. I thank Charles Thorpe for posing this question.

23. Halperin and Hoppe, *War on Sex,* 6.

24. David M. Halperin, *What Do Gay Men Want? An Essay on Sex, Risk, and Subjectivity* (Ann Arbor: University of Michigan Press, 2007), 11.

25. While my approach may be somewhat different, I am indebted to Heather Love's insights on the limits of the "heroic anti-normativity" found in much queer theory. See Heather Love, "Doing Being Deviant: Deviance Studies, Description, and the Queer Ordinary," *Differences: A Journal of Feminist Cultural Studies* 26, no. 1 (2015): 74–95; Heather Love, *Underdogs: Social Deviance and Queer Theory* (Chicago: University of Chicago Press, 2021). Similarly, Robyn Wiegman and Elizabeth Wilson have asked, "What objects of study, analytic perspectives, and understanding of politics might emerge if we suspend antinormativity's axiomatic centrality?" Robyn Wiegman and Elizabeth A. Wilson, "Introduction: Antinormativity's Queer Conventions," *Differences: A Journal of Feminist Cultural Studies* 26, no. 1 (2015): 1–25, esp. 10; see also Annamarie Jagose, "The Trouble with Antinormativity," *Differences: A Journal of Feminist Cultural Studies* 26, no. 1 (2015): 26–47.

26. Eunjung Kim, "How Much Sex Is Healthy? The Pleasures of Asexuality," in *Against Health: How Health Became the New Morality,* ed. Jonathan M. Metzl and Anna Kirkland (New York: NYU Press, 2010), 157–69, esp. 157.

27. Irwin Goldstein et al., "Hypoactive Sexual Desire Disorder: International Society for the Study of Women's Sexual Health (ISSWSH) Expert Consensus Panel Review," *Mayo Clinic Proceedings* 92, no. 1 (2017): 114–28. On

distinctions between asexuality and HSDD, see Andrew Hinderliter, "How Is Asexuality Different from Hypoactive Sexual Desire Disorder?," *Psychology & Sexuality* 4, no. 2 (2013): 167–78.

28. Home page, Asexual Visibility and Education Network, https://www.asex uality.org/. See also Lori A. Brotto and Morag Yule, "Asexuality: Sexual Orientation, Paraphilia, Sexual Dysfunction, or None of the Above?," *Archives of Sexual Behavior* 46, no. 3 (2016): 619–27.

29. These include people who are aromantic, demisexual ("who can only experience sexual attraction or desire after an emotional bond has been formed"), and gray-sexual (who fall somewhere within the "asexual spectrum"), along with others considered to fall under the "asexual umbrella." "General FAQ," Asexual Visibility and Education Network, https://www .asexuality.org/?q=general.html.

30. Brenna Conley-Fonda and Taylor Leisher, "Asexuality: Sexual Health Does Not Require Sex," *Sexual Addiction & Compulsivity* 25, no. 1 (2018): 6–11, esp. 10.

31. Angela Jones, "Sex Is Not a Problem: The Erasure of Pleasure in Sexual Science Research," *Sexualities* 22, no. 4 (2019): 643–68, esp. 661.

32. Barcelos, *Distributing Condoms*, 142.

33. Lynn Barclay, interviewed by author, 22 July 2019.

34. Eli Coleman, interviewed by author, 11 July 2019.

35. Kane Race, *Pleasure Consuming Medicine: The Queer Politics of Drugs* (Durham, NC: Duke University Press, 2009), ix.

36. Laura M. Carpenter and Monica J. Casper, "A Tale of Two Technologies: HPV Vaccination, Male Circumcision, and Sexual Health," *Gender & Society* 23, no. 6 (2009): 790–816, esp. 809.

37. Joan Morgan, "Why We Get Off: Moving toward a Black Feminist Politics of Pleasure," *Black Scholar* 45, no. 4 (2015): 36–46, esp. 44.

38. On neoliberalism, see chapter 8, note 21.

39. Barry Adam, "Constructing the Neoliberal Sexual Actor: Responsibility and Care of the Self in the Discourse of Barebackers," *Culture, Health & Sexuality* 7, no. 4 (2005): 333–46, esp. 339.

40. Ibid., 345.

41. Jorge Fontdevila, "Framing Dilemmas during Sex: A Micro-Sociological Approach to HIV Risk," *Social Theory & Health* 7, no. 3 (2009): 241–63; Héctor Carrillo, *Pathways of Desire: The Sexual Migration of Mexican Gay Men* (Chicago: University of Chicago Press, 2017), 272–75.

42. I am grateful to Héctor Carrillo for suggesting this formulation.

43. Therefore I consider the broader notion of being "against health," as described by Jonathan Metzl and Anna Kirkland, to be a useful provocation and thought experiment but not a direct pathway to politics. Jonathan M. Metzl and Anna Kirkland, eds., *Against Health: How Health Became the New Morality* (New York: NYU Press, 2010).

44. See chapter 2, note 53.

45. Angela Jones, *Camming: Money, Power, and Pleasure in the Sex Work Industry* (New York: NYU Press, 2020).

46. Sharon Elaine Preves, "Negotiating the Constraints of Gender Binarism: Intersexuals' Challenge to Gender Categorization," *Current Sociology* 48, no. 3 (2000): 27–50; Steffie Goodman, "Venturing Beyond the Binary Sexual Health Interview," *American Journal of Public Health* 108, no. 8 (2018): 965; Steven Hobaica, Kyle Schofield, and Paul Kwon, "'Here's Your Anatomy . . . Good Luck': Transgender Individuals in Cisnormative Sex Education," *American Journal of Sexuality Education* 14, no. 3 (2019): 358–87; J. E. Sumerau, Lain A. B. Mathers, and Dawne Moon, "Foreclosing Fluidity at the Intersection of Gender and Sexual Normativities," *Symbolic Interaction* 43, no. 2 (2019): 205–34; Nik M. Lampe and Alexandra C. H. Nowakowski, "New Horizons in Trans and Non-Binary Health Care: Bridging Identity Affirmation with Chronicity Management in Sexual and Reproductive Services," *International Journal of Transgender Health* 22, nos. 1–2 (2021): 141–53.

47. James Horley, "Sexuality and Sexual Health in Prisons," *Sexuality & Culture* 23 (2019): 1372–86, esp. 1382.

48. Brian Mustanski, Amy Johnson, and Robert Garofalo, "At the Intersection of HIV/AIDS Disparities: Young African American Men Who Have Sex with Men," in *Social Work with African American Males: Health, Mental Health, and Social Policy*, ed. Waldo E. Johnson Jr. (New York: Oxford University Press, 2010), 226–42; Triana Kazaleh Sirdenis et al., "Toward Sexual Health Equity for Gay, Bisexual, and Transgender Youth: An Intergenerational, Collaborative, Multisector Partnerships Approach to Structural Change," *Health Education & Behavior* 46, no. 1 (suppl.) (2019): 88S–99S. More generally, and borrowing from the work of activists who promote the "decolonizing of contraception," much thinking and work is required in order to decolonize sexual health. Home page, Decolonising Contraception, https://www.decolonisingcontraception.com.

49. Nita Bhalla, "LGBT+ Delegates Say Sidelined at 'Inclusive' Global Sexual Health Summit," *Reuters*, 14 November 2019, https://www.reuters.com/article/us-global-lgbt-health-trfn/lgbt-delegates-say-sidelined-at-inclusive-global-sexual-health-summit-idUSKBN1XO31Q.

50. See chapter 3, note 26.

51. Race, *Pleasure Consuming Medicine*, 162–63.

52. For a useful example, see Ana Amuchástegui Herrera and Azucena Ojeda Sanchez, "'If You Aren't Married Yet, You'll Be Married to Your Treatment from Now On': Embodied Mediations in a Women's HIV Peer Advisory Project in Mexico," *Culture, Health & Sexuality*, advance online publication, 4 January 2021, https://doi.org/10.1080/13691058.2020.1852312.

53. Kath Albury, "Young People, Digital Media Research and Counterpublic Sexual Health," *Sexualities* 21, no. 8 (2018): 1331–36, esp. 1334.

54.   Sonia Corrêa, Rosalind Petchesky, and Richard Parker, *Sexuality, Health and Human Rights* (London: Routledge, 2008), 220.
55.   Ibid.
56.   Barcelos, *Distributing Condoms*, 22.
57.   Ibid., 232–33.

Index

Page numbers in italics refer to figures.

Rockefeller Foundation, 167
Roen, Philip R., 49
Rofes, Eric, 355n93
Ronen, Shelly, 222
Roo chatbot, 193
Roosth, Sophia, 30
"Root 100," 242
rope play, 221
Rose, Nikolas, 13, 134, 213–14, 317n36
Rosen, David, 177
Rosenberg, Charles, 39, 326n17, 343n92
Royal College of Obstetricians and
    Gynaecologists (UK), 130
Rubin, Gayle, 159, 200–201, 385n74
Rubio-Aurioles, Eusebio, 93

sadomasochism, 152
safer sex, 111, 195, 197, 215, 258. *See also*
    HIV/AIDS: prevention
safety, 5, 44, 102, 108, 276
salud sexual, 31, 78, 257, 334n8
same-sex desires, 151–52, 177. *See also*
    homosexuality; LGBTQ
same-sex marriage. *See* marriage:
    same-sex
same-sex relationships, 108. *See also*
    homosexuality; LGBTQ
Sandfort, Theo, 14, 28, 44, 82, 330n82,
    333n3
San Diego Sexual Medicine, 67
Sandset, Tony, 355n84, 404n123
San Francisco, 111, 195–96, 221–22
San Francisco AIDS Foundation, 195
San Francisco Public Health Depart-
    ment, 228–29
San Francisco Sex Information, 383n47
Sanger, Margaret, 35
santé sexuelle, 31, 78, 334n8
Saperstein, Aliya, 172
Satcher, David, 234, 238–41, 245, 248,
    260–61, 281, 354n74, 397n31
satisfaction, 40, 80, 83, 107–8, 172–73,
    203, 226. *See also* sexual satisfaction
Savage, Dan, 189–90
Say, Lale, 150

scales. *See* sexual inventories
Schaffer, Simon, 373n130
Schilt, Kristen, 392n79
Schlessinger, Laura, 189–90
Schmidt, Gunter, 97
Schüll, Natasha, 215
science, 3, 9, 11, 26, 40–42, 47–52, 64,
    66, 69, 80, 94, 130; attitudes toward,
    252–54; authority of, 403n110; au-
    tonomy of, 163; communication, 142;
    fields, 88, 185; infrastructure, 78;
    invoking, 271–73; and legitimacy, 97,
    252; overlay mapping, 381n13; poli-
    tics of, 167; promissory, 87; termi-
    nology, 38; and values, 103; working
    objects, 202
science (and technology) studies, 26–
    28, 380n1, 385n76; and sexuality
    studies, 27
scientific research. *See* biomedical re-
    search; sex research; survey research
scientization. *See* health: scientizing
    sexuality; morality: scientizing
Seely, Stephen, 103
Segal, Judy, 126, 318n46, 359n3
seksuelle gesondheid, 31
self: -actualization, 69, 71, 117, 119,
    212; -classification, 204; -defense,
    277; -determination, 97, 104, 116–
    17, 278; -empowerment, 215, 222;
    -expression, 70–71, 119; -formation,
    21; -fulfillment, 70, 231; -governance,
    46–47, 235–37, 244, 287; -help, 85,
    189, 213; -hood, 3, 134;
    -improvement, 207, 211–12, 231, 288;
    -investment, 215; -knowledge, 246;
    -management, 240; -optimization
    (*see* optimization); -pleasure, 196 (*see
    also* masturbation); -representation,
    44; -surveillance, 214–15, 230
sex addiction, 70, 154–55, 245, 272,
    371n101. *See also* sexual compulsivity
sex advice, 38–41, 43, 47, 49, 59, 123,
    174, 182, 326n11, 326n13; Christian,
    265–74; diversification of, 188–200,

9 780226 818221